AF770799

Handbook of Toxicology

Volume I

Handbook of Toxicology
Volume I

Edited by **Abby Calvin**

FOSTER ACADEMICS

New Jersey

Published by Foster Academics,
61 Van Reypen Street,
Jersey City, NJ 07306, USA
www.fosteracademics.com

Handbook of Toxicology: Volume I
Edited by Abby Calvin

© 2015 Foster Academics

International Standard Book Number: 978-1-63242-219-4 (Hardback)

This book contains information obtained from authentic and highly regarded sources. Copyright for all individual chapters remain with the respective authors as indicated. A wide variety of references are listed. Permission and sources are indicated; for detailed attributions, please refer to the permissions page. Reasonable efforts have been made to publish reliable data and information, but the authors, editors and publisher cannot assume any responsibility for the validity of all materials or the consequences of their use.

The publisher's policy is to use permanent paper from mills that operate a sustainable forestry policy. Furthermore, the publisher ensures that the text paper and cover boards used have met acceptable environmental accreditation standards.

Trademark Notice: Registered trademark of products or corporate names are used only for explanation and identification without intent to infringe.

Printed in China.

Contents

Preface

The scientific and medical field of study known as Toxicology derives its name from the Greek word 'toxicos' which means poisonous. It is a branch of medicine as well as biology and chemistry but more specifically of pharmacology. Toxicology is concerned with study of the harmful effects of chemical on living organisms. This field specializes in the study of the symptoms, treatments and mechanisms as well as detection of toxins and venoms, especially in humans. These harmful chemicals can include drugs as well. The main goal is the study of such effects and the safe amelioration of these effects. There are many sub divisions of toxicology, ranging from regulatory and clinical toxicology to forensic toxicology and risk assessment. The research done in this field involves the study and focus on the structure and mechanism of toxins and is strongly multidisciplinary. It spans computational chemistry, bioinformatics, molecular epidemiology as well as drug discovery and drug metabolism. The need for more qualified and skilled research scientists in this discipline is great as the rate of discovery of harmful substances is almost the same as that of recovery from it. The future of this scientific discipline is promising and is a great area to learn the intricacies of toxins and venoms as well as its sister discipline, pharmacology.

This book attempts to collate all available research and data on toxicology. I am thankful to those who put their efforts and hard work behind these researches. I am also grateful to my family and friends for their support in this endeavour.

Editor

Potassium Channels Blockers from the Venom of *Androctonus mauretanicus mauretanicus*

Marie-France Martin-Eauclaire and Pierre E. Bougis

Aix-Marseille University, CNRS, UMR 7286, CRN2M, Faculté de Médecine secteur Nord, CS80011, Boulevard Pierre Dramard, 13344 Marseille Cedex 15, France

Correspondence should be addressed to Marie-France Martin-Eauclaire, marie-france.eauclaire@univmed.fr and Pierre E. Bougis, pierre-edouard.bougis@univmed.fr

Academic Editor: Maria Elena de Lima

K^+ channels selectively transport K^+ ions across cell membranes and play a key role in regulating the physiology of excitable and nonexcitable cells. Their activation allows the cell to repolarize after action potential firing and reduces excitability, whereas channel inhibition increases excitability. In eukaryotes, the pharmacology and pore topology of several structural classes of K^+ channels have been well characterized in the past two decades. This information has come about through the extensive use of scorpion toxins. We have participated in the isolation and in the characterization of several structurally distinct families of scorpion toxin peptides exhibiting different K^+ channel blocking functions. In particular, the venom from the Moroccan scorpion *Androctonus mauretanicus mauretanicus* provided several high-affinity blockers selective for diverse K^+ channels (SK_{Ca}, $K_v4.x$, and $K_v1.x$ K^+ channel families). In this paper, we summarize our work on these toxin/channel interactions.

1. The Scorpion Venom Content

Scorpion venoms are very complex mixtures of molecules, constituting a diverse, naturally occurring peptide library, with most peptides displaying different kinds of biological activity [1, 2]. These peptides can specifically bind to a variety of pharmacological targets, in particular ion channels, resulting in neurotoxic effects. Toxins modulating Na^+, K^+, Ca^{++}, and Cl^- currents have been described in scorpion venoms [2].

Toxins that are highly lethal for mammals modify voltage-gated Na^+ (Na_v) currents in excitable cells and are referred to as "Na_v channel long-chain toxin." These toxins are single-chain, small, basic peptides (60- to 75-amino-acid residue chain generally folded by four disulfide bridges). They have been described as α- or β-toxins due to their binding site on Na_v channels as well as to their pharmacological effects [1, 3]. α-Toxins bind in a voltage-dependent manner on the voltage sensor of the Na_v channel domain IV and inhibit the inactivation phase of the action potential. β-Toxins act on the channel activation phase by binding to extracellular loops located preferentially on the voltage sensor of the Na_v channel domain II (but also occasionally of domain III) [1, 3–6].

Another class of scorpion toxins has also been widely studied, even if these toxins are devoid of serious lethal effect. They block different K^+ channel subtypes (some of them in the picomolar range) and are so-called "K^+ channel toxins" [1, 2, 7]. They are usually shorter than Na_v channel toxins but are structurally closely related to them. These Na_v and K^+ channels toxins share a common dense scaffold typically formed by an α-helix and a β-sheet stabilized by disulfide bridges [8].

Several components of scorpion venom that act on Cl^- and Ca^{++} channels have also been described [2]. However, they have little or no influence on the venom toxicity for mammals.

This overview will focus, in particular, on our work done on the K^+ channel blockers purified from the *Androctonus mauretanicus mauretanicus* venom, which were among the first K^+ channel blockers characterized from scorpion venoms.

2. K^+ Channel Blockers from Scorpion Venoms

K^+ channels constitute a ubiquitous family of transmembrane proteins which play a key role in the regulation of a wide variety of physiological processes involved in cell excitability, including regulation of heart beat, muscle contraction, neurotransmitter release, hormonal secretion, signal transduction, and cell proliferation [9]. Multiple combinations of K^+ channels result from the ability of their subunits to coassemble as tetramers, thus considerably increasing the total number of functionally distinct K^+ channels. According to their functional and gating properties, K^+ channels have been first divided into four groups: voltage-activated, Ca^{2+}-activated, inward rectifier, and two-pore K^+ channels [10]. Their 3D architecture has now been depicted by X-ray crystallography [11].

K^+ channel blocker's toxins (KTxs) from scorpion venoms are short peptides, which are made usually of about 28–40-amino-acid residues reticulated by three or four disulfide bridges, forming compact and resistant molecules [7]. They have been invaluable tools for understanding the physiological role of K^+ channels and have been exploited to gain insights into the structure of the channel pore that they occlude via electrostatic and hydrophobic interactions [12, 13]. They block K^+ channels from the extracellular side and bind to their outer vestibules. In most cases, they possess at least two functionally crucial residues: examples include a lysine residue that plugs the channel pore with its side chain and a hydrophobic residue that strengthens the interaction between the toxin and its target. These residues are found in very low concentrations in the venoms (from 0.01 to 1% by weight of crude venom) and have almost no toxic effects in mice when injected by subcutaneous route. However, some of them could be very toxic following direct intracerebroventricular injection.

Based on primary amino acid sequences and cysteine pairing, KTxs have been classified into four families, the α-, β-, γ-, and κ-KTx [2, 7]. So far more than 120 KTxs, ranging from 23 to 64 amino acids, have been isolated and sequenced. Most of their structures exhibit a common minimal motif, named the "Cystein-Stabilized-Helix" (CSH). As found in Buthidae scorpions, long and short toxins consist of one α-helix and two or three β-strands, in which two disulfide bridges covalently link a segment of the α-helix with one strand of the β-sheet structure [8]. Even if their amino acid sequences are different, the conserved peptide fold allows insertions, deletions, and mutations conferring to the toxins diverse selectivity and affinity for their target. Only the recently characterized κ-KTxs are formed by two parallel α-helices linked by two disulfide bridges [14].

The α-KTx family is the largest one and is divided into at least 22 subfamilies, defined according to the primary sequence alignments of the toxins. Each member has diverse, specific blocking activities against voltage-gated (K_V) and calcium-activated (K_{Ca}) channels. Most of the α-KTxs bind to the ion channel vestibule through the β-sheet side of their structure.

Other, longer peptides, with 45- to 68-amino acid residues and cross-linked by three disulfide bridges, have been characterized and classified as the β-KTx family. They possess two structural and functional domains: an N-terminal α-helix (with cytolytic or antimicrobial activity like the insect defensins) and a tightly folded C-terminal region with the CSH motif (displaying K^+ channel-blocking activities [15]). Finally, the γ-KTx family was described as specifically targeting hERG channels [16].

3. The *Androctonus mauretanicus mauretanicus* Venom

Scorpion stings in Morocco are the primary cause of envenomation and constitute a largely underestimated health problem. An epidemiologic study of four regions of the Moroccan Kingdom, where scorpion stings are prevalent, showed that the stings are mainly due to the black scorpion *Androctonus mauretanicus mauretanicus* (83% of the reported cases). Children, in desert areas far from medical centers, were the primary victims, with casualty rates up to 8% in those under ten years old. The *Androctonus mauretanicus mauretanicus* venom is one of the most toxic Buthidae venoms ever described (its median lethal dose ranges from 0.05 to 0.2 mg/kg by subcutaneous injection in mice) and immunotherapy remains the treatment of choice [17].

Previous fractionation studies of the venom allowed identification of several toxins that are active on different Na_V or K_V channels [18–22]. At least several major proteins, considered highly toxic to mice, have already been purified and chemically and pharmacologically characterized as classical α-toxins [18, 19]. All together, these toxins represent about 28% of the absorbance (wavelength 280 nm) of the crude venom and 73% of the total lethality for mice. The most represented and the most lethal classical α-toxin Amm V alone constitutes 11% of the absorbance and 47% of the total lethality.

However, other toxins isolated from the *Androctonus mauretanicus mauretanicus* venom gained popularity as powerful tools because they have displayed some of the highest binding affinity and specificity for K^+ channels. They have been extensively used to investigate the mechanisms of ion conduction and channel selectivity, as well as the architecture of the pore region. Finally, significant advances have been made by using solid-state NMR data to construct 3D structures from Kaliotoxin (KTX) in complex with a chimeric K^+ channel KcsA-K_V1.3 [13]. These studies allowed direct investigation of the molecular rearrangements associated with KTX binding on both the channel selectivity filter and the KTX itself.

A recent MALDI-TOF mass spectrometry (MS) study has provided new information about the molecular composition of scorpion venom [23]. Through the developments in proteomics, MS is now widely used for accurate and sensitive determinations of molecular masses and identification of heterogenous complex mixtures such as crude venoms. Using an offline MALDI-TOF/MS analysis, we were able to determine the molecular masses of about 70 to 80 different compounds ranging between 3000 and 8000 Da in an *Androctonus mauretanicus mauretanicus* venom obtained under manual stimulation from a pool of animals kept alive at the "Pasteur Institute" of Casablanca, Morocco. Figure 1 presents the snapshot of this crude venom.

4. The Smallest Toxins Identified so Far in the *Androctonus mauretanicus mauretanicus* Venom: P01 (α-KTx8) and P05 (α-KTx5), Ligands of SK_{Ca} Channels

P01 (α-KTx 8.1 subfamily, 3177 Da) is devoid of significant toxicity in mouse [26]. This toxin of 28-amino-acid residues, which is the smallest K^+ channels ligand in the *Androctonus mauretanicus mauretanicus* venom, is slightly negatively charged with acidic amino acids localized at the beginning of the β-turn and extending along the α-helix (Figure 2(a)). Surprisingly, P01 presents exactly the same sequence in *Androctonus mauretanicus mauretanicus, Androctonus australis, Androctonus amoreuxi*, and *Buthus occitanus* venoms. Usually, the polymorphism among scorpion toxins is so high that their sequences vary from a scorpion subspecies to another, even in the same structural, pharmacological, and immunological family. P01 is a poor-affinity ligand (300 nM) for the apamin-binding site on rat brain synaptosomes. In comparison, apamin purified from the bee venom displays a very high affinity ($K_d = 8$ pM) for its target, that is, the small-conductance calcium-activated K^+ channel (SK_{Ca}) channel so-called apamin-sensitive channel. Since the first P01 characterization, other closely related analogs have been purified from other Buthidae venoms. Among them, one is particularly interesting because it shares 89% of identity with P01. This analog, called OdK1, was purified from the Iranian scorpion *Odontobuthus doriae* (α-KTx 8.5 subfamily). OdK1 is able to block $K_v1.2$ channels expressed in oocytes with a median inhibition concentration (IC_{50}) value of 183 nM and has no effect on $K_v1.1$, $K_v1.3$, $K_v1.4$, $K_v1.5$, and the *Shaker* channels [27]. It is important to mention that P01 has not been tested yet on $K_v1.2$ channels in electrophysiological experiments. P01 was only shown unable to compete with ^{125}I-KTX (a $K_v1.1$ and $K_v1.3$ and not $K_v1.2$ blocker) bound to its receptor on rat brain synaptosomes. Thus, we cannot totally exclude that P01 could exhibit a poor $K_v1.2$ blocking activity. In the same line, OdK1 activity on SK_{Ca} channels has not been tested yet either.

In contrast to P01, P05, another toxin from *Androctonus mauretanicus mauretanicus*, is a high-affinity selective ligand ($K_d = 100$ pM) for the apamin-binding site on rat brain synaptosomes, and it has no effects on BK_{Ca} or K_v channels. P05 is a 31-amino-acid long peptide (3415 Da), which belongs to the α-KTx5.x's family (as Leiurotoxin1 or Scyllatoxin from the venom of the scorpion *Leiurus quinquestriatus Hebraeus*) (Figure 2(b)) [29, 30]. The toxins from this family have only two-stranded β-sheet because of their short N-terminal side [28]. P05 is highly toxic (14 ng, i.e., 4 pmols for a 20 g mouse) and leads to an epileptic behavior when injected in mouse by the intracerebroventricular route. P05 possesses a short stretch of four amino acids similar to the one in the apamin sequence, which constitutes a highly positively charged region in the

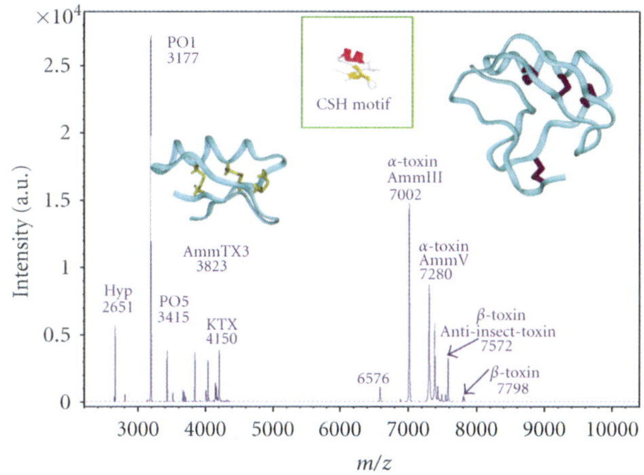

FIGURE 1: MALDI-TOF mass spectra of pool venom manually extracted from *Androctonus mauretanicus mauretanicus*. K^+ channel blockers and voltage-gated Na^+ channels modulators are indicated. P01 and P05, blockers of SK_{Ca} channels; AmmTX3, blockers of K_v4 and hERG channels; KTX, $K_v1.1$, and $K_v1.3$ blockers. Amm III and Amm V are major lethal α-toxins; β-toxins specific for insects are also mentioned. The 3D structure of KTX (left) and of the α-toxin of reference AaH II from *Androctonus australis* (right) are shown [13, 24, 25]. The Cys-Stabilized-Helix (CSH) motif is shown in inset [8].

α-helix (containing in particular two Arg residues, Arg_7 and Arg_9) exposed to solvent. Extensive structure-function studies using chemically synthesized analogs revealed that these two Arg were critical for P05's interaction with its target as described for apamin [31]. When Arg were replaced by Lys, the activity dropped by a factor of one hundred, and when they were replaced by Ile, the affinity decreased even more to a Kd value in the micromolar range. Moreover, α-amidation of His in P05 C-terminal conferred a large gain of function leading to an almost irreversible binding to its receptor [21]. When the apamin C-terminal residue is in the free carboxylic form, only 0.06% of the pharmacological activity of the native C-amidated apamin is retained [32]. Both Arg and C-terminal His create a strong positive electrostatic potential, which drives the toxin to negative residues (Asp) of the channel pore. Using homology-modeling models of SK channels (rsk1, rsk2, and rsk3) and Brownian dynamics methods, the recognition between P05 and its targets was investigated [33]. It was found that the rsk2 channel, presenting the highest frequencies and lowest electrostatic interaction energies, was the most favorable target for P05 binding, while rsk3 was intermediate, and rsk1 was the least favorable. From the P05-rsk2 complex model, it was shown that P05 probably locates around the extracellular pore of SK channels and assures the contact with rsk2 channel using critical basic amino acid residues in its α-helix: Arg_6 (P05)-Asp_{364} (SK), Arg_7 (P05)-Asn_{368} (SK), and Arg_{13} (P05)-Asp_{341} and Asp_{364} (SK). Further refinements of P05-rsk2 complex model using molecular mechanics showed that six hydrogen bonding interactions exist between P05 and the rsk2 channel. These simulation results were in good agreement with our previous *in vivo* binding experiments and could explain

VSCEDCPEHCSTQAKCDNDKCVCEP

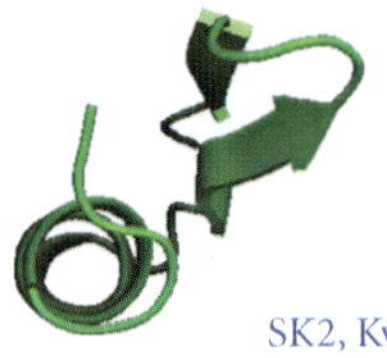

(a)

TVCNLRRCQLSCRSCRSLGLLGKCIGVKCECVKH
CNCKAPETALCARRCQQH–NH_2 (Apamin)

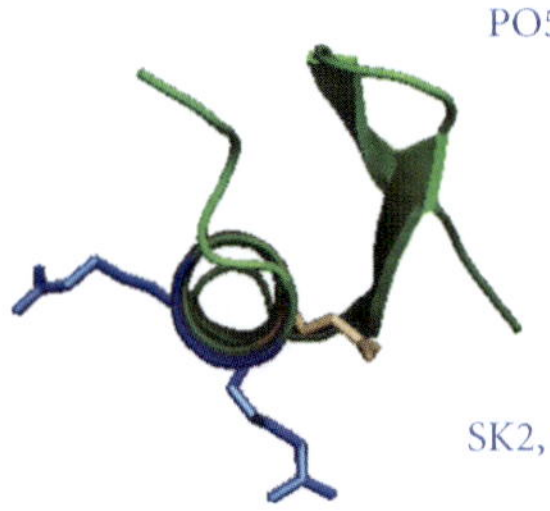

(b)

FIGURE 2: Amino acid sequences and 3D structures of P01 and P05. (a) Amino acid sequence (single letter notation) and 3D structure of P01 [26, 28]. (b) Amino acid sequence (single letter notation) of P05 compared to that of the bee venom apamin (18 mers peptide). Amino acids common to P05 and apamin and crucial for the SK_{Ca} blockade are in blue. These amino acids are materialized on the 3D structure of P05, view by the α-helix axe. The two positive Arg are in blue and the neutral Gln is in brown.

the interaction between P05 and SK channels at the level of the molecular structure.

5. The Most Noted K^+ Channel Blocker Characterized in the *Androctonus mauretanicus mauretanicus* Venom: Kaliotoxin (α-KTx3 Subfamily)

The Kaliotoxin (KTX, 4150 Da) purified from the venom of the *Androctonus mauretanicus mauretanicus* was the first identified member of the α-KTx3.1 subfamily, which is currently composed of 13 highly homolog members sharing more than 75% sequence identity. KTX was first described as a BK_{Ca} low-affinity blocker [20], but further analysis showed that KTX blocked more specifically $K_v1.3$ channels with a very high affinity ($K_d = 10$ pM) and $K_v1.1$ with a much weaker affinity (in the 10 nM range). KTX also exhibited a functional blockade of Ca^{2+}-activated K^+ Gardos channel from rabbit or human red blood cells with a median inhibition concentration value of 5 nM. Interaction between this channel and other peptide toxins indicated that the Gárdos channel was pharmacologically different in several interesting ways from the other Ca^{2+}-activated K^+ channels [34]. Interestingly, KTX was not toxic in mice by subcutaneous injection up to 500 micrograms (100 nmols), but intracerebroventricularly injected mice showed tremor, paralysis, and death with a median lethal dose of only 24 ng of KTX (about 6 pmol for a 20 g mouse).

KTX was then widely used by different international groups to probe the vestibule topology from the lymphocyte $K_v1.3$ channel. The homotetrameric $K_v1.3$ channel controls the resting potential membrane in T cells and plays a crucial role in human T-lymphocyte activation [35]. Its inhibition causes depolarization and an attenuation of the rise in the intracellular Ca^{2+} concentration that is required for T-cell activation. Accordingly, $K_v1.3$ channel is a good therapeutic target for the development of immunosuppressant drugs. It is important to note that $K_v1.3$ channel is a key mediator of multiple sclerosis, type 1 diabetes mellitus, and rheumatoid arthritis pathologies [36]. In experimental autoimmune encephalomyelitis (EAE) rat, animal model for multiple sclerosis, KTX was capable of immunosuppressant activity *in vivo*. Addition of KTX during Antigen/T-cell activation led to a large reduction of the T-cell proliferative response, a decreased encephalitogenicity of T cells, and finally improved the symptoms of EAE [37].

A new therapeutic approach for inflammatory bone resorption by targeting $K_v1.3$ was also investigated and the potential effect of KTX was tested on inflammatory lesions of periodontal disease. These lesions contain abundant activated/memory T and B cells, which control immunological interactive networks and accelerate bone resorption. Systemic KTX administration finally resulted in an 84% decrease of the bone resorption. These results suggested that KTX could also constitute a potential therapy to prevent alveolar bone loss in periodontal disease [38].

Monoiodinated derivative of KTX (^{125}I-KTX) binds specifically to rat brain total membranes with a maximal binding capacity of about 14 fmol/mg of protein and with a high affinity ($K_d = 80$ pM). The distribution of ^{125}I-KTX binding sites in rat brain was first studied using quantitative autoradiography on adult brain tissue sections. A comparison with the distribution of $K_v1.1$ and $K_v1.3$ α-subunits by immunohistochemistry or *in situ* hybridization suggested that KTX recognizes channels containing these subunits [39]. Further, we used KTX injected by intracerebroventricular route to rat brain in order to investigate the involvement of K_v channels containing $K_v1.1$ and $K_v1.3$ α-subunits in olfactory associative learning and memory. KTX facilitated cognitive processes as learning, in particular in a reference representation [40]. Therefore, it is likely that KTX-sensitive K_v channels contribute to the repolarization of action potentials at presynaptic terminals of hippocampal inhibitory neurons and induce facilitation of the transmission.

Concerning the KTX structure-function relationship studies, they were first performed using synthetic analogs such as $KTX_{(1-37)}$, $KTX_{(1-37)\text{-amide}}$ and short peptides including $KTX_{(27-37)}$, $KTX_{(25-32)}$, and $KTX_{(1-11)}$. Concerning the short peptides, which corresponded to secondary structural elements, only $KTX_{(27-37)}$ and $KTX_{(25-32)}$were able to compete with ^{125}I-KTX for its receptor on rat brain synaptosomes and act as antagonists of KTX. These results demonstrated for the first time that the C-terminal region, particularly the toxin β-sheet, was involved in the interaction with the

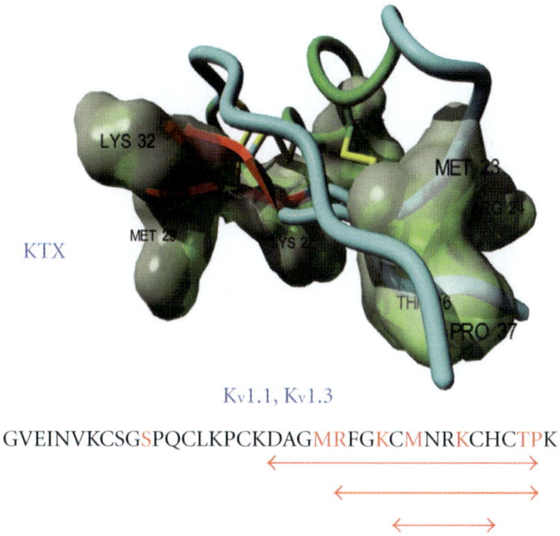

FIGURE 3: Amino acid sequence and 3D structure of KTX. The crucial amino acid residues involved in the receptor recognition are in red and are materialized on the 3D structure according to Lange et al., 2006 [13]. The α-helix is in green, the β-sheet in red. Arrows in red indicate the three peptides able to compete ($K_d = 100$ nM) with the ^{125}I-KTX bound to its binding site on rat brain synaptosomes [41].

receptor and the channel blockade [41]. Figure 3 summarizes these results.

Several international groups also produced KTX and numerous mutants using chemical synthesis or heterologous expression, in order to identify KTX residues implicated in the specific interaction with $K_v1.3$ channels. It was found that the side chain of Lys_{27} of the toxin enters deeply into the channel pore and interacts with the Asp_{402} residue of each subunit [24]. Briefly, the KTX residues involved in the interaction with the channel were Arg_{24}, Phe_{25}, Lys_{27}, Met_{39}, Asn_{30}, Arg_{31}. All these residues were present in the short peptides that we first used to demonstrate the β-sheet importance in the channel blockade. A model also predicted that Ser_{11} of the KTX made steric contacts with His_{404} and Pro_{405} of the α-subunit IV of the $K_v1.3$ and Thr_{36} with His_{404} of the opposing $K_v1.3$ α-subunit [42].

KTX binding to a chimeric K^+ channel (KcsA-$K_v1.3$) in proteoliposomes was investigated using solid-state nuclear magnetic resonance (ssNMR) [13]. Upon complex formation, significant chemical shift changes of the residues implicated in the specific interaction were observed for both KTX and chimeric channel. For KTX, the conformational changes involved mainly β-sheet contacts between the first and third β-strand and for the chimeric channel it affected the conformation of both the pore helix and the selectivity filter. The backbone conformation of Kcsa-$K_v1.3$ selectivity filter adopted a novel structure with features of both the conducting and collapsed conformation of the KcsA. The ssNMR data directly showed that Asp_{64} in the KcsA-$K_v1.3$ vestibule represented an important interaction site for KTX. Large chemical shift changes were seen for Gly_{77}, Tyr_{78}, and Gly_{79} in the selectivity filter and also for the side chains of Glu_{71} and Asp_{80} that form carboxyl-carboxylate pairs on the backside of the filter [13]. Finally, an enhanced backbone mobility was detected for two glycine residues within the selectivity filter that are highly conserved amongst potassium channels and are of core relevance to the filter structure and ion selectivity [43, 44].

Combination of additional ssNMR studies, dynamic simulations, and electrophysiological measurements finally revealed the complete mechanism of KTX binding to its receptor site and showed a structural link between inactivation and block of the channel. A mechanism of cooperative toxin-induced conformational changes that are structurally and functionally related to recovery from C-type inactivation, would be the consequence of the very tight interaction between KTX and Kcsa-$K_v1.3$. The KTX affinity was lowered by about 20-fold when the $K_v1.3$ channels entered in C-type inactivation probably due to changes of the interaction surface between the toxin and the channel [43–45].

All these recent ssNMR data obtained between the chimeric KcsA-$K_v1.3$ channel and KTX have largely contributed to decrypt the intimate interaction between a K^+ channel blocker and its target, as well as to better understand the blockade of the K^+ conduction.

6. The α-KTx_{15} Subfamily: Janus $K_v4.x$ and hERG Blockers

The first member of the α-KTx_{15} subfamily characterized was Aa1 from the *Androctonus australis* venom (3869 Da) [46]. At the primary sequence level, the toxin has an unusual N-terminal pyroglutamic acid, like Charybdotoxin and Iberiotoxin, but the rest of its sequence was totally original. Aa1 completely blocked a fast I_A-type K^+ current from cerebellum granular cells. Using whole-cell patch clamp recording on striatal neurons in culture, we selected another novel toxin, BmTX3 from *Buthus martensii*, which was also able to block a fast I_A-type K^+ current. The sustained current was unaffected with a micromolar dose of toxin whereas the I_A-type K^+ current completely disappeared independently of the membrane potential. Autoradiograms of adult rat brain sections demonstrated a highly heterogeneous distribution of ^{125}I-BmTX3 binding sites throughout the adult rat brain. High density of receptors was found in the striatum, the CA1 and CA3 field of the hippocampus, the superior colliculus, and in the granular layer of the cerebellum [47]. We then purified AmmTX3 (3827 Da), an analog of Aa1 and BmTX3, from the venom of *Androctonus mauretanicus mauretanicus* [22]. Latter, several cDNAs encoding two Aa1 isoforms, AaTX1 (3867 Da) and AaTX2 (3853 Da), were identified by PCR amplification from a venom gland cDNA library of *Androctonus australis* [48]. Also, another oligonucleotide sequence, AamTX (3751 Da), was amplified from a venom gland cDNA library of *Androctonus amoreuxi* [49]. Altogether these toxins constitute the first members of the α-KTx_{15} subfamily (Figure 4). From a pharmacological point of view, theses toxins were unable to compete with any other already described toxins purified from animal venom. However, they were toxic in mouse at high doses by intracerebral injections and induced epileptic status, which

Aa1	ZNETNKKCQGGS-CASVCRRVIGVAAGKCINGRCVCYP
BmTX3	ZVETNVKCQGGS-CASVCRKAIGVAAGKCINGRCVCYP
AmmTX3	ZIETNKKCQGGS-CASVCRKVIGVAAGKCINGRCVCYP
AamTX*	ZVQTNKKCKGGS-CASVCAKVIGVAAGKCINGRCVCYP
AaTX1*	ZIETNKKCQGGS-CASVCRRVIGVAAGKCINGRCVCYP
AaTX2*	ZVETNKKCQGGS-CASVCRRVIVVAAGKCINGRCVCYP
Discr.	ZIDTNVKCSGSSKCVKICIDRYNTRGAKCINGRCTCYP

Figure 4: Amino acid sequences of the toxins from the α-KTx$_{15}$ subfamily. Aa1 [46], AaTX1, and AaTX2 [48] are from *Androctonus australis*; BmTX3 [47] is from *Buthus martensii*; AmmTX3 [22] is from *Androctonus mauretanicus*; AamTX [49] is from *Androctonus amoreuxi*. Discrepin [54] is from the Venezuelan scorpion *Tityus discrepans*. Single letter notation is used for amino acid sequences. Z is pyroglutamic acid. *Indicates putative amino acid sequence deduced from cloned cDNA oligonucleotide sequence. The β-sheet consensus sequence is in grey.

could last 24 to 48 hours. Also, they all shared the same target on rat brain synaptosomes because they competed with each other for the same binding site. The nature of the K^+ channels blocked by AmmTX3 was assessed by performing whole-cell patch recording of the K^+ currents of striatal neurons and of cerebellum granular cells in culture. In all cases, AmmTX3 inactivated the transient A-current without affecting the sustained K^+ current, as observed for Aa1 and BmTX3. As well described, A-type K^+-currents result mainly from the expression of voltage-dependent K_v α-subunits (K_v1.4, 3.4, 4.1, 4.2, 4.3) or from the association of K_v β-subunit with K_v1 α-subunits [50, 51]. In the cerebellum granular cells, the voltage-gated K^+ channels K_v4 of the Shal subfamily elicits A-type currents. These channels are fast transient K^+ channels that regulate the kinetics of the action potential [51, 52]. The localizations of K_v4 subunits and their auxiliary subunits were similar to the distribution of BmTX3 binding sites in numerous regions of the brain. For example, the high density of BmTX3 binding sites in the CA1 field and CA3 field followed K_v4.2 and K_v4.3 immunostaining patterns. In the molecular layer of the dendate gyrus, the BmTX3 binding pattern was also similar to the immunoreactivity pattern of K_v4 and KChIP subunits, with a higher density in distal dendrites of the granular layer than in the more proximal dendrite areas [53].

Finally, electrophysiological analysis of mammalian cells expressing different A-type channels showed that BmTX3 completely inhibited the rapidly activating and inactivating K_v4.1 current in a voltage-independent manner. This inhibition was less effective on K_v4.2 and K_v4.3 channels and the toxin did not show any effects on other transient currents elicited by K_v1.4 and K_v3.4 [53]. Recent electrophysiological studies using acute coronal midbrain slices and AmmTX3 confirmed that the targets of the α-KTx$_{15}$ subfamily are K_v4 channels [55, Rudy B, personal communication]. Interestingly, the radioiodinated α-KTx$_{15}$ toxins bound to their receptor on rat brain neurons were not displaced by any spider toxin, which block K_v4 channels. This result suggests that these scorpion and spider K_v4 blockers have different binding sites. The α-KTx$_{15}$ toxins most probably block the K_v4 channel pore because tarantula toxins inhibit K_v4 channels by binding to the voltage-sensor paddles (crucial helix-turn-helix motifs within the voltage-sensing domains composed of the S3b and S4 helices) [56]. Moreover, deletions of the last two BmTx3 C-terminal residues (α-KTx$_{15}$ subfamily) were made to assess the role of the penultimate Tyr residue in the receptor recognition. This Tyr resembled to the canonical dyad previously proposed as necessary to block the K^+ channel conduction with high efficacy. Our results showed that the truncated toxin bound to its receptor less efficiently than the wild-type toxin (by a factor of about 10^5) and had no more channel blocking activity [57]. All these results suggest that the K_v4 channels blocked by the α-KTx$_{15}$ subfamily might have a canonical K^+ channel pore structure.

Moreover, we also described a significant hERG-blocking activity from the α-KTx$_{15}$ toxins, as previously shown for the γ-KTx peptides. AmmTx3 induced a hERG channel block with no alteration of the gating kinetics. According to a model of the γ-KTx toxin BeKm-1 from *Buthus eupeus* docked on hERG channels, the toxin BeKm-1 is above the pore entrance and none of its side chains penetrate deeply into the pore. While α-KTx members usually interact with channels through their β-sheets, γ-KTxs modulate hERG in a different way than the one proposed for the interaction between Charybdotoxin and the Shaker channel or between KTX and the K_v1.3, in which the critical Lys$_{27}$ protrudes into the pore of the channel. BeKm-1 uses its α-helix and the following turn (possessing two basic residues Lys$_{18}$ and Arg$_{20}$), to interact with hERG channel [58, 59]. In contrast to the other α-KTx$_{15}$ members, a new toxin of this subfamily isolated from the Venezuelan scorpion *Tityus discrepans*, called Discrepin (α-KTx$_{15-6}$), was also able to block an A-type K^+ current in cerebellum granular cells in culture, but was ineffective to block the hERG channel. Its amino acid sequence displays only 50% identity with the other members purified mainly from Old-World scorpion venoms (Figure 4). Discrepin C-terminal β-sheet, supposed to interfer with the K_v4 channel pore, presented a consensus amino acid sequence similar to those found in the other members (in grey on Figure 4), but its "hot spot" for hERG channel blockade was altered. After several point mutations in AmmTX3 and introduction of positive charged residues in Discrepin, it was finally demonstrated that a common "hot spot" composed of two basic residues (Arg$_{18}$ and Lys$_{19}$ near the end of the α-helix) conferred hERG blockade activity of α-KTx$_{15}$ peptides [54]. From a structural point of view, we proposed that two separate functional surfaces (A and B) could coexist on the α-KTx$_{15}$ toxins, and were responsible for two different K^+-current-blocking functions [60].

To extend our theory to other members from α-KTx subfamily, the effects of a "hot spot-" bearing toxin were tested on hERG channels and compared to the results obtained with a toxin without the "hot spot." From these studies, it was concluded that only the α-KTxs possessing the "hot spot" were able to interact with the pore of hERG channels. This pharmacophore could either be -CKKX- or -CKXK- or -CXKKX-, with C being the third Cys, X being any nonpositively charged amino acid, and K being Lys or Arg [54].

7. Conclusion

Scorpion venom still remains a proven resource for the discovery of novel biologically active compounds, especially for the pharmacologists involved in research on ionic channels. A total of about 210 α-KTx oligonucleotide or amino acid sequences are now referenced in the UniProtKB data bank, but only some of these α-KTx peptides have really been shown able to block K^+ currents. Unfortunately, very often, there is no direct evidence described for the function of the reported peptides. Some of them represent new analogs of well-known families with described channel selectivity, but others exhibit novel structural features or activities. Majority of the α-KTx effects were determined on the $K_v1.x$ subfamily or in a less extent on the Ca^{2+}-activated K^+ channels (SK_{Ca} sensitive to the bee venom apamin or BK_{Ca}). During the last two decades, we obtained a lot of results that provided new insight into the targets and the mode of action of some α-KTxs isolated from different potent North African *Androctonus* venoms. In particular, numerous studies on the *Androctonus mauretanicus mauretanicus* venom "manually" extracted, which can be considered as the physiological venom secretion, have greatly contributed to the chemical, immunological, structural, and pharmacological characterization of some highly specific K^+ channel blockers. With AmmTX3, we have enlarged the α-KTx_{15} subfamily and defined more properly its target, the K_v4 channels. KTX, from the α-KTx_3 subfamily, was finally proven to be a powerful tool used by several international teams to depict the molecular mechanisms of interaction between K^+ channels and peptide inhibitors, as well as to demonstrate that the binding of K^+ channel specific scorpion toxins does not take place only on the outer vestibule of the channel pore but also deeper into the selectivity filter. The binding involves a combination of hydrophobic, hydrogen bonding and electrostatic interactions, which induces significant structural rearrangements in both interacting molecules. It was then proposed that structural flexibility of the K^+ channel and the toxin represent an important determinant of the high specificity of toxin/K^+ channel interactions [13].

Acknowledgments

The authors wish to thank Drs. N. Abbas, F. Bosmans, B. Card, C. Legros, J. Tytgat, and H. Vacher, H for their contribution at a moment or another in the purification, pharmacological or electrophysiological characterization and cloning and mutagenesis of the *Androctonus mauretanicus* toxins blocking K^+ channels.

References

[1] M. F. Martin-Eauclaire and F. Couraud, "Scorpion neurotoxins: effects and mechanisms," in *Handbook Neurotoxicology*, L. W. Chang and R. S. Dyer, Eds., pp. 683–716, Marcel Dekker, New York, NY, USA, 1995.

[2] L. D. Possani, E. Merino, M. Corona, F. Bolivar, and B. Becerril, "Peptides and genes coding for scorpion toxins that affect ion-channels," *Biochimie*, vol. 82, no. 9-10, pp. 861–868, 2000.

[3] R. C. Rodríguez De La Vega and L. D. Possani, "Overview of scorpion toxins specific for Na^+ channels and related peptides: biodiversity, structure-function relationships and evolution," *Toxicon*, vol. 46, no. 8, pp. 831–844, 2005.

[4] S. Cestèle and W. A. Catterall, "Molecular mechanisms of neurotoxin action on voltage-gated sodium channels," *Biochimie*, vol. 82, no. 9-10, pp. 883–892, 2000.

[5] F. Bosmans, M. F. Martin-Eauclaire, and K. J. Swartz, "Deconstructing voltage sensor function and pharmacology in sodium channels," *Nature*, vol. 456, no. 7219, pp. 202–208, 2008.

[6] F. Bosmans, M. Puopolo, M. F. Martin-Eauclaire, B. P. Bean, and K. J. Swartz, "Functional properties and toxin pharmacology of a dorsal root ganglion sodium channel viewed through its voltage sensors," *Journal of General Physiology*, vol. 138, no. 1, pp. 59–72, 2011.

[7] J. Tytgat, K. G. Chandy, M. L. Garcia et al., "A unified nomenclature for short-chain peptides isolated from scorpion venoms: α-KTx molecular subfamilies," *Trends in Pharmacological Sciences*, vol. 20, no. 11, pp. 444–447, 1999.

[8] F. Bontems, C. Roumestand, B. Gilquin, A. Ménez, and F. Toma, "Refined structure of charybdotoxin: common motifs in scorpion toxins and insect defensins," *Science*, vol. 254, no. 5037, pp. 1521–1523, 1991.

[9] O. Pongs, *Regulation of Excitability by Potassium Channels. Inhibitory Regulation of Excitatory Neurotransmission*, vol. 44 of *Results and Problems in Cell Differentiation*, Springer, Heidelberg, Germany, 2007.

[10] G. A. Gutman, K. G. Chandy, S. Grissmer et al., "International Union of Pharmacology. LIII. Nomenclature and molecular relationships of voltage-gated potassium channels," *Pharmacological Reviews*, vol. 57, no. 4, pp. 473–508, 2005.

[11] S. B. Long, E. B. Campbell, and R. MacKinnon, "Crystal structure of a mammalian voltage-dependent Shaker family K^+ channel," *Science*, vol. 309, no. 5736, pp. 897–903, 2005.

[12] C. S. Park and C. Miller, "Interaction of charybdotoxin with permeant ions inside the pore of a k^+ channel," *Neuron*, vol. 9, no. 2, pp. 307–313, 1992.

[13] A. Lange, K. Giller, S. Hornig et al., "Toxin-induced conformational changes in a potassium channel revealed by solid-state NMR," *Nature*, vol. 440, no. 7086, pp. 959–962, 2006.

[14] K. N. Srinivasan, V. Sivaraja, I. Huys et al., "kappa-Hefutoxin1, a novel toxin from the scorpion Heterometrus fulvipes with unique structure and function. Importance of the functional diad in potassium channel selectivity," *Journal of Biological Chemistry*, vol. 277, no. 33, pp. 30040–30047, 2002.

[15] E. Diego-García, Y. Abdel-Mottaleb, E. F. Schwartz, R. C. R. De La Vega, J. Tytgat, and L. D. Possani, "Cytolytic and k^+ channel blocking activities of β-KTx and scorpine-like peptides purified from scorpion venoms," *Cellular and Molecular Life Sciences*, vol. 65, no. 1, pp. 187–200, 2008.

[16] M. Corona, G. B. Gurrola, E. Merino et al., "A large number of novel Ergtoxin-like genes and ERG k^+-channels blocking peptides from scorpions of the genus Centruroides," *FEBS Letters*, vol. 532, no. 1-2, pp. 121–126, 2002.

[17] N. Oukkache, M. F. Martin-Eauclaire, F. Chgoury et al., "Identification des paramètres influençant la prise en charge de l'envenimation scorpionique au Maroc," in *Toxines et Cancer, Rencontres en Toxinologie*, pp. 295–300, LAVOISIER, 2006.

[18] J. P. Rosso and H. Rochat, "Characterization of ten proteins from the venom of the Moroccan scorpion Androctonus mauretanicus mauretanicus, six of which are toxic to the mouse," *Toxicon*, vol. 23, no. 1, pp. 113–125, 1985.

[19] H. Zerrouk, P. E. Bougis, B. Ceard, A. Benslimane, and M. F. Martin-Eauclaire, "Analysis by high-performance liquid chromatography of Androctonus mauretanicus mauretanicus (black scorpion) venom," *Toxicon*, vol. 29, no. 8, pp. 951–960, 1991.

[20] M. Crest, G. Jacquet, M. Gola et al., "Kaliotoxin, a novel peptidyl inhibitor of neuronal BK-type Ca^{2+}-activated k^+ channels characterized from Androctonus mauretanicus mauretanicus venom," *Journal of Biological Chemistry*, vol. 267, no. 3, pp. 1640–1647, 1992.

[21] J. M. Sabatier, H. Zerrouk, H. Darbon et al., "P05, a new leiurotoxin I-like scorpion toxin: synthesis and structure-activity relationships of the α-amidated analog, a ligand of Ca^{2+}-activated k^+ channels with increased affinity," *Biochemistry*, vol. 32, no. 11, pp. 2763–2770, 1993.

[22] H. Vacher, M. Alami, M. Crest, L. D. Possani, P. E. Bougis, and M. F. Martin-Eauclaire, "Expanding the scorpion toxin α-KTX 15 family with AmmTX3 from Androctonus mauretanicus," *European Journal of Biochemistry*, vol. 269, no. 24, pp. 6037–6041, 2002.

[23] N. Oukkache, J. P. Rosso, M. Alami et al., "New analysis of the toxic compounds from the Androctonus mauretanicus mauretanicus scorpion venom," *Toxicon*, vol. 51, no. 5, pp. 835–852, 2008.

[24] J. Aiyar, J. M. Withka, J. P. Rizzi et al., "Topology of the pore-region of a k^+ channel revealed by the NMR-derived structures of scorpion toxins," *Neuron*, vol. 15, no. 5, pp. 1169–1181, 1995.

[25] J. C. Fontecilla-Camps, C. Habersetzer-Rochat, and H. Rochat, "Orthorhombic crystals and three-dimensional structure of the potent toxin II from the scorpion Androctonus australis Hector," *Proceedings of the National Academy of Sciences of the United States of America*, vol. 85, no. 20, pp. 7443–7447, 1988.

[26] H. Zerrouk, F. Laraba-Djebari, V. Fremont et al., "Characterization of PO15 a new peptide ligand of the apamin-sensitive $Ca2^+$ activated k^+ channel," *International Journal of Peptide and Protein Research*, vol. 48, no. 6, pp. 514–521, 1996.

[27] Y. Abdel-Mottaleb, E. Clynen, A. Jalali et al., "The first potassium channel toxin from the venom of the Iranian scorpion Odonthobuthus doriae," *FEBS Letters*, vol. 580, no. 26, pp. 6254–6258, 2006.

[28] H. Darbon, E. Blanc, and J. M. Sabatier, "Three-dimensional structure of scorpion toxins: toward a new model of interaction with potassium channels," *Perspectives in Drug Discovery and Design*, vol. 16, pp. 41–60, 1999.

[29] P. Auguste, M. Hugues, B. Grave et al., "Leiurotoxin I (scyllatoxin), a peptide ligand for Ca^{2+}-activated k^+ channels. Chemical synthesis, radiolabeling, and receptor characterization," *Journal of Biological Chemistry*, vol. 265, no. 8, pp. 4753–4759, 1990.

[30] G. G. Chicchi, G. Gimenez-Callego, E. Ber, M. L. Garcia, R. Winquist, and M. A. Cascieri, "Purification and characterization of a unique, potent inhibitor of apamin binding from Leiurus quinquestriatus hebraeus venom," *Journal of Biological Chemistry*, vol. 263, no. 21, pp. 10192–10197, 1988.

[31] C. Labbe-Jullie, C. Granier, F. Albericio et al., "Binding and toxicity of apamin. Characterization of the active site," *European Journal of Biochemistry*, vol. 196, no. 3, pp. 639–645, 1991.

[32] C. Devaux, M. Knibiehler, M. L. Defendini et al., "Recombinant and chemical derivatives of apamin. Implication of post-transcriptional C-terminal amidation of apamin in biological activity," *European Journal of Biochemistry*, vol. 231, no. 3, pp. 544–550, 1995.

[33] M. Cui, J. Shen, J. M. Briggs et al., "Brownian dynamics simulations of the recognition of the scorpion toxin P05 with the small-conductance calcium-activated potassium channels," *Journal of Molecular Biology*, vol. 318, no. 2, pp. 417–428, 2002.

[34] C. Brugnara, C. C. Armsby, L. De Franceschi, M. Crest, M. F. Martin Euclaire, and S. L. Alper, "Ca^{2+}-activated k^+ channels of human and rabbit erythrocytes display distinctive patterns of inhibition by venom peptide toxins," *Journal of Membrane Biology*, vol. 147, no. 1, pp. 71–82, 1995.

[35] E. Honore, E. Guillemare, F. Lesage, J. Barhanin, and M. Lazdunski, "Injection of a k^+ channel ($K_V1.3$) cRNA in fertilized eggs leads to functional expression in cultured myotomal muscle cells from Xenopus embryos," *FEBS Letters*, vol. 348, no. 3, pp. 259–262, 1994.

[36] M. D. Cahalan and K. G. Chandy, "The functional network of ion channels in T lymphocytes," *Immunological Reviews*, vol. 231, no. 1, pp. 59–87, 2009.

[37] C. Beeton, J. Barbaria, P. Giraud et al., "Selective blocking of voltage-gated k^+ channels improves experimental autoimmune encephalomyelitis and inhibits T cell activation," *Journal of Immunology*, vol. 166, no. 2, pp. 936–944, 2001.

[38] P. Valverde, T. Kawai, and M. A. Taubman, "Selective blockade of voltage-gated potassium channels reduces inflammatory bone resorption in experimental periodontal disease," *Journal of Bone and Mineral Research*, vol. 19, no. 1, pp. 155–164, 2004.

[39] C. Mourre, M. N. Chernova, M. F. Martin-Eauclaire et al., "Distribution in rat brain of binding sites of kaliotoxin, a blocker of $K_V1.1$ and $K_V1.3$ α-subunits," *Journal of Pharmacology and Experimental Therapeutics*, vol. 291, no. 3, pp. 943–952, 1999.

[40] S. Kourrich, C. Mourre, and B. Soumireu-Mourat, "Kaliotoxin, a $K_V1.1$ and $K_V1.3$ channel blocker, improves associative learning in rats," *Behavioural Brain Research*, vol. 120, no. 1, pp. 35–46, 2001.

[41] R. Romi, M. Crest, M. Gola et al., "Synthesis and characterization of kaliotoxin. Is the 26-32 sequence essential for potassium channel recognition?" *Journal of Biological Chemistry*, vol. 268, no. 35, pp. 26302–26309, 1993.

[42] G. M. Lipkind and H. A. Fozzard, "A model of scorpion toxin binding to voltage-gated k^+ channels," *Journal of Membrane Biology*, vol. 158, no. 3, pp. 187–196, 1997.

[43] C. Ader, R. Schneider, S. Hornig et al., "A structural link between inactivation and block of a k^+ channel," *Nature Structural and Molecular Biology*, vol. 15, no. 6, pp. 605–612, 2008.

[44] C. Ader, O. Pongs, S. Becker, and M. Baldus, "Protein dynamics detected in a membrane-embedded potassium channel using two-dimensional solid-state NMR spectroscopy," *Biochimica et Biophysica Acta*, vol. 1798, no. 2, pp. 286–290, 2010.

[45] U. Zachariae, R. Schneider, P. Velisetty et al., "The molecular mechanism of toxin-induced conformational changes in a potassium channel: relation to C-type inactivation," *Structure*, vol. 16, no. 5, pp. 747–754, 2008.

[46] M. Pisciotta, F. I. Coronas, C. Bloch, G. Prestipino, and L. D. Possani, "Fast k^+ currents from cerebellum granular cells are completely blocked by a peptide purified from Androctonus australis Garzoni scorpion venom," *Biochimica et Biophysica Acta*, vol. 1468, no. 1-2, pp. 203–212, 2000.

[47] H. Vacher, R. Romi-Lebrun, C. Mourre et al., "A new class of scorpion toxin binding sites related to an A-type k^+ channel: pharmacological characterization and localization in rat brain," *FEBS Letters*, vol. 501, no. 1-3, pp. 31–36, 2001.

[48] C. Legros, P. E. Bougis, and M. F. Martin-Eauclaire, "Characterisation of the genes encoding Aa1 isoforms from

the scorpion Androctonus australis," *Toxicon*, vol. 41, no. 1, pp. 115–119, 2003.

[49] T. Chen, B. Walker, M. Zhou, and C. Shaw, "Molecular cloning of a novel putative potassium channel-blocking neurotoxin from the venom of the North African scorpion, Androctonus amoreuxi," *Peptides*, vol. 26, no. 5, pp. 731–736, 2005.

[50] M. C. Sanguinetti, J. H. Johnson, L. G. Hammerland et al., "Heteropodatoxins: peptides isolated from spider venom that block $K_v4.2$ potassium channels," *Molecular Pharmacology*, vol. 51, no. 3, pp. 491–498, 1997.

[51] W. A. Coetzee, Y. Amarillo, J. Chiu et al., "Molecular diversity of k^+ channels," *Annals of the New York Academy of Sciences*, vol. 868, pp. 233–285, 1999.

[52] H. Vacher and J. S. Trimmer, "Diverse roles for auxiliary subunits in phosphorylation-dependent regulation of mammalian brain voltage-gated potassium channels," *Pflugers Archiv European Journal of Physiology*, vol. 642, no. 5, pp. 631–643, 2011.

[53] H. Vacher, S. Diochot, P. E. Bougis, M. F. Martin-Eauclaire, and C. Mourre, "K_v4 channels sensitive to BmTX3 in rat nervous system: autoradiographic analysis of their distribution during brain ontogenesis," *European Journal of Neuroscience*, vol. 24, no. 5, pp. 1325–1340, 2006.

[54] Y. Abdel-Mottaleb, G. Corzo, M. F. Martin-Eauclaire et al., "A common "hot spot" confers hERG blockade activity to α-scorpion toxins affecting k^+ channels," *Biochemical Pharmacology*, vol. 76, no. 6, pp. 805–815, 2008.

[55] J. Amendola, A. Woodhouse, M. F. Martin-Eauclaire, and J. M. Goaillard, "Ca^{2+}/cAMP-Sensitive co-variation of IA and IH voltage dependences tune rebound firing in dopaminergic neurons," *The Journal of Neuroscience*, vol. 32, no. 6, pp. 2166–2181, 2012.

[56] L. R. Phillips, M. Milescu, Y. Li-Smerin, J. A. Mindell, J. I. Kim, and K. J. Swartz, "Voltage-sensor activation with a tarantula toxin as cargo," *Nature*, vol. 436, no. 7052, pp. 857–860, 2005.

[57] H. Vacher, R. Romi-Lebrun, M. Crest et al., "Functional consequences of deleting the two C-terminal residues of the scorpion toxin BmTX3," *Biochimica et Biophysica Acta*, vol. 1646, no. 1-2, pp. 152–156, 2003.

[58] G. N. Tseng, K. D. Sonawane, Y. V. Korolkova et al., "Probing the outer mouth structure of the hERG channel with peptide toxin footprinting and molecular modeling," *Biophysical Journal*, vol. 92, no. 10, pp. 3524–3540, 2007.

[59] R. C. Rodríguez De La Vega, E. Merino, B. Becerril, and L. D. Possani, "Novel interactions between k^+ channels and scorpion toxins," *Trends in Pharmacological Sciences*, vol. 24, no. 5, pp. 222–227, 2003.

[60] I. Huys, C. Q. Xu, C. Z. Wang et al., "BmTx3, a scorpion toxin with two putative functional faces separately active on A-type k^+ and HERG currents," *Biochemical Journal*, vol. 378, no. 3, pp. 745–752, 2004.

2

Reconstructing Organophosphorus Pesticide Doses Using the Reversed Dosimetry Approach in a Simple Physiologically-Based Pharmacokinetic Model

Chensheng Lu[1] and Leo Andres[2]

[1] *Department of Environmental Health, Harvard School of Public Health, 401 Park Drive, Boston, MA 02215, USA*
[2] *Atlanta Clinical and Translational Science Institute, School of Medicine, Emory University, 1440 Clifton Road, Atlanta, GA 30322, USA*

Correspondence should be addressed to Chensheng Lu, cslu@hsph.harvard.edu

Academic Editor: Marina V. Evans

We illustrated the development of a simple pharmacokinetic (SPK) model aiming to estimate the absorbed chlorpyrifos doses using urinary biomarker data, 3,5,6-trichlorpyridinol as the model input. The effectiveness of the SPK model in the pesticide risk assessment was evaluated by comparing dose estimates using different urinary composite data. The dose estimates resulting from the first morning voids appeared to be lower than but not significantly different to those using before bedtime, lunch or dinner voids. We found similar trend for dose estimates using three different urinary composite data. However, the dose estimates using the SPK model for individual children were significantly higher than those from the conventional physiologically based pharmacokinetic (PBPK) modeling using aggregate environmental measurements of chlorpyrifos as the model inputs. The use of urinary data in the SPK model intuitively provided a plausible alternative to the conventional PBPK model in reconstructing the absorbed chlorpyrifos dose.

1. Introduction

A physiologically based pharmacokinetic (PBPK) model would allow for simulating the dynamics of pesticide absorption, distribution, metabolism, and elimination (ADME) from different routes of exposures and, in theory, could be used as a tool for evaluating biomarker measurements (e.g. blood or urine levels) associated with the exposures [1–4]. The mechanistic representation of biological processes embedded in the PBPK model allows systematic route, dose, and species extrapolation, and for these reasons, PBPK models have been applied in pesticide risk assessments that are relevant for the interpretation of biomarker data [5–12].

Although the interpretation of PBPK model outputs could provide a link to the regulatory metrics in the form of reference dose, its application remains problematic due to the fundamental limitations resulting from the potential measurement errors associated with the aggregate exposure measurements [11, 13]. Although those aggregate exposure data are needed in order to simulate the dynamics of ADME for a specific pesticide, the uncertainties, mainly the temporal and spatial variations, associated with the measurements may inadvertently be carried over to the model outcomes. Those uncertainties, however, are merely explicit statements of underlying assumption applied in the analysis of urinary biomarker data.

A simple pharmacokinetic (SPK) model incorporating reverse dosimetry and PBPK modeling approach, on the other hand, only requires urinary biomarker data as inputs and the a-priori knowledge of the exposure pathways for individuals [14, 15]. The use of urinary biomarker data in the SPK simulation might be advantageous over the traditional PBPK model because urinary excretion is a primary route of elimination for many compounds, and urine samples are relatively easy to collect from individuals comparing to the aggregate environmental samples. The SPK model allows for the estimation of absorbed dose from a dominated route of exposure while reducing the number of inputs into the model

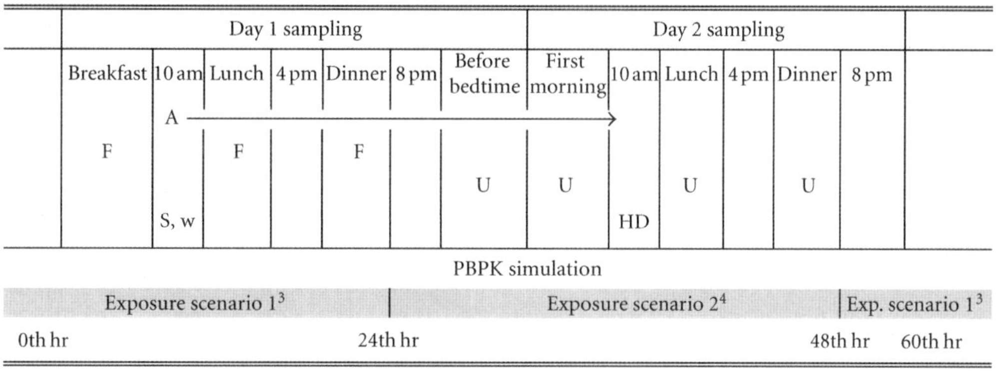

Figure 1: Sampling schedule for the 1998 study[1] and the corresponding PBPK model simulation[2].

and could potentially minimize the uncertainties. Therefore, the development of SPK model may be important in the field of PBPK model by reducing the resources needed to model the dose metrics of certain chemicals.

In this paper, we illustrated the development of an SPK model adapted from a previously published PBPK model and the performance of the exploratory analysis using urinary biomarker data as inputs to the SPK model. The effectiveness of the SPK model in the pesticide risk assessment was evaluated by comparing the dose estimates among three different composites of biomarker data.

2. Methods

The development of the SPK model began with the pharmacokinetic equations that are used in previously developed PBPK models for animal and human data [2, 11, 16, 17]. While the solution of a conventional PBPK model results in a uniquely determined excretion profile of urinary biomarker, the "reverse" dosimetry analysis in this SPK model development, which uses urinary biomarker concentrations as input, does not lead to a unique solution. It is, therefore, necessary to constrain the dose profile with additional information to reach an optimum dosing profile. We assumed that the predominant exposure pathway for organophosphorus (OP) pesticides is via foods and, therefore, constructed the SPK model focusing on oral ingestion. Such assumption was based on the results of aggregate exposure assessment, and the previous PBPK model outputs which shows very little OP residues in the environment [18] and suggests dietary intakes of OP pesticides constitute the majority of urinary metabolite concentrations [11], respectively.

2.1. Urinary Biomarker Data. Data employed in this SPK model simulation were collected from a cross-sectional study with repeated biological and environmental sampling conducted in Washington State in 1998. Results for the environmental measurements of several OP pesticides and their respective urinary metabolites, as well as for absorbed dose reconstruction using a conventional PBPK model, were published previously [11, 18–20]. In brief, the study was conducted in the homes of 13 children ages 3–6, who either lived in an urban/suburban (nonagricultural) area or in the agricultural region in which OPs have been used in the nearby fruit tree orchards. Each home was sampled for two 24-hour periods (over 3 days) in summer and fall of 1998. Environmental and biological sample collections included 24-hour indoor air, drinking water; outdoors soil, house dust, toy wipes, 24-hour duplicate diets, and 4 spot urine samples over a 24-hour period (Figure 1). The 1998 study was designed to capture the aggregate OP exposures in the subsequent 4 spot urines over the course of a 24-hour period. These were the before bedtime voids on the first day and the first morning lunch, and dinner voids on the second day. Chlorpyrifos (CPF) was selected as the modeled pesticide in this study because it was commonly detected in the environmental matrices, and its specific metabolite, 3,5,6-trichlorpyridinol (TCPY), was frequently measured in the urine samples, as compared to other OP pesticides.

Urinary data from the 1998 study, including TCPY concentrations, urine void volumes, and urine sample collection times, were used as inputs into the SPK model to estimate the absorbed dose of CPF. The study protocol and procedures to obtain the assent of the children and informed consent of their parents or guardians were reviewed and approved by the University of Washington Institutional Review Board (IRB). The use of those data in the PBPK model analysis was reviewed and approved by Emory University IRB.

2.2. Model Development and Validation

2.2.1. Input File Construction. A database was created in Microsoft Access 2002 to hold study variables and data. Tables in the database were structured in the same form as the raw study data to allow for easier manipulation of the data later in the analysis. There were missing values (not collected), including the void and exposure times, values for void volumes, and values for the weight of the study subjects that were necessary to create the data file. Values for the default void and exposure times were chosen based on a previous data file for the Matlab PK model script. Values for the default void volume were taken from a study by Voorhess [21] which examined urinary catecholamine excretion by healthy children. Lastly, values for the default weights of children were taken from table 7-3 of the Exposure Factors Handbook [22]. Tables were created to hold these values specific to sample, age, or sex depending on the measure.

Queries were written in SQL to create the data files for input into the SPK model. SQL was used to join data from separate data tables into one query output, to make logic and arithmetic transformations to the data for input into the model, and to allow for dynamic creation of data files simplifying modification of data input file creation. Since some of the data that are necessary to create the input file were missing, default values had to be calculated. This was done according to the type of data that was available and which data would provide values that would best represent the inputs. The script would first try to determine values based on data that would yield the most representative values. If this data was not available, then it would try other data that would yield less representative values successively based on availability of the relevant data until it reached the least representative values.

The main query that produced the data file was qry_createdata. This query pulled data from database tables and other queries. These queries were qry_calcttime and qry_urinesampcalc. The qry_calcttime query was used to calculate the previous and current void times using available data and default values depending on the data that was available. The qry_urinesampcalc query was used to calculate the urinary excretion rate from metabolite concentrations, sample void volumes, and times from qry_calcttime. Once these queries produced the correct data for input into the model, the main query was used to export the data from Access into Excel 97–2002 format.

Once constructed, each of the input file for the Matlab SPK model script (see supplementary material available online at doi:10.1155/2012/131854) had nine variables. The first variable held the subject ID and study period. The subject ID was the part before the separator, and the study period was the part after the separator. For the study period, 1 signified the summer period, and 2 signified the fall period. For example, the identifier 114.1 denoted subject ID 114 in the summer study period. The second variable reflected whether the subject resided in an agricultural area. The third variable held the average metabolite urinary excretion rate that was calculated using the urinary metabolite concentration, the volume of the void, and the times for the previous and current void

$$\mathrm{UER}_{\mathrm{avg}}\ (\mathrm{mmoL/hr}) = \frac{C_u V_u}{\left(t_c - t_p\right)}. \tag{1}$$

In this formula, $\mathrm{UER}_{\mathrm{avg}}$ is the average urinary excretion rate between the current void and the previous void, C_u is the measured metabolite concentration in the urine, V_u is the volume of the void, t_c is the time of the current void, and t_p is the time of the previous void [1]. The fourth variable held the body weight of the child in kilograms. The fifth variable denoted the route of the exposure and scenario, where 1 is an inhalation exposure, 2 is a dermal exposure, and 3 through 7 are bolus events. In this analysis, 3 was the first morning void on the second day, 4 was the lunchtime void, 5 was the before bedtime void on the first day, and 6 was the dinnertime void on the second day. The sixth variable held the start time of the exposure event on a 24-hour clock with 0 at midnight before the exposure event. The seventh variable held the end time of the exposure event. However, for the current analysis, this variable was not used since the exposures that were analyzed were bolus events. The eighth variable held the time of the previous urine void before the exposure event on a 24-hour clock. The ninth variable held the time of the current urine void sample before the exposure event on a 24-hour clock.

2.2.2. Data Processing. Once input files were created, the SPK model was run using Matlab version 7.0.1. Each input into the simple SPK model was able to calculate an estimated absorbed dose for CPF by fitting the input variables to a generalized dose absorption curve. It then calculated the absorbed dose by finding the area under the curve over the course of a day. Due to the construction of the script, the model was only able to compute one dose estimate from one exposure rather than from a collection of exposures. Using the output from the SPK model script, we composited four spot urine samples in three different ways in order to estimate the daily absorbed doses of CPF in three different scenarios.

For the first composite (SPK I) scenario, only TCPY concentrations from the first morning void were used to calculate the dose estimate. This void was suggested to be an accurate measure of TCPY metabolite because it was assumed that TCPY concentrations in the urine were 0 after the before bedtime void [20]. Urine would then be formed and held during the night and voided in the morning, which would give the sample greater accuracy in determining metabolite concentrations since a long period of time had elapsed before the void.

For the second composite (SPK II) scenario, dose estimates from the before bedtime void and the first morning void were averaged normalized by the volume of each void. This was done because the SPK model was only able to analyze one sample at a time rather than taking a collection of samples and computing a dose from them. In this calculation, it was assumed that metabolite concentrations from the before bedtime void and the first morning void were both due to exposure from dinner on the first day. Since metabolite concentrations were assumed to be caused by the same exposure event (dinner event), they should compute to the same absorbed dose. Therefore, the two dose estimates were averaged to provide a fair measure based on both outputs.

In order to determine the times used to calculate the urinary excretion rate for the before bedtime sample of SPK II, we used the volume of the void sample to estimate the time that the urine was allowed to collect in the bladder. This estimate was based on the average daily void volume of children of the same age and gender over a 24-hour period [21]. By dividing the sample void volume by the average daily void volume, the time that the urine was allowed to collect in the bladder was estimated using (2), in which $(t_c - t_p)$ is the difference in hours from the time of the current void (t_c) to the time of the previous void (t_p), V_u is the volume of the urine sample, and $\mathrm{V}_{\mathrm{avg24}}$ is the volume of the average daily void over the span of 24 hours:

$$\left(t_c - t_p\right) \approx \left(\frac{V_u}{\mathrm{V}_{\mathrm{avg24}}}\right) * 24 \tag{2}$$

For the third composite (SPK III) scenario, dose estimates from the before bedtime void on the first day, and the first morning void, the lunchtime void, and the dinner void on the second day were averaged to reach a single absorbed dose estimate. For this calculation, the beginning exposure time for the lunch and dinner voids on the second day was set at dinner time on the first day. We assumed that part of the urinary metabolite measurements from the lunchtime and dinner voids on the second day may come from dinnertime exposure on the first day. Since absorbed dose estimates could not be calculated using more than one exposure, a composite meal exposure was created using urinary metabolite measurements from the before bedtime void on the first day, the first morning void, the lunchtime void, and the dinnertime void on the second day. The time of the composite meal exposure was set at dinnertime on the first day. The results from the four estimates were then averaged to get an overall absorbed dose estimate. Again, the times used to calculate the urinary excretion rate were estimated from dividing the sample void volume by the average daily void volume using (2).

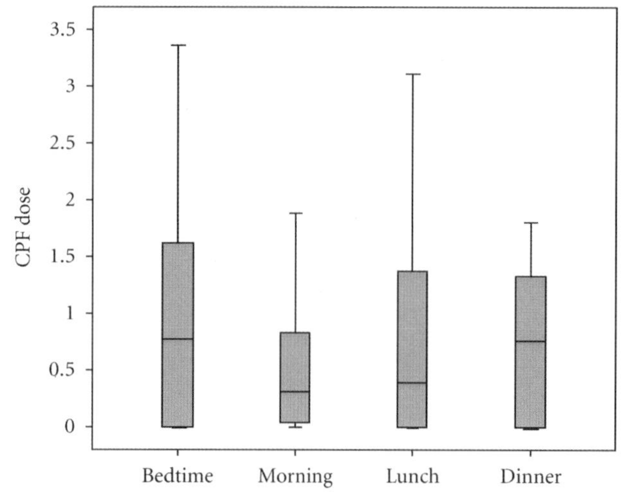

FIGURE 2: The dose estimates (CPF_DOSE, μg/kg/day) for chlorpyrifos using 3,5,6-trichlorpyridinol concentrations in the spot urine samples collected at before bedtime in Day 1 and the first morning, lunch, and dinner voids in Day 2 as the SPK model inputs.

3. Results and Discussion

The PBPK model was developed to quantitatively integrate the physiological, metabolic, and biochemical factors associated with ADME. Although the initial model validation has proven the accuracy of predicting CPF exposures, it was found later that the effectiveness of the PBPK model was highly dependent on the model parameters and the limitation of the input exposure data [2]. This limitation has been highlighted in a recent study in which the PBPK model failed to predict TCPY excretion as compared to TCPY levels measured in urine collected from study subjects [11]. Such failure exposes the vulnerability of employing PBPK models in risk assessment without sufficient knowledge or assurance of the quality of exposure data that are used as PBPK model inputs. Therefore, we were prompted to develop this simple pharmacokinetic model in order to improve the ability for estimating absorbed dose using urinary metabolite data as the model inputs. Should TCPY levels measured in urine be considered the gold standard in reflecting the exposure to CPF (by subtracting the preformed portion of TCPY), the use of urinary TCPY data in the pharmacokinetic analysis would provide more reliable dose estimates of CPF than using aggregate exposure data.

The SPK model simulation yielded to a total of 88 CPF dose estimates, separated by summer and fall seasons. The dose estimates resulted from the first morning void measurements appeared to be lower than but not significantly different to those using before bedtime, lunch, or dinner voids (Figure 2). Those estimates were modeled assuming that the exposure to CPF occurred during dinner meal (at 7 pm) on the first day. Knowing that the biological half-life for orally ingested CPF is approximately 16 hours [23], the estimated absorption curve for the first morning void may mostly reflect the intake of CPF from dinner last night. Dose estimates for spot urine samples collected later in the 2nd day were increasingly larger, suggesting additional CPF exposures from earlier in the day (breakfast and lunch). Dose estimates from before bedtime void samples were likely to be representative of CPF exposures that occurred throughout the first day rather than intakes from dinner, as was modeled.

The disparity among the dose estimates using spot urinary TCPY measurements in different time points raises the concern of the validity of using single spot urinary measurement as the basis of dose estimation in risk assessment. The magnitude of such uncertainty would be considerably larger under the circumstance in which spot urine samples are collected at different time points within a predetermined time period (e.g., 24 hours) from individuals. For instance, the National Health and Nutrition Examination Survey (NHANES) conducted by the Center for Disease Control and Prevention (CDC) collected single spot urine samples from subjects based on their appointments. If TCPY data from NHANES were used in the SPK model simulation, the interpretation and the conclusions of the estimated doses for CPF in NHANES subjects should therefore be cautiously made. Georgopoulos et al. [13] also raised this issue in their case study involving the use of a physiologically based toxicokinetic modeling in conjunction with numerical "inversion" techniques for reconstructing CPF exposure using TCPY data measured in the National Human Exposure Assessment Survey (NHEXAS). As authors stated "Although the NHEXAS data set provides a significant amount of supporting exposure-related information, especially when compared to national studies such as the NHANES, this information is still not adequate for detailed reconstruction of exposures under several conditions," as demonstrated in the paper.

We estimated the daily absorbed CPF doses for individual children using three different composites of the 4 spot urine biomarker measurements (Table 1). Dose estimates for SPK I, II and III were not significantly different (one-way ANOVA); however, the box plot in Figure 3 showed that

TABLE 1: Descriptive statistics for the estimated daily dose (μg/kg/day) of chlorpyrifos in thirteen children ages 2–5 using the simple pharmacokinetic model.

Overall	SPK I	SPK II	SPK III
Mean (St. Dev.)	0.98 (1.95)	0.97 (1.19)	0.87 (0.81)
Median	0.37	0.82	0.92
N	21	23	26
95% confidence interval (lower, upper)	(0.09, 1.86)	(0.43, 1.51)	(0.51, 1.24)
Min–max	(0, 9.13)	(0, 5.5)	(0, 3.65)
Summer season			
Mean (St. Dev.)	0.55 (0.58)	0.8 (1.0)	0.73 (0.68)
Median	0.34	0.27	0.52
N	10	11	13
95% confidence interval (lower, upper)	(0.19, 0.91)	(0.24, 1.37)	(0.37, 1.09)
Min–max	(0, 1.89)	(0, 3.36)	(0, 2.5)
Fall season			
Mean (St. Dev.)	1.3 (2.53)	1.32 (1.42)	1.13 (0.9)
Median	0.42	0.97	0.94
N	11	12	13
95% confidence interval (lower, upper)	(0, 2.67)	(0.55, 2.09)	(0.66, 1.6)
Min–max	(0.05, 9.13)	(0.2, 5.5)	(0.23, 3.65)
Urban/suburban children			
Mean (St. Dev.)	0.48 (0.52)	0.67 (0.64)	0.63 (0.55)[1]
Median	0.35	0.48	0.45
N	11	12	12
95% confidence interval (lower, upper)	(0.19, 0.77)	(0.31, 1.03)	(0.32, 0.94)
Min–max	(0.04, 1.88)	(0.02, 2.27)	(0.01, 1.97)
Agricultural children			
Mean (St. Dev.)	1.53 (2.73)	1.51 (1.58)	1.19 (0.92)[1]
Median	0.88	1.06	1.04
N	10	11	14
95% confidence interval (lower, upper)	(0.1, 2.96)	(0.91, 2.11)	(0.68, 1.7)
Min–max	(0, 9.12)	(0, 5.5)	(0, 3.65)

[1] Marginally significantly different (one-way ANOVA, $P = 0.077$).

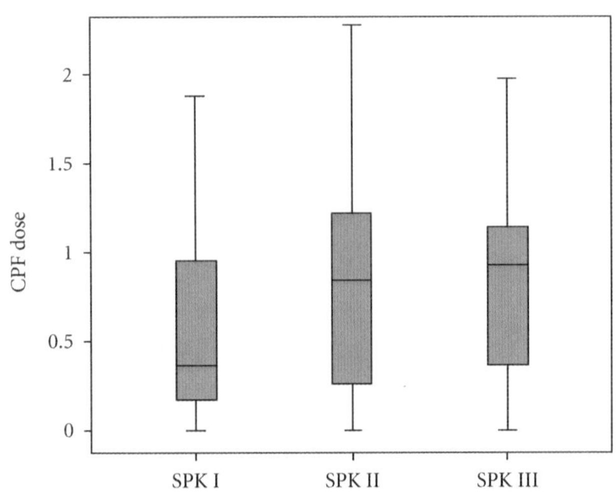

FIGURE 3: The dose estimates (CPF_DOSE, μg/kg/day) for chlorpyrifos using urinary 3,5,6-trichlorpyridinol concentrations in three different spot urine sample composite methods; SPK_I, SPK_II, and SPK_III.

the median dose estimate from SPK I model simulation are lower than those of SPK II and III, consistent to the trend for the individual void simulations. While this may suggest that dose estimates between models reflect similar CPF exposure among subjects, it is also possible that the similarity among dose estimates is merely the result of the dose estimation being based on shared data. For instance, SPK II was based on the average between SPK I and the dose estimates using the before bedtime voids, and SPK III was based on the estimates that comprised the SPK II estimate and estimates from the lunch and dinner samples. The SPK II dose estimates seemed to be more accurately representative of the daily exposure to CPF simply because it takes into account the excretion of TCPY in before bedtime voids in day 1 and the first morning voids in day 2. The additional CPF exposure between lunch and dinner, if any, captured in the SPK III dose estimates did not significantly increase the overall daily dose estimates would support the validity of using SPK II as the benchmark for daily CPF absorbed dose. Comparing the dose estimates by seasonality and the

TABLE 2: The dose estimates (μg/kg/day) for chlorpyrifos using PBPK, SPK I, SPK II and SPK III model simulations.

Subject ID[1]	Season	Body wt. (kg)	PBPK	SPK I[2]	SPK II[3]	SPK III[4]
R1	Summer	15.5	0.004	0.546	0.273	1.140
R2	Summer	21.4	0.003	0.281	0.246	0.380
R3	Summer	14.5	0.004	0.043	0.022	0.014
R4	Summer	16.8	0.003	0.831	1.439	0.987
R5	Summer	13.4	0.004	0.338	0.213	0.158
R6	Summer	19.6	0.003	n.a.[5]	0.840	0.520
S1	Summer	17.3	0.003	0	0	0
S2	Summer	18.2	0	0.224	0.112	0.488
S3	Summer	15	0	n.a.[5]	3.357	2.497
S4	Summer	15.5	0	1.881	1.450	1.282
S5	Summer	16.8	0.004	n.a.[5]	n.a.[5]	0.326
S6	Summer	22.7	0.440	0.808	0.820	0.672
S7	Summer	14.5	0	n.a.[5]	n.a.[5]	1.056
R1	Fall	15.5	0.004	1.881	2.274	1.973
R2	Fall	21.4	0.003	0.051	0.204	0.229
R3	Fall	14.5	0.012	0.347	0.980	0.944
R4	Fall	16.8	0.003	0.366	0.541	0.603
R5	Fall	13.4	0.018	0.082	0.483	0.368
R6	Fall	19.6	0.005	0.476	0.476	0.250
S1	Fall	17.3	2.302	9.125	5.496	3.647
S2	Fall	18.2	0.003	0.172	0.949	1.110
S3	Fall	15	0.004	1.060	1.060	1.219
S4	Fall	15.5	0	0.956	1.260	1.017
S5	Fall	16.8	0	1.028	1.184	0.922
S6	Fall	22.7	0.001	0.041	0.969	0.934
S7	Fall	14.5	0.006	n.a.[5]	n.a.[5]	1.513

[1]"R" for children living in agricultural community and "S" for children living in urban/suburban community.
[2]Significantly different to PBPK dose estimates (paired t-test, $P < 0.001$).
[3]Significantly different to PBPK dose estimates (paired t-test, $P = 0.02$).
[4]Significantly different to PBPK dose estimates (paired t-test, $P < 0.001$).
[5]Missing data due to missing spot urine samples.

community where children lived in 1998, we found that children living in urban/suburban have higher CPF exposure than those lived in agricultural community, and their CPF exposure was higher in fall than in summer season.

The SPK dose estimates for individual children participating in the 1998 study were significantly higher than those using the conventional PBPK model approaching, as published earlier [11]. The highest PBPK predicted CPY dose of 2.3 μg/kg/day resulted from the consumption of a food item containing 350 ng/g of CPF remained as the highest in the SPK I, II, and III simulations with the estimated CPF doses of 9.1, 5.5, and 3.7 μg/kg/day, respectively (Table 2). The striking difference of dose estimates between these two pharmacokinetic models may be primarily due to the differences of input data. The use of aggregate exposure assessment as the input variables in the PBPK models targeted at chemicals with short biological half-lives, such as CPF, is prone to significant spatial and temporal variations associated with exposures that would lead to inaccurate outcome measurements. This is evident by the fact that the majority of the data collected from the environment (Figure 1) where the children lived were nondetectable for CPF residue, while spot urine samples collected from those same children frequently contained TCPY. By taking into account the degradation of CPF in the environment (or in foods) in the PBPK model simulation as described in previous studies [11, 24, 25], the PBPK model predicted that TCPY excretion was still not within a reasonable range of accuracy to the measured TCPY levels which are used in the SPK model simulation. It is apparent that the 24-hr aggregate exposure assessment is not capable of capturing CPF exposure in those children. This leads to the serious doubt of the validity of applying aggregate exposure measurements to the PBPK model simulation and subsequently in the risk assessment. The use of urinary TCPY data in the SPK model simulation intuitively provided a plausible alternative to PBPK model in reconstructing the absorbed CPF dose. In theory, the dose estimates resulting from either PBPK or SPK approach should yield to numerical values that are not significantly different to each other, particularly in this case in which both models were constructed using identical parameters, and the input data were collected from a study that is designed specifically for validating the PBPK model simulation. However, the problem of significant under estimation of CPY doses using the traditional PBPK, as identified in this paper, would be even more prevalent and dramatic under other circumstances in which less-structured environmental exposure data are collected and used as the PBPK model inputs.

4. Study Limitations

Similar to other PBPK model applications, assumptions are needed in the SPK models in order to facilitate the model simulation. The unique assumptions for SPK model simulation include the prior knowledge of the predominant exposure pathway (such as dietary intake in this project) and the default time of exposure (dinner in Day 1). Without detail information of the exposure, those assumptions have to be made either arbitrarily (time of exposure) or by interpretation of study observations (dietary ingestion). A mischaracterization of the predominant exposure pathway (such as dietary intake versus inhalation) will lead to completely different SPK simulation and outcomes.

Due to the limitation in constructing the script files, the SPK model is only able to compute one dose estimate from one urinary biomarker data input, instead of from a series of urinary biomarker data input within 24 hours. In order to overcome this limitation, we used the average dose estimates in SPK II and SPK III to incorporate more urinary biomarker data that is related to the interest of a specific exposure event in the simulation. It is likely that we would introduce unknown uncertainties to the overall simulation because urinary TCPY levels measured in the dinner time may include CPF exposure in Day 2 which is not the interest of the analysis. Although the magnitude of such uncertainty is relatively minimal in this study, by further examining the data for SPK II and SPK III, we acknowledge the existence of such uncertainty.

Acknowledgment

This work was supported by the U.S. Environmental Protection Agency under the Science to Achieve Results research assistance program (R-832244 and R-829364). The authors would like to thank Dr. Miles S. Okino and Christina Holbrook for their assistance with the PBPK model development. Authors declare no competing financial interests in this work.

References

[1] M. L. Rigas, M. S. Okino, and J. J. Quackenboss, "Use of a pharmacokinetic model to assess chlorpyrifos exposure and dose in children, based on urinary biomarker measurements," *Toxicological Sciences*, vol. 61, no. 2, pp. 374–381, 2001.

[2] C. Timchalk, R. J. Nolan, A. L. Mendrala, D. A. Dittenber, K. A. Brzak, and J. L. Mattsson, "A physiologically based pharmacokinetic and pharmacodynamic (PBPK/PD) model for the organophosphate insecticide chlorpyrifos in rats and humans," *Toxicological Sciences*, vol. 66, no. 1, pp. 34–53, 2002.

[3] X. Zhang, A. M. Tsang, M. S. Okino et al., "A physiologically based pharmacokinetic/pharmacodynamic model for carbofuran in sprague-dawley rats using the exposure-related dose estimating model," *Toxicological Sciences*, vol. 100, no. 2, pp. 345–359, 2007.

[4] C. A. Ellison, J. N. Smith, P. J. Lein, and J. R. Olson, "Pharmacokinetics and pharmacodynamics of chlorpyrifos in adult male Long-Evans rats following repeated subcutaneous exposure to chlorpyrifos," *Toxicology*, vol. 287, no. 1–3, pp. 137–144, 2011.

[5] J. N. Blancato, "Pharmacokinetics, chemical interactions, and toxicological risk assessment in perspective," *Environmental Health Perspectives*, vol. 102, supplement 9, pp. 133–137, 1994.

[6] H. J. Clewell, P. R. Gentry, J. M. Gearhart, B. C. Allen, and M. E. Andersen, "Comparison of cancer risk estimates for vinyl chloride using animal and human data with a PBPK model," *Science of the Total Environment*, vol. 274, no. 1–3, pp. 37–66, 2001.

[7] J. B. Knaak, C. C. Dary, M. S. Okino et al., "Parameters for carbamate pesticide QSAR and PBPK/PD models for human risk assessment," *Reviews of Environmental Contamination and Toxicology*, vol. 193, pp. 53–212, 2008.

[8] A. Campbell, "Development of PBPK model of molinate and molinate sulfoxide in rats and humans," *Regulatory Toxicology and Pharmacology*, vol. 53, no. 3, pp. 195–204, 2009.

[9] P. L. Mosquin, A. C. Licata, B. Liu, S. C. Sumner, and M. S. Okino, "Reconstructing exposures from small samples using physiologically based pharmacokinetic models and multiple biomarkers," *Journal of Exposure Science & Environmental Epidemiology*, vol. 19, no. 3, pp. 284–297, 2009.

[10] S. J. Godin, M. J. DeVito, M. F. Hughes et al., "Physiologically based pharmacokinetic modeling of deltamethrin: development of a rat and human diffusion-limited model," *Toxicological Sciences*, vol. 115, no. 2, pp. 330–343, 2010.

[11] C. Lu, C. M. Holbrook, and L. M. Andres, "The implications of using a physiologically based pharmacokinetic (PBPK) model for pesticide risk assessment," *Environmental Health Perspectives*, vol. 118, no. 1, pp. 125–130, 2010.

[12] R. Tornero-Velez, A. Mirfazaelian, K. B. Kim et al., "Evaluation of deltamethrin kinetics and dosimetry in the maturing rat using a PBPK model," *Toxicology and Applied Pharmacology*, vol. 244, no. 2, pp. 208–217, 2010.

[13] P. G. Georgopoulos, A. F. Sasso, S. S. Isukapalli et al., "Reconstructing population exposures to environmental chemicals from biomarkers: challenges and opportunities," *Journal of Exposure Science & Environmental Epidemiology*, vol. 19, no. 2, pp. 149–171, 2009.

[14] Y. M. Tan, K. Liao, R. Conolly, B. Blount, A. Mason, and H. Clewell, "Use of a physiologically based pharmacokinetic model to identify exposures consistent with human biomonitoring data for chloroform," *Journal of Toxicology and Environmental Health A*, vol. 69, no. 18, pp. 1727–1756, 2006.

[15] H. J. Clewell, Y. M. Tan, J. L. Campbell, and M. E. Andersen, "Quantitative interpretation of human biomonitoring data," *Toxicology and Applied Pharmacology*, vol. 231, no. 1, pp. 122–133, 2008.

[16] C. Timchalk, T. S. Poet, M. N. Hinman, A. L. Busby, and A. A. Kousba, "Pharmacokinetic and pharmacodynamic interaction for a binary mixture of chlorpyrifos and diazinon in the rat," *Toxicology and Applied Pharmacology*, vol. 205, no. 1, pp. 31–42, 2005.

[17] J. N. Blancato, F. W. Power, R. N. Brown, and C. C. Dary, ") Exposure Related Dose Estimating Model (ERDEM)

a Physiologically-Based Pharmacokinetic and Pharmacodynamic (PBPK/PD) model for assessing human exposure and risk," Tech. Rep. EPA/600/R-06/061, U.S. Environmental Protection Agency, Washington, DC, USA, 2006, (NTIS PB2006-114712).

[18] C. Lu, G. Kedan, J. Fisker-Andersen, J. C. Kissel, and R. A. Fenske, "Multipathway organophosphorus pesticide exposures of preschool children living in agricultural and nonagricultural communities," *Environmental Research*, vol. 96, no. 3, pp. 283–289, 2004.

[19] R. A. Fenske, C. Lu, G. Kedan, J. Fisker-Andersen, and C. Curl, "Assessment of organophosphorous pesticide exposures in the diets of preschool children in Washington State," *Journal of Exposure Analysis and Environmental Epidemiology*, vol. 12, no. 1, pp. 21–28, 2002.

[20] J. C. Kissel, C. L. Curl, G. Kedan et al., "Comparison of organophosphorus pesticide metabolite levels in single and multiple daily urine samples collected from preschool children in Washington State," *Journal of Exposure Analysis and Environmental Epidemiology*, vol. 15, no. 2, pp. 164–171, 2005.

[21] M. L. Voorhess, "Urinary catecholamine excretion by healthy children. I. Daily excretion of dopamine, norepinephrine, epinephrine, and 3-methoxy-4-hydroxymandelic acid," *Pediatrics*, vol. 39, no. 2, pp. 252–257, 1967.

[22] United States Environmental Protection Agency (USEPA). Exposure Factor Handbook, 1997, http://rais.ornl.gov/documents/EFH_Final_1997_EPA600P95002Fa.pdf.

[23] P. Griffin, H. Mason, K. Heywood, and J. Cocker, "Oral and dermal absorption of chlorpyrifos: a human volunteer study," *Occupational and Environmental Medicine*, vol. 56, no. 1, pp. 10–13, 1999.

[24] M. K. Morgan, L. S. Sheldon, C. W. Croghan et al., "Exposures of preschool children to chlorpyrifos and its degradation product 3,5,6-trichloro-2-pyridinol in their everyday environments," *Journal of Exposure Analysis and Environmental Epidemiology*, vol. 15, no. 4, pp. 297–309, 2005.

[25] C. Lu, R. Bravo, L. M. Caltabiano, R. M. Irish, G. Weerasekera, and D. B. Barr, "The presence of dialkylphosphates in fresh fruit juices: implication for organophosphorus pesticide exposure and risk assessments," *Journal of Toxicology and Environmental Health A*, vol. 68, no. 3, pp. 209–227, 2005.

3

Metal Toxicity at the Synapse: Presynaptic, Postsynaptic, and Long-Term Effects

Sanah Sadiq, Zena Ghazala, Arnab Chowdhury, and Dietrich Büsselberg

Weill Cornell Medical College in Qatar, Qatar Foundation—Education City, P.O. Box 24144, Doha, Qatar

Correspondence should be addressed to Dietrich Büsselberg, dib2015@qatar-med.cornell.edu

Academic Editor: David O. Carpenter

Metal neurotoxicity is a global health concern. This paper summarizes the evidence for metal interactions with synaptic transmission and synaptic plasticity. *Presynaptically* metal ions modulate neurotransmitter release through their interaction with synaptic vesicles, ion channels, and the metabolism of neurotransmitters (NT). Many metals (e.g., Pb^{2+}, Cd^{2+}, and Hg^{+}) also interact with intracellular signaling pathways. *Postsynaptically*, processes associated with the binding of NT to their receptors, activation of channels, and degradation of NT are altered by metals. Zn^{2+}, Pb^{2+}, Cu^{2+}, Cd^{2+}, Ni^{2+}, Co^{2+}, Li^{3+}, Hg^{+}, and methylmercury modulate NMDA, AMPA/kainate, and/or GABA receptors activity. Al^{3+}, Pb^{2+}, Cd^{2+}, and As_2O_3 also impair *synaptic plasticity* by targeting molecules such as CaM, PKC, and NOS as well as the transcription machinery involved in the maintenance of synaptic plasticity. The multiple effects of metals might occur simultaneously and are based on the specific metal species, metal concentrations, and the types of neurons involved.

1. Introduction

Metals and their compounds are distributed in ecosystems as a result of natural processes as well as anthropogenic activities. Metals are used in their elementary form as well as in compounds for various human needs. Therefore, a number of these metals enter our environment as a consequence of their widespread use in preservatives, biocides, and paints [1]. They are taken up by organisms through inhalation or by ingestion of food and water contaminated with these metals. For living systems, metals can be divided in those which are essential for life, such as cobalt (Co), copper (Cu), zinc (Zn), manganese (Mn), and iron (Fe); which are potentially toxic only at higher concentration, and those which have no known biological function, which can be toxic at all concentrations such as cadmium (Cd), chromium (Cr), mercury (Hg), and *lead* (Pb) [13] (for all abbreviations used in the review please refer to the abbreviations section; to facilitate reading, the names of the specific metals discussed are given in *italics*).

Since the uptake mechanisms of the body are not able to distinguish between "physiologically required" and harmful metals, the toxic metals absorbed consequently might interact with the functions of the central nervous system (CNS), liver, kidneys, and hematopoietic system, thus presenting a significant health hazard. In this review, we will examine the effects of these metals in the CNS, specifically at the synapse.

The human brain has about 10^{11} neurons, which interconnect and "communicate" with each other through synapses. It is estimated that each neuron has approximately 7000 synapses. At the presynaptic side of the synapse the incoming electrical signal, in from of action potentials, is transformed to a chemical signal in the form of neurotransmitter release. Synaptic transmission depends on the timely opening of membrane channels, the precise functioning of intracellular signaling pathways, and metabolic pathways involved in the synthesis and the release of neurotransmitters. Postsynaptically the binding of neurotransmitters changes the membrane potential, resulting in a hyper- or depolarization of the neuron and in the generation of an action potential when the threshold potential is reached. These are crucial process and the basis of all higher cognitive functions including learning and memory.

Therefore, we highlight the mechanisms by which metals and their compounds interfere with the processes of synaptic transmission and synaptic plasticity. This review covers the effects of metals on signal transmission from the presynaptic to the postsynaptic membrane, as well as the effects on synaptic plasticity with an emphasis on learning and memory, since subtle alterations in synaptic transmission due to the interaction of metals may have profound toxic effects in the CNS [14].

Some metals, which have already been shown to alter synaptic transmission, are discussed in this review. The metals are listed in an alphabetical order below with a short description of their neurotoxic effects, to show their relevance to this study (for more details regarding the neurotoxicity of these metals see [15]).

Aluminum was found present in high concentrations in brains of patients with Alzheimer's disease, Parkinson's disease, and dialysis encephalopathy and could contribute to neurogenerative disorders [21]. In animals the administration of *aluminum* salts results in neurofibrillary degeneration, a condition similar to the encephalopathy in Alzheimer's disease [3].

Arsenic, one of the oldest known poisons, due to its cholera-like symptoms, became a favorite poisoning agent and earned the title the "Poison of Kings" [15]. An acute ingestion of *arsenic* affects many systems of the body including gastrointestinal, cardiovascular, respiratory, and the nervous system. Even today, chronic low-dose exposure to *arsenic* is very common in countries like Bangladesh, India, Taiwan, and other parts of South East Asia due to contamination of groundwater by *arsenic*. It is a major cause of infant mortality in Bangladesh [8]. Chronic manifestations of *arsenic* poisoning are pigmentation changes, gastrointestinal problems, anemia, liver disease, black foot disease, and Mees' lines on the nails. Central neuropathy due to *Arsenic* poisoning usually manifests as impairment of learning, short-term memory and concentration. However, peripheral neuropathy is more frequently observed and this might last for several years. It manifests as a rapid and severe ascending weakness and sometimes these patients require mechanical ventilation [8, 15].

Cadmium and *manganese* also have neurotoxic effects, where *cadmium* damages cells of the cerebellar cortices of young rats as well as rabbits and chronic *manganese* poisoning causes extrapyramidal symptoms much like those of Wilson's disease and Parkinsonism [9]. Moreover, increased total *cadmium* levels in human hair were associated with mental retardation and impairment in visual motor abilities [4]. Similar toxicities also occur in humans.

Lead, whose mechanisms of neurotoxicity have been extensively studied, was discovered more than 5000 years ago and was used in the ancient world for lead water piping, as utensils, to sweeten food and wine, and as a constituent of eye paints [2]. It was discovered that acute exposure to *Pb* could cause lead colic and mental disturbances and even chronic exposure to low concentrations of lead in children caused several cognitive and behavioral disturbances. Since *Pb* crosses the placenta, prenatal exposure to lead can have especially severe consequences [4, 5, 15].

Exposure to dietary *methylmercury* leads to Minamata disease, which manifested in patients as paresthesias followed by irreversible impairment of vision, hearing, speech, gait, and ultimately leads to death. In addition, cognitive impairment ensued with prenatal exposure to *methylmercury* [4].

Organo-tins are industrially produced in large quantities for applications as PVC stabilizers, glass coverings, silicone, wood preserver additives, and antifouling paints. Moreover, considerable amounts of *organo-tins* are released in the environment causing large concern about their impact on human health. Due to their lipophilicity *organo-tins* are taken up by humans and distributed in different tissues. In mammalian organs such as brain, liver, and kidneys, *organo-tins* are biotransformed and this process may increase their toxicity [7]. Specifically *alkyl-tins* have been shown to cause neurotoxicity [15].

Even though metals are well known for their various toxicities, they are also used as therapeutic agents. *Lithium* salts have been used in the treatment and prophylaxis of bipolar affective disorder [10, 16]. *Arsenic* in the form of *arsenic trioxide* is used for the treatment of leishmaniasis, leukemia, and trypanosomiasis [8, 15]. The specific toxicities of some metals are actually being used to man's benefit, especially for the treatment of cancers. *Cisplatin* (*cis-diammine-dichloro-platin* = *CDDP*) is used as an anticancer drug and testicular cancer, endometrial cancer, prostatic tumors, bladder carcinoma, and small cell bronchial carcinoma [17] are successfully treated with this drug.

With the wide description of harmful effects of metals as well as their irreplaceability in modern life and medicine, it becomes essential to demarcate the level at which metals become toxic. This includes concentrations of metals as well as their targets of actions. Recognizing the targets sites at which metals interact can serve as a stepping-stone for the development of therapeutic agents to counteract metal toxicity as well as the side effects of anticancer drugs such as *arsenic* and *cisplatin* compounds.

This paper aims to review the literature available of the mechanisms of actions of metals at targets presynaptically, postsynaptically, and on long-term potentiation (LTP) and summarizes the findings in a logical and easily comprehensible manner. In the first part the toxic effects of organic and inorganic metals on the ***pre***synaptic part will be described (Section 2), followed by a review of their ***post***synaptic actions (Section 3), and the review finally looks at the impairment of ***synaptic plasticity*** (Section 4) before concluding remarks are made (Section 5).

2. Presynaptic Targets of Toxic Metals

Presynaptically, the action potential, which is an electrical signal, is transduced to a chemical signal in the form of neurotransmitter release. Generally, the action potential induces a membrane depolarization, which opens voltage gated calcium channels allowing the influx of Ca^{2+}. Ca^{2+} activates calmodulin (CaM) and therefore CaM kinases (CamK) are activated, which leads to the phosphorylation of synaptic vesicle associated proteins and the conversion of the reserve pool of synaptic vesicles to a readily releasable pool of vesicles. Ca^{2+} also binds synaptotagmin, a calcium sensor protein in the vesicle membrane and triggers neurotransmitter vesicle fusion and the release of neurotransmitter [18] (Figure 1).

Metals interact with specific targets in these pathways and the same metals might even interact with various targets simultaneously. For instance, *aluminum* blocks voltage gated calcium channels, decreases the biological activity of CaM, and also inhibits Ca^{2+} ATPase [19, 20]. In addition, if a metal interacts with an upstream target of a pathway, it may influence all the processes succeeding it. For example, *cadmium* reduces voltage activated calcium channel currents, therefore, it can influence the intracellular calcium concentration and consequently the activation of CaM and calcium-dependent intracellular signaling pathways [6, 11]. Notably, *cadmium* caused a decrease in release of excitatory neurotransmitters glutamate and aspartate while it caused an increase in the release of inhibitory neurotransmitters GABA and glycine [12].

The upcoming sections (Sections 2.1 to 2.6) highlight the literature relating to the toxic effects of metals on presynaptic targets including voltage-activated ion channels (Section 2.1), signaling cascades (Section 2.2), transporters (Section 2.3), synaptic vesicle associated proteins (Section 2.4), neurotransmitters (Section 2.5), and neurofilaments and microtubules (Section 2.6). For ease of access, wherever possible metals are described in alphabetical order in each Section.

2.1. Voltage-Activated Channels

2.1.1. Voltage-Activated Calcium Channels. Voltage activated calcium channels open by a depolarization. They are subdivided into high- and low-voltage activated channels. The high-voltage activated channels, which have to be depolarized to more positive voltages than −30 mV for activation, include the L-type, P/Q-type, N-type, and R-type, where the L-type has a "long-lasting" current. The other types are divided on the basis of their inactivation and their susceptibility to various peptide toxins. There are also low-voltage activated channels which are mainly composed of the T-type channels which have a small, fast inactivating and therefore transient current [22].

Aluminum (Al^{3+}) blocked N- and L-type voltage activated calcium channels in cultured rat dorsal root ganglions, with a threshold concentration of 20 μM and a Hill's coefficient of 3 (Table 1). It also required an open channel for its actions thereby indicating that the possible site of action of Al^{3+} was inside the channel. The current-voltage relation was shifted to depolarizing voltages in the presence of Al^{3+} [19]. *Aluminum* also blocked voltage-activated calcium channels *in vivo* in rats when given 10 mg per kg body weight per day intraperitoneally for 4 weeks. Inhibition was nearly 85% in the corpus striatum, 58% in the cerebral cortex, and 46% in the hippocampus [20].

Cadmium (Cd^{2+}) effectively reduced voltage-activated calcium channel currents, which were high threshold and fast inactivating types in cultured chick dorsal root ganglion cells, at concentrations of 20 μM. This block was released at hyperpolarizing voltages, which may be due to shifts in gating and permeability of the channels. When the membrane potential was hyperpolarized, the channels conducted transiently, as Cd^{2+} exited the channels, but closed again thereafter. The channels can close with Cd^{2+} in the channel pore, therefore implying that Cd^{2+} does not affect the closing mechanisms of the channels [6]. Similar results were obtained in squid giant fiber neurons. In addition, a kinetic model was created and the binding site for Cd^{2+} was determined to be near the outer end of the pore, and the entry of Cd^{2+} into the pore was voltage independent while its exit was voltage dependent [11].

Lead (Pb^{2+}) is a potent blocker of voltage-activated calcium channels in invertebrate *Aplysia* neurons as well as in mammalian neurons [19, 23, 25, 27, 28, 30]. There is no change in the voltage dependence of activation or inactivation of the channels in mammalian neurons, which suggests an external binding site for Pb^{2+} [25, 27, 28]. In mammals Pb^{2+} blocked N-, L- and T-type voltage activated calcium channels [19, 27, 28, 30]. The block of L- and T-type channels was concentration dependent and reversible in N1E-115 mouse neuroblastoma cells [30]. The concentration for 50% inhibition (IC_{50}) of L-type channels was 30 nM, and for N-type channels it was 80 nM free Pb^{2+} where 10 mM Ba^{2+} was used as the charge carrier in cultured E-18 rat hippocampal neurons [28]. Some contradictory data were obtained in a study of mouse N1E-115 neuroblastoma cells, where in five of the fifteen cells studied, 2.3 μM Pb^{2+} enhanced L-type calcium channel currents and also enhanced the inactivation of L-type channels at holding potentials of −60 to −40 mV [30]. A study on human neuroblastoma cells SH-SY5Y determined that *lead acetate* at concentrations of 1 to 30 μM blocked voltage-activated calcium channels, both N- and L-types in a concentration-dependent and reversible way. More importantly, the concentrations used in the study were inclusive of the blood level concentrations at which children present with neuropsychological disorders (between 1.5–2.5 μM) [29].

Mercury (Hg^{2+}) blocked voltage-activated calcium channels with an IC_{50} of 1.1 μM *in vitro* in rat pup dorsal root ganglion cells, and it required a partially open channel for its block [24]. *Mercury (Hg^{2+})* blocked neuronal N- and R-type calcium channels transiently expressed in human embryonic kidney 293 cells with an IC_{50} of 2.2 and 0.7 μM. This effect was partially reversible in N-type but not in R-type channels [26]. *Mercury* also blocked T-type calcium channel currents in the concentration range of 0.5–2 μM in cultured rat dorsal root ganglion cells. In addition the current-voltage relation was shifted to positive voltages implying that *mercury* may have an effect on channel gating [40].

Platinum in the form of *cis-diammine-dichloro-platin (CDDP)* reduced voltage-activated calcium channel currents in dorsal root ganglion cells of rats *in vitro*. *CDDP* reduced peak *calcium* current with an IC_{50} of 23.9 ± 4.5 μM and sustained current with an IC_{50} of 38.8 ± 6.1 μM in small

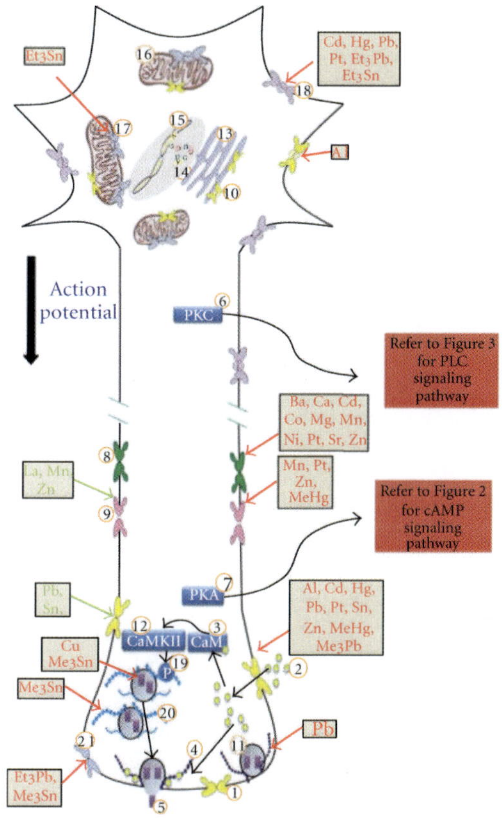

No.	Symbol	Target	No.	Symbol	Target	No.	Symbol	Target
1		Voltage-gated calcium channels	8		Voltage-gated sodium channels	15		DNA
2		Calcium ions	9		Voltage-gated potassium channels	16		Mitochondria
3	CaM	Calmodulin	10	ATPase	Ca^{2+} ATPase	17	ATPase	Mitochondrial ATPase
4		Synaptotagmin	11		Neurotransmitter vesicle	18	ATPase	$Na^{+}K^{+}$ ATPase
5		Neurotransmitter	12	CaMKII	Calmodulin kinase	19	P	Phosphate
6	PKC	PKC	13		Endoplasmic reticulum	20		Synapsin
7	PKA	PKA	14		mRNA	21		Transporter for neurotransmitter reuptake

FIGURE 1: Presynaptic targets of neurotoxic metals. Events at the synapse from the arrival of the action potential which results in the membrane depolarization-induced opening of voltage-activated calcium channels and the entry of calcium which activates CaM, which activates CaM kinases and causes the phosphorylation of synaptic vesicle-associated proteins and an increase in readily releasable neurotransmitter vesicles. Calcium also binds synaptotagmin and causes exocytosis of neurotransmitter from the vesicles. Shown in boxes are the metals and the targets at which they act in the synaptic transduction pathway. A table at the end indicates the symbols and what they indicate. Green indicates activation or upregulation while red indicates inhibition or downregulation. Please refer to the section of Abbreviations and metals.

Table 1: Effects of metals on voltage-activated ion channels (↑—activation/upregulation, ↓—inhibition/downregulation).

Target		Voltage-gated channels										
		Calcium channels						Sodium channels			Potassium channels	
		L	N	T	R	All(ii)		Tetrodotoxin sensitive	Tetrodotoxin resistant	All(i)		
Al	Effect	↓	↓			↓						
	Conc	20 μM	20 μM			50 μM						
	Ref	[1]	[1]			[2]						
Cd	Effect		↓			↓		↓	↓			
	Conc		20 μM			2.2, 125 μM		5 mM	0.2 mM			
	Ref		[3]			[4], [5]		[6]	[6]			
Co	Effect					↓						
	Conc					500 μM						
	Ref					[7]						
Hg	Effect		↓	↓	↓	↓						
	Conc		2.2 μM	0.5–2 μM	0.7 μM	1.1 μM						
	Ref		[8]	[9]	[8]	[10]						
La	Effect										↑	
	Conc										10 μM	
	Ref										[11]	
Mn	Effect										↓	↑
	Conc										10 mM	1 mM
	Ref										[12]	[12]
Pb	Effect	↓	↓	↓		↓						
	Conc	30 nM(i), 0.7, 0.64, 0.1 μM	80 nM(i), 0.64, 0.1 μM	1.3 μM, 6 μM, 6 μM		1, 1, 0.6, (1–30) μM						
	Ref	[13], [14], [15], [1]	[13, 15] [1], [5], [1]	[14], [15], [4]		[16], [15], [4], [17]						
Pt	Effect					↓				↓	↓	
	Conc					23.9 μM				10 μM	10 μM, 100 μM	
	Ref					[18]				[18]	[18], [18]	
Sn	Effect					↓	↑					
	Conc					50 μM	50 μM					
	Ref					[19]	[20]					
Zn	Effect	↓	↓	↓		↓		↓	↓		↑	
	Conc	5,69 μM	5,69 μM	20 μM		2 mM, 69 μM		2 mM	50 μM		30 μM	
	Ref	[1, 21]	[1, 21]	[21]		[10, 16]		[6]	[6]		[22]	

(i) Extent of block and EC_{50} differ based on concentration of charge carrier used.
(ii) Paper does not describe which sub-type is affected.

neurons with a diameter of $\leq 20\,\mu m$. Surprisingly, in large neurons with a cross-sectional diameter of $\geq 25\,\mu m$, the peak calcium current was only reduced by 14.1 ± 2.3% even with a concentration of $100\,\mu M$ *CDDP*. It is unlikely that the voltage-activated calcium channel currents were blocked directly since the small and large cells were unequally affected and the Hill's coefficient was not 1. *CDDP* probably decreases voltage-activated calcium channel currents by acting through an intracellular pathway more prominent in small neurons, possibly through IP_3 receptor activation as described later [17].

Tin (Sn^{2+}) used as *stannous chloride* ($SnCl_2$) decreased voltage-activated calcium channel currents *in vitro* in rat dorsal root ganglion cells in a concentration-dependent manner with a threshold of $1\,\mu M$. These effects were found to be irreversible [41]. However, contradictory results were obtained in a study of motor nerve terminals of frog, where nerve muscle preparations were exposed to $50\,\mu M$ $SnCl_2$, which caused an increased inward Ca^{2+} current [34].

Zinc (Zn^{2+}) blocked voltage-activated calcium channels in cultured rat dorsal root ganglion cells [19, 24, 31]. The IC_{50} for this effect on N- and L-type channels was $69\,\mu M$ Zn^{2+} while the Hill's coefficient was 1. T-type currents were more sensitive, and the block was partly reversible in 50% of the neurons [31]. *Zinc* did not require an open channel for this blocking effect [24]. The current voltage relationship shifted to more depolarizing voltages in the presence of Zn^{2+}, implying that the mechanism of action of Zn^{2+} may involve the screening of charges in the vicinity of the channels [19].

Methylmercury (MeHg) caused an increase in calcium influx and therefore $[Ca^{2+}]_i$ through nifedipine and ω-conotoxin sensitive mechanisms, that is, through either, L-, N-, or Q-type calcium channels [36]. However, *methylmercury* caused an irreversible time and concentration dependent block of calcium channel currents at concentrations between 0.25 and $1\,\mu M$ *in vitro* in rat cerebellar granule neurons. The block did not require depolarization, indicating that it did not require an open channel. Increasing the frequency of stimulation of cells increased the magnitude of block at $0.25\,\mu M$ and $0.5\,\mu M$ but not at $1\,\mu M$, which may suggest the presence of other counteracting effects. None of the calcium channel antagonists used—ω-conotoxin GVIA, ω-conotoxin MVIIC, ω-agatoxin IVA, calcicludine, and nimodipine, were able to decrease the *MeHg*-induced block of calcium channel currents [38]. *MeHg* blocked N-, R-, and L-type voltage-activated calcium channels [26, 39]. *MeHg* blocked human neuronal N- and R- type calcium channel currents transiently expressed in human embryonic kidney 293 cells with an IC_{50} of $1.3\,\mu M$ and $1.1\,\mu M$ respectively (Table 4). This block was determined to be irreversible [26].

Trimethyl lead blocked voltage-activated calcium channels with a threshold concentration of $0.5\,\mu M$ *in vitro* in rat dorsal root ganglion cells. This block was irreversible and concentration dependent but not voltage dependent. It required an open channel and the IC_{50} was between $1\text{–}5\,\mu M$ [33].

2.1.2. Voltage-Activated Sodium Channels. There are 9 subtypes of voltage-activated sodium channels Na_v 1.1–Na_v 1.9 distinguished by their sensitivity to tetrodotoxin and their rate of inactivation. Na_v 1.8 and Na_v 1.9 have relatively slower inactivation [35]. Na_v 1.1, Na_v 1.2, Na_v 1.3, and Na_v 1.7 are expressed in neurons and are highly sensitive to tetrodotoxin. Na_v 1.5, Na_v 1.8, and Na_v 1.9 are relatively tetrodotoxin resistant and are found in heart and dorsal root ganglion neurons. Na_v 1.4 and Na_v 1.6 are mostly expressed in skeletal muscle and the CNS, respectively [37].

Zinc (Zn^{2+}) and *cadmium* (Cd^{2+}) reduced both tetrodotoxin-sensitive and tetrodotoxin-insensitive voltage-activated sodium channel currents in voltage clamp experiments in neuronal, cardiac, and skeletal muscle cells [42]. Tetrodotoxin-resistant channels were more sensitive to Zn^{2+} and Cd^{2+} with IC_{50} of the block being $50\,\mu M$ and 0.2 mM, respectively; tetrodotoxin-sensitive channels were less resistant with IC_{50} of the block being 2 mM and 5 mM for Zn^{2+} and Cd^{2+}, respectively [42] (compare effects in Table 1). It was suggested that the site of action of Zn^{2+} contains cysteine sulfhydryl groups in or near the saxitoxin binding site since Zn^{2+} was able to relieve the saxitoxin-induced block of the channel in a competitive manner, and the blocking action of *zinc* was inhibited by sulfhydryl-specific alkylating reagents. These experiments were done in voltage-activated sodium channels taken from the hearts of dogs or calves [32].

$SnCl_2$ had an effect on voltage-activated sodium channel currents of the mollusk *Lymnaea stagnalis in vitro* where it shifted the current voltage curve to the left. $SnCl_2$ increased voltage-activated sodium channel currents at a concentration of $10\,\mu M$, but caused a depression in current at concentrations above $25\,\mu M$. Organic tin in the form of $(CH_3)_3SnCl$ decreased significantly the Na current only at high concentrations above $100\,\mu M$. Additionally the current voltage curve was shifted to the left. These effects were time dependent and irreversible [43].

Cobalt, manganese, nickel, calcium, magnesium, strontium, and *barium* in divalent cation form blocked both tetrodotoxin-sensitive and tetrodotoxin-insensitive channels in channels incorporated into planar bilayers in the presence of batrachotoxin. The block was voltage dependent and the sequence of affinity to block was $Co^{2+} \cong Ni^{2+} > Mn^{2+} > Ca^{2+} > Mg^{2+} > Sr^{2+} > Ba^{2+}$. The suggested mechanisms of block included a specific divalent cation binding site and surface charge screening [44]. Also $10\,\mu M$ of the anticancer drug *CDDP* reduced voltage-activated sodium channel currents by 9.2% ± 7.2% in rat dorsal root ganglions *in vitro* [17].

2.1.3. Voltage-Activated Potassium Channels. The family of voltage-activated potassium channel includes K_v1–6, K_v 8, and K_v 9, where the principal subunit of the channels contains 6 transmembrane domains. All these channels are expressed in brain tissue [45]. Whole cell patch-clamp measurements of transient voltage-dependent potassium currents in rat suprachiasmatic nucleus neurons showed that Zn^{2+} potentiated current when activated from a holding potential of −60 mV (approximately the resting membrane potential). This potentiation was voltage dependent and arose from a shift of the inactivation current to more positive voltages. Zn^{2+} ($30\,\mu M$) shifted the half-inactivation voltage by 20 mV from −80 mV to −60 mV [46]. Kuo and

Chen showed that at hyperpolarized voltages Zn^{2+} inhibited voltage-dependent transient K^+ currents which can be accounted for by the selective binding of Zn^{2+} to closed K^+-channels with a dissociation constant of approximately 3 μM, which kept the channels closed and slowed the activation of the current [47].

Whole cell patch clamp studies in central neurons of Drosophila third instar larvae showed that millimolar Ca^{2+} and Mg^{2+} concentrations and micromolar concentrations of Zn^{2+} increased the peak inactivation current and shifted the steady-state inactivation curve of voltage gated potassium channels to more positive voltages, but had no effect on the voltage dependence of activation. A micromolar concentration Cd^{2+} had the same effect; however, millimolar concentrations of Cd^{2+} had an effect on both steady state inactivation and activation curves, where the midpoint of the activation curve was shifted more positively. The potency of effect on the inactivation current in terms of amount of shift of steady state inactivation curves was Zn^{2+} (2 mM) $>Cd^{2+}$ (2 mM) $>Ca^{2+}$ (20 mM) $>Mg^{2+}$ (20 mM). The mechanism of action was most likely through specific binding to the channels at extracellular sites [48].

10 μM *cisplatin* in the form of *CDDP* reduced voltage-gated potassium channel currents by 20.9 $\pm$ 4.8% in small dorsal root ganglion neurons while 100 μM *CDDP* reduced the peak current by 12.8 $\pm$ 3.4% [17]. Micromolar concentrations of *lanthanum* (La^{3+}) enhanced outward voltage-gated potassium channel currents evoked by depolarization steps from −50 mV in rat cerebellar granule neurons. 10 μM La^{3+} shifted the steady state inactivation curve by approximately 40 mV in the depolarizing direction and increased the slope factor slightly [49].

Mayer and Sugiyama showed that fast activating transient potassium channel currents were reduced by 10 mM *manganese* (Mn^{2+}) in cultured rat sensory neurons. This reduction was due to a depolarizing shift of the activation curve and a slight reduction in maximum conductance. At the same concentration, steady state inactivation curves were also shifted to depolarizing voltages. The positive shift of steady state inactivation and activation curves were obtained for other metals as well, where the potency of shift was $Cd^{2+} > Mn^{2+} = Co^{2+} > Ca^{2+} > Mg^{2+}$. Lower concentrations of Mn^{2+} (1 mM), however, increased the amplitude of fast inactivating transient potassium channel currents at prepulse potentials from −50 to −70 mV, which was due to a shift of the inactivation curve with no significant shift in the activation curve. These effects may have been due to binding to a specific site within the channel or to phospholipids in close proximity of the gating apparatus [50].

Organic metals also affect voltage-gated potassium channels. *Methylmercury (MeHg)* blocked voltage-gated potassium channels irreversibly, with an IC_{50} of 2.2 $\pm$ 0.3 μM in a concentration-dependent manner. The Hill's coefficient for this block was ~1 [51].

2.2. Signaling Cascades

2.2.1. The cAMP System. G-protein-coupled receptors (GPCR) are coupled to G_s or $G_{i/o}$, where G_s acts as a stimulator of adenylate cyclase and the Gα subunit of $G_{i/o}$ acts as an inhibitor of PKA (Figure 1). PKA phosphorylates Ca^{2+}-channels, thereby enhancing the influx of Ca^{2+} and this increases the release of neurotransmitters [52]. Also PKA phosphorylates SNAP-25 and this leads to a larger pool of readily releasable vesicles [52]. The cAMP-system appears to enhance the release of neurotransmitter in response to a stimulus (Figure 2).

In vitro and *in vivo* exposure to *lead acetate* decreased cAMP-dependent synaptic vesicle protein phosphorylation in rat brain which is most likely a contributing mechanism of *lead* toxicity [53].

Gs. Rodrigues and colleagues determined the effect of *lead acetate* on rat cerebral cortex membranes using 5′ Guanylylimidodiphosphate (Gpp(NH)p). Gpp(NH)p is a nucleotide phosphorylase-resistant GTP analogue, which is known to stimulate adenylate cyclase by saturating Gs. On preincubation of membranes with *lead acetate*, the stimulatory effect of Gpp(NH)p on the adenylate cyclase activity was inhibited [10].

Adenylate Cyclase. The same group [10] also determined the effects of *lead* acetate on adenylate cyclase activity in the cerebral cortex membranes and found that *lead* caused a concentration-dependent inhibition of adenylate cyclase activity with an IC_{50} of 2.5 $\pm$ 0.1 μM (Table 2) [10].

In another series of experiments, Ewers and Erbe [54] determined the effects of *lead, cadmium, and mercury* on adenylate cyclase of the cerebrum, cerebellum, and the brain stem, *in vitro* and *in vivo*. Adenylate cyclase activity was determined in terms of the number of moles of cAMP formed. Concentrations between 0.1 and 30 μM *lead nitrate, cadmium nitrate,* or *mercury nitrate* inhibited adenylate cyclase activity *in vitro* in homogenates of the cerebrum, brain stem, and the cerebellum. *In vivo* studies were performed on rats, which received *lead acetate* dissolved in sterile demineralized water, cAMP formation was determined 1 hour, 4 hours, and 24 hours after treatment. In the cerebellum, and brainstem, adenylate cyclase activity increased after one hour by about 25% but was unaffected in the cerebrum. After four hours, adenylate cyclase declined by 29%, 33%, and 21% in the cerebrum, cerebellum, and brainstem respectfully. By 24 hours adenylate cyclase activity had returned to normal in the cerebrum and brainstem but not in the cerebellum [54]. These differences in the effects of *lead* acetate on adenylate cyclase in different parts of the brain may be an indicator of the varied effects of *lead* on different isoforms of adenylate cyclase.

Zinc (Zn^{2+}) inhibited adenylate cyclase with an IC_{50} of 1-2 μM and a Hill's coefficient of 1.33, which was not competitive with Mg^{2+} or Mg^{2+}ATPase [82]. Both the CI and the CII domains of adenylate cyclase bind Zn^{2+} with high affinity which is correlated with Zn^{2+} inhibition of enzyme activity [83].

2.2.2. The PLC System. The PLC system consists of GPCRs coupled to Gq, which activate DAG and IP_3 through PLC.

TABLE 2: Effects of metals on presynaptic signaling pathways (↑—activation/upregulation, ↓—inhibition/downregulation).

Target		Pathways							
		PKC		Adenylate cyclase		Phosphodiesterase	CaM	IP3	Intracellular calcium
Al	Effect	[illegible]	↑				↓		↑
	Conc	0–100 μM					0–1000 microM		0–1000 μM
	Ref	[2]	[23]				[2]		[2]
As	Effect								↑
	Conc								1 μM
	Ref								[24]
Cd	Effect				↓	↓			↑
	Conc				0.4, 0.9, 1.4$^{(i)}$ μM				0.1–1 mM
	Ref				[25], [25], [25]	[25]			[26]
Hg	Effect				↓	↓			
	Conc				0.8, 0.5, 0.9$^{(i)}$ μM				
	Ref				[25], [25], [25]	[25]			
Ni	Effect	↓							
	Conc	30 μM							
	Ref	[27]							
Pb	Effect			NC	↓	↓			
	Conc			1500–10000 ppm	2.5, 8.6,1.9, 8.0$^{(i)}$ μM				
	Ref			[25]	[28], [25], [25], [25]	[25]			
Pt	Effect							↑	↑
	Conc							1 nM–10 μM	1 nM–10 μM
	Ref							[29]	[29]
Zn	Effect				↓				
	Conc				1-2 μM				
	Ref				[30]				

$^{(i)}$The three different concentrations indicate actions in different areas of the brain—cerebrum, cerebellum, and brainstem.

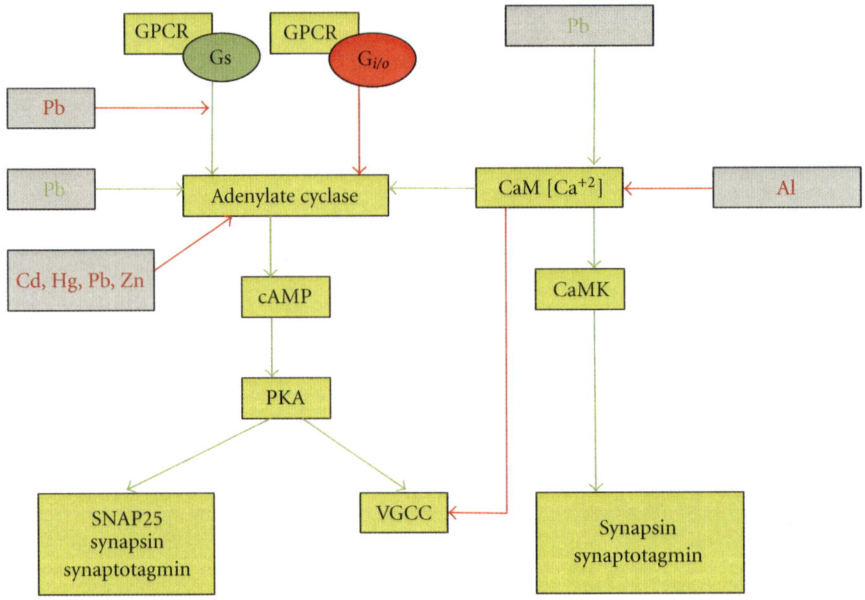

FIGURE 2: Effects of Metals on the cAMP Signaling Pathway at the Presynaptic Terminal (green: activation/increase, red: inhibition/decrease). GPCR's are coupled to G_s or $G_{i/o}$, where G_s stimulates adenylate cyclase and $G_{i/o}$ inhibits PKA. PKA phosphorylates Ca^{2+}-channels, thereby enhancing the influx of Ca^{2+} and this increases the release of neurotransmitters. PKA phosphorylates SNAP-25 and this leads to a larger pool of readily releasable vesicles. The cAMP-system appears to enhance the release of neurotransmitter in response to a stimulus. Metals act at different points in this pathway either enhancing certain processes or inhibiting some. A green color indicates an activation or an increase, and a red color indicates an inhibition or a decrease.

IP_3 causes an increase of intracellular calcium ($[Ca^{2+}]_i$) and the activation of DOC2 and synaptotagmin which leads to increased evoked release and readily releasable pool size. DAG through PKC causes an activation of voltage-gated calcium channels. PKC phosphorylates Munc 18, which negatively regulates syntaxin and synaptic vesicle fusion [52, 84]. PKC activation eventually leads to an increase of spontaneous and evoked neurotransmitter release and more readily releasable pool of vesicles (Figure 3) [52].

PKC. Metals that inhibit PKC include *lead, aluminum,* and *nickel.* Pb^{2+} inhibits PKC enzymes through interactions with its catalytic domains [85]. The effect of *aluminum* on PKC is debated: Julka and Gill demonstrated that *aluminum* lactate given to male albino rats for four weeks, caused an inhibition of PKC at all concentrations used (up to 100 μM). This was shown both *in vivo* and *in vitro.* The largest inhibition was observed in the cerebral cortex (47.73%) followed by the hippocampus (45.95%) and the corpus striatum (38.74%) [20]. However, contrasting findings were determined by Johnson and coworkers who showed that *aluminum* sulfate, when given orally for a period of 4 months to male Sprague-Dawley rats, showed an increase in PKC specific activity by 60% and total activity by 70% in the soluble fraction of cerebral cortex homogenates [69]. The different effects of *aluminum* could be attributed to the mode of intake reflecting differences in concentration of *aluminum* absorbed and its distribution to the brain or the duration of exposure.

Microarray analysis in neuronal PC12 cells indicated that exposure to *Nickel* (Ni^{2+}) caused a decline in the transcription of two isoforms of PKC- prkcc, prkz, and two regulatory binding proteins prkcbp1 and prkcdbp, and also caused temporary upregulation and downregulation of prkcq at 24 hours and 72 hours, respectively [86]. These effects are important in terms of the events at the synapse because PKC activates voltage-activated calcium channels, and increases the secretion of neurotransmitter through effects on proteins involved in neurotransmitter exocytosis-Munc-18, and SNAP25 (a SNARE protein) [87].

IP_3. Increase of $[Ca^{2+}]_i$ in human cervix adenocarcinoma cells by *cisplatin* (0.001–10 μM) was dependent on extracellular Ca^{2+} and was blocked by an IP_3 receptor blocker. The types 1–3 IP_3 receptors were at the cellular membrane of these cells, which suggests a possible mechanism of *cisplatin*-induced calcium entry through IP_3 receptor activation. This was supported by the observation that the same results were not obtained in human osteosarcoma cells, which in addition did not show the presence of types 1–3 IP_3 receptors at cell membrane [88]. *Arsenic trioxide (As_2O_3)* similarly caused an increase in intracellular calcium which was dependent on calcium release from the intracellular calcium stores through the activation of IP_3receptors [88]. *MeHg* also causes an increase in intracellular calcium, which may be due to release from intracellular stores through inositol phosphate. *MeHg* doubled intracellular inositol phosphate levels at concentrations above 3 μM *in vitro* in rat cerebellar granule neurons [89].

2.2.3. Intracellular Calcium ($[Ca^{2+}]_i$). Aluminum (Al^{3+}) caused an increase of $[Ca^{2+}]_i$ in rat synaptosomes, which

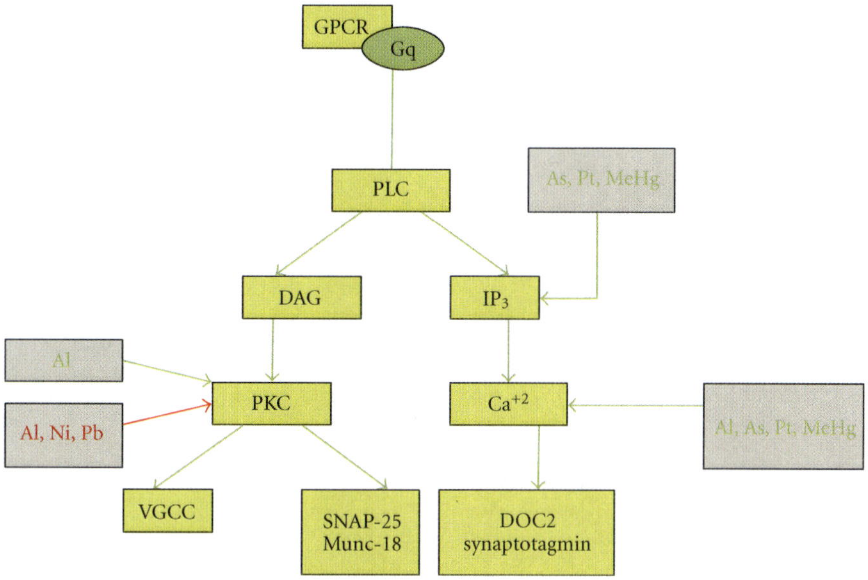

FIGURE 3: Effects of metals on the PLC signaling pathway at presynaptic terminal (green: activation/increase, red: inhibition/decrease). The PLC system consists of GPCRs coupled to Gq, which activate PLC, which activates DAG and IP_3. IP_3 increases intracellular calcium ($[Ca^{2+}]_i$) and activates DOC2 and synaptotagmin which leads to increased evoked release and readily releasable pool size. DAG activates PKC, which activates voltage-gated calcium channels. PKC phosphorylates Munc 18, which negatively regulates vesicle fusion and syntaxin. PKC activation leads to the increased spontaneous and evoked neurotransmitter release. The effects of metals on this pathway are shown in this figure where a green color indicates an activation/upregulation and a red color indicates an inhibition/downregulation.

could be a consequence of the inhibition of the Ca^{2+}-ATPase [20]. 1 μM *arsenic* trioxide (As_2O_3) caused an irreversible increase in $[Ca^{2+}]_i$ in human neuroblastoma cells (SY-5Y) and in human embryonic kidney 293 cells. This rise of $[Ca^{2+}]_i$ was independent of extracellular calcium, but dependent on intracellular calcium stores. Blocking of IP_3 receptor and ryanodine receptors with their specific blockers reduced the increase in $[Ca^{2+}]_i$ indicating their involvement in this process [88]. *Cisplatin* also increased $[Ca^{2+}]_i$ in a concentration-dependent manner in human cervix adenocarcinoma cells but not in human osteosarcoma cells. It is unlikely that the increase in $[Ca^{2+}]_i$ is induced by entry of extracellular calcium, but more likely through activation of IP_3 receptor as described above [88].

In addition, $[Ca^{2+}]_i$ could indirectly be affected by several mechanisms. For example, *$[cis\text{-}(NH_3)_2Pt(H_2O)_2]^{2+}$*, a form of platinum, caused an uncoupling of oxidative phosphorylation one minute after exposure in a concentration-dependent manner, which resulted in a release of Ca^{2+} from the mitochondria. *Cisplatin* did not produce the same effect even at a concentration of 500 μM [90]. However, another study by Gemba et al. showed that mitochondrial uptake of Ca^{2+} in rat kidney cortical mitochondria was decreased 24 hours after exposure to 500 μM *cisplatin* [91].

Methyl-mercury (*MeHg*) 0.5–1 μM caused an increase in $[Ca^{2+}]_i$ *in vitro* in rat cerebellar granule neurons, which decreased cell viability (Table 4). This increase in cell death was prevented 3.5 hours after exposure by using two calcium channel blockers (ω-conotoxin and nifedipine) and a calcium chelator (1,2-bis(2-aminophenoxy) ethane-N,N,N9,N9-tetracetic acid tetrakis (acetoxymethyl) ester (BAPTA)). The effect of the calcium channel blockers could indicate that they inhibit the *MeHg* interaction with the target site or block of the entry of *MeHg* in addition to the effects on $[Ca^{2+}]_i$. BAPTA may have reduced calcium-induced cell death at 3.5 hours after exposure but was unable to prevent *methylmercury*-induced cell death at 24.5 hours. That may indicate that calcium-independent pathways of cell death are involved [92]. The increase of $[Ca^{2+}]_i$ by *methylmercury* is caused by release from intracellular stores and through an influx of Ca^{2+} into the cell [89].

In HeLa cells, *trimethyl-tin* caused spikes in $[Ca^{2+}]_i$ as well as sustained increases. The spikes were of variable size and duration and required 0.25 μM *trimethyl tin*. The sustained increase in intracellular calcium was partially reversible and dependent on the concentration of *trimethyl tin* used, where a 5 μM concentration caused an 8% increase in $[Ca^{2+}]_i$. These effects were independent of external calcium concentrations; however, the increase in $[Ca^{2+}]_i$ was reduced when the internal calcium stores were compromised [7].

Overall, any of the metals affecting any channel or active transport mechanism that involves calcium, at the cellular membrane or the internal stores (as described above) could potentially change $[Ca^{2+}]_i$.

2.2.4. Calmodulin (CaM). Calmodulin is a calcium binding protein. Ca^{2+}/calmodulin activates CaMK, which phosphorylates synapsin I and opens voltage-activated calcium channels by phosphorylation. Thereby Ca^{2+}-influx is increasing which is crucial for releasing the neurotransmitter from vesicles [52, 93].

Aluminum (*Al^{3+}*) decreased the biological activity of CaM both *in vitro* and *in vivo* where inhibition *in vivo* is largest in the hippocampus (36.56%), followed by the cerebral cortex (31.76%) and the corpus striatum (22.49%) [20]. *Lead*, however, had an opposite effect as *lead acetate* enhanced CaM activity both *in vitro* and *in vivo* resulting in an increase in CaM-dependent synaptic vesicle protein phosphorylation including the phosphorylation of proteins such as synapsin I. This was proposed as a mechanism for increased spontaneous release of neurotransmitter and depletion of neurotransmitters norepinephrine and acetylcholine following exposure to *lead* [53].

2.3. Transporters

2.3.1. Ca^{2+}-ATPase. Ca^{2+}-ATPase activity in male albino rat synaptic plasma membranes was reversibly inhibited by *Al^{3+}* (up to100 μM). This inhibition was concentration dependent with an IC_{50} of 10 μM and resulted in an increase of $[Ca^{2+}]_i$ [20] (Table 3).

2.3.2. Na^+/K^+-ATPase. Cisplatin caused a concentration and time-dependent decrease in Na^+-K^+ATPase activity in liver and kidney cells [90]. *Lead* also affected Na^+-K^+ATPase activity, and one study showed lowered RBC membrane Na^+/K^+-ATPase activity below 60% in 77% of patients with Pb-Rbc $\geq$ 40 μg/100 mL while only 40% had the same decrease in activity who had a Pb-Rbc $\leq$ 40 μg/100 mL [94]. *Mercury* compounds, *cadmium, triethyltin, and trimethyltin* also inhibit Na^+-K^+ATPase activity [95–97]. *Triethyl lead* altered the microviscosity of the plasma membrane of ascites tumor cell and also completely inhibited Na^+-K^+-ATPase at concentrations 5–20 μM possibly through direct interaction with its catalytic subunit [98].

2.3.3. Mitochondrial ATPase. Mitochondrial ATPase was inhibited in adult rat brain homogenates with an IC_{50} of 260 μM by *triethyltin* [99]. *Trimethyl tin* has also been shown to affect mitochondrial ATPases *in vitro* [97].

2.4. Synaptic Vesicle Associated Proteins

2.4.1. Synaptotagmin I. Synaptotagmin I is a membrane protein, which is hypothesized to be a Ca^{2+}-sensor in Ca^{2+}-dependent neurotransmitter exocytosis. It has a short intravesicular N-terminus and the cytoplasmic part is composed mostly of two C2 domains, C2A and C2B. The C2A domain is known to bind two Ca^{2+}-ions and the binding affinity shows a correlation with the Ca^{2+} dependence of exocytosis [100]. Synaptotagmin I binds phospholipids and syntaxin in a Ca^{2+}-dependent manner. The binding to syntaxin is associated with exocytosis. The C2B domain of synaptotagmin I also has Ca^{2+} binding sites and is involved in the Ca^{2+} dependent self-association of synaptotagmin I into multimers [100].

Synaptotagmin I was recently described as a target site for *lead*. Bouton and coworkers suggested a competitive interaction between *Pb^{2+}* and Ca^{2+} for the Ca^{2+} binding sites in the C2A domain of synaptotagmin I. At nanomolar concentrations *Pb^{2+}* induced the binding of synaptotagmin I to phospholipids with an EC_{50} of 8 nM. This made it a thousand times more potent than Ca^{2+} at increasing phospholipid binding to synaptotagmin I. Binding of *Pb^{2+}* also increased the stability of the secondary structure of synaptotagmin I. A concentration of 2 μM free *Pb^{2+}* protected a 32 kDa fragment of synaptotagmin I from proteolytic degradation. It required 11 μM free Ca^{2+} to protect the same size of synaptotagmin I. The same authors showed that *Pb^{2+}*, unlike Ca^{2+}, did not induce the interaction of synaptotagmin I and syntaxin. Overall, the interaction of *Pb^{2+}* was competitive with Ca^{2+} and nanomolar concentrations of *Pb^{2+}* could inhibit the ability of micromolar concentrations of Ca^{2+} to induce the interaction of synaptotagmin I and syntaxin [101].

Four binding sites of *Cu^{2+}* in the cytoplasmic C2A domains of synaptotagmin I are discussed, three of which are common to Ca^{2+}, and one of which is unique to *Cu^{2+}*. It was suggested that *Cu^{2+}* has a competitive interaction with Ca^{2+}, but *Cu^{2+}* has a greater affinity for the binding sites common to these metals. Also it was determined that *Cu^{2+}* caused a conformational change in the protein, which may make it less susceptible to trypsin cleavage [102]. Kathir and colleagues looked at the interactions between *Cu^{2+}* and the C2B domain of p40 synaptotagmin I, which is formed by an alternative translation of the synaptotagmin I gene at the Met103 of the p65 synaptotagmin I. They determined that these interactions stabilized synaptotagmin I bound to phosphatidyl serine vesicles [103].

2.4.2. Synapsin I and p38. Synaptic vesicle associated proteins, synapsin I and p38, in rat CNS decreased on acute exposure of rat to *trimethyl tin*. This decrease was both concentration and time dependent; however, 12 weeks after the exposure, the levels returned to normal. The decline was not a result of loss of tissue which also occurs with *trimethyl tin* exposure but was significantly greater that the reduction in tissue [104].

2.5. Neurotransmitters. Release of neurotransmitters is modulated by multiple mechanisms. How metals interfere with some of these pathways has been described above. The following paragraph focuses how metals modulate neurotransmitter levels, their release, and uptake in the presynaptic button.

2.5.1. Effect on Neurotransmitter Metabolism. Treatment of PC-12 dopaminergic neuronal cells with 10 μg/mL *copper* nanoparticles (Ø 90 nm) caused a decrease in dopamine and its metabolites 3.4-dihydroxyphenylacetic acid (DOPAC) and homovanillic acid (HVA). This indicates that the decrease in dopamine may be attributed to a decrease in production and an increase in the breakdown of dopamine [105].

In the same cell line, 10 μg/mL *manganese* nanoparticles (Ø 40 nm) caused a suppression of the tyrosine hydroxylase gene expression, which is involved in the synthesis of dopamine [105]. *Aluminum* has been shown to decrease

TABLE 3: Effects of metals on transporters, neurotransmitters, and neuropeptides (↑—activation/upregulation, ↓—inhibition/downregulation).

Target		Transporters			Neurotransmitters						Neuropeptides
		Ca^{2+} into mitochondria	Ca^{2+} ATPase	Dopamine transporter	Glutamate	Aspartate	GABA	Glycine	Dopamine	Acetylcholine	Substance P, neuropeptide K, and neurokinin
Al	Effect		↓								
	Conc		0–100 μM								
	Ref		[2]								
Cd	Effect				↓(v)	↓(v)	↑(v)	↑(v)			↓
	Conc				10–30 μM	10–30 μM	10–30 μM	10–30 μM			5(iii) μM
	Ref				[31]	[31]	[31]	[31]			[32]
Cu	Effect								↓		
	Conc								10(i) μg m^{-1}		
	Ref								[33]		
Hg	Effect			NC					h		
	Conc			400 μM					6 mg/kg, 400 μM		
	Ref			[34]					[35], [34]		
Mn	Effect				↓	↓	↓		↓		
	Conc				20–200 nm(iv)	20–200 nm	20–200 nm		10(ii) μg mL^{-1}		
	Ref				[36]	[36]	[36]		[33]		
Ni	Effect								↑		
	Conc										
	Ref								[37]		
Pb	Effect				↑		↑			↑	
	Conc						50 μmol L^{-1}			100 μmol L^{-1}	
	Ref				[38]		[39], [38]			[39]	
Pt	Effect	↓	NC								
	Conc	0.5 mM	500 μM								
	Ref	[40]	[41]								
Sn	Effect									↑	
	Conc									10–100 μM	
	Ref									[42]	

(i) Upregulates expression of monoamine oxidase, decreases production, and increases depletion
(ii) Downregulates expression of tyrosine hydroxylase gene
(iii) Reduces expression of precursor gene
(iv) Another study shows that uptake of glutamate into astrocytes is reduced through the decreased expression of glutamate aspartate transporter; this may result in increase in glutamate levels in the synapse [43]
(v) Shows effect on neurotransmitter release.

TABLE 4: Effects of organic metals on presynaptic targets (↑—activation/upregulation, ↓—inhibition/downregulation).

Target			MeHg			Me_3Pb			Et_3Pb			Me_3Sn			Et_3Sn		
			Effect	Conc	Ref	Effect	Conc	Ref	Effect	Conc	Ref	Effect	Conc	Ref	Effect	Conc	Ref
Voltage-gated channels	Calcium channels	L															
		N	↓	1.3 μM	[8]												
		T															
		R	↓	1.1 μM	[8]												
	All[(i)]		↓	0.25–1 μM	[44]	↓	0.5–50 μM	[45]									
	Potassium channels		↓	2.2 μM	[46]												
ATPases															↓	260 μM	[47]
	Na$^+$K$^+$ATPase								↓	5–20 μM	[48]	↓	5–20 μM	[48]	↓		
Transporters	Na$^+$-dependent GABA transporter								↓	10 μM	[49]	↓	10 μM	[49]	↓		
Pathways		IP_3	↑	3 μM	[50]												
		Intracellular Calcium	↑	(0.5–1) μM	[51]												
		Synapsin I										↓		[52]			
		p38										↓		[52]			
Neurotransmitters		GABA							↑[(iii)]	10 μM	[49]	↑[(ii)]	75 μM	[53]	↓		
		Dopamine										↓		[54]			
		Norepinephrine										↑[(ii)]	43 μM	[53]	↓		
		Serotonin										↑[(ii)]	24 μM	[53]	↓		

[(i)] Paper does not describe which subtype is affected
[(ii)] Decreases uptake of neurotransmitter into synaptosomes, thereby probably increasing the amount in cleft
[(iii)] Release of neurotransmitter from vesicles is being measured.

striatal dopamine content and inhibit the enzyme dopamine-β-hydroxylase, which converts dopamine to norepinephrine [106].

Among organic metals, *trimethyl tin* hydroxide treatment of rats on alternate days from days 2–29 of life was shown to decrease the amount of dopamine in the striatum without affecting dopamine metabolites homovanillic acid and dihydroxyphenylacetic acid [107].

2.5.2. Effect on Neurotransmitter Release. *Stannous chloride* increased the amplitude of end-plate potentials in frog neuromuscular junction. A concentration of 10–100 μM *$SnCl_2$* increased the quantum of end plate potentials (EPP). However, the miniature end plate potential (MEPP) was not affected. Hattori and Maehashi (1988) suggested that this was due to an increase in the evoked neurotransmitter release while there was no effect on spontaneous release of neurotransmitter. Also, *$SnCl_2$* did not increase MEPP amplitude or acetylcholine (Ach) potential, indicating that the sensitivity to ACh was not altered [108].

Lead (Pb^{2+}) in concentrations of at least 100 nM was found to increase the spontaneous release of glutamate and GABA from the presynaptic terminal of rat hippocampal neurons. This effect was found to be concentration dependent and partially reversible and the suggested mechanism of action was through an intracellular signaling pathway [109]. Similarly, it is likely that other metals also affect neurotransmitter release through their interaction with the voltage-gated ion channels, intracellular signaling pathways, and synaptic vesicle associated proteins.

One study looked at the effects of *cadmium* on synaptic transmission by perfusing the amygdala of rats with 10–30 μM *$CdCl_2$*. There was an inhibitory effect on the release of excitatory neurotransmitters glutamate and aspartate while the release of inhibitory neurotransmitters glycine and GABA was stimulated [12]. *Aluminum*, as described in previous chapters, affects $[Ca^{2+}]_i$ and, therefore, as expected, inhibits the release and uptake of GABA from synaptosomes by inhibiting Ca^{2+}/calmodulin-dependent calcineurin. It also inhibited pyruvate-supported calcium-evoked acetylcholine release in synaptosomes while in differentiated SN56 cells it decreased acetylcholine release on short-term exposure and increased release on long-term exposure [106].

2.5.3. Effect on Neurotransmitter Reuptake. *Trimethyl tin, in vitro,* inhibited the uptake of neurotransmitters GABA, norepinephrine and serotonin, with an IC_{50} of 75, 43, and 24 μM in a concentration-dependent manner in mouse forebrain synaptosomes. *In vivo*, at 2 and 14 hours after *trimethyl tin* exposure, uptake of GABA, and serotonin was decreased whereas there was no significant decline in norepinephrine. These changes in uptake of neurotransmitters could explain their altered levels in the synaptic cleft [110]. However, unlike *trimethyl tin, triethyl tin sulfate* had no effect on the levels of dopamine, GABA or acetylcholine in rat brain on exposure for 6 days a week from days 2 to 29 of life in mice [107].

Triethyl lead caused a concentration-dependent inhibition of Na^+-dependent high-affinity GABA uptake with an IC_{50} of 10 μM in rat brain synaptosomes. These results were not dependent on Na^+ and GABA concentration-indicating that competition with Na^+ and GABA were not the mechanism of action. Triethyl lead also caused a time- and chloride-dependent decrease in ATP [111]. Skilleter showed that *trialkyl lead* at 1 μM causes a decrease in pyruvate uptake by mitochondria in a KCl medium which could possible explain the decline in ATP [112]. However, since the inhibition of GABA uptake occurs before a significant decline in ATP, Seidman and Verity suggested that the inhibition could be due to a defect in GABA binding to uptake site [111].

2.6. Neurofilaments and Microtubules. *In vivo* exposure of Wistar rats to *arsenic* caused a dose-dependent decrease in neurofilament M and L proteins in the sciatic nerve [113]. These components are required for the formation of a heteropolymer in the cytoskeleton. Since the mRNA expression of these proteins was unaffected, it is possible that the decrease was a consequence of proteolysis. Caplain, which is a calcium-activated cytoplasmic protease, has been implicated in this phenomenon due to the increase in cytoplasmic calcium caused by trivalent *arsenic* [8].

Triethyl lead also affects microtubules [114–116] and neurofilaments [117]. 50 μM *triethyl lead* caused an inhibition of assembly and a disassembly of microtubules *in vitro* in porcine brain [114]. *Triethyl lead* also caused a reversible perinuclear coil formation of neurofilaments *in vivo* in mouse neuroblastoma cells, which was not associated with a significant change in the microtubules. *In vitro, triethyl lead* caused bulging and constriction of isolated neurofilaments from porcine spinal cord, and an unraveling of fibers in preformed filaments [117].

2.7. Summary of Presynaptic Effects of Metals. To summarize, presynaptically, voltage-gated sodium, potassium and calcium ion channels are affected by metals such as *Al^{3+}, $Cd^{2+}Pb^{2+}$, Hg^{2+}, cisplatin, Sn^{2+}, Zn^{2+}, Co^{2+}, Ni^{2+}, Mn^{2+}, Ca^{2+}, Mg^{2+}, Sr^{2+}, Ba^{2+},* and *La^{3+}*. Mechanisms of effect included binding to a specific target, charge screening, shift of current-voltage curves, and competitive inhibition with the physiological ion or a combination of mechanisms [6, 11, 17, 19, 20, 23–32, 34, 41, 42, 44, 46–50]. Metals also interact with intercellular signaling pathways to modulate synaptic transmission. *Lead* modulated Gs, adenylate cyclase, PKC, and CaM [10, 53, 54, 85]. Adenylate cyclase activity was also modulated by *cadmium, mercury, and zinc* [54, 82, 83] while PKC was inhibited by *lead, aluminum, and nickel,* [20, 69, 85, 86], and IP_3 was inhibited by *cisplatin and arsenic* [88]. Intracellular calcium was affected through interference with several targets including voltage-gated calcium channels, Ca^{2+} ATPases, and intracellular pathways. *Al^{3+}, As_2O_3,* and *cisplatin* modulated intracellular calcium [20, 88, 90, 91], and *aluminum,* and *lead* affected Calmodulin activity [20, 53]. Ca^{2+}-ATPase activity was inhibited by *aluminum* and Na^+/K^+-ATPase activity was modulated by *lead, cisplatin, mercury,* and *cadmium* [20, 90, 94–96]. Synaptotagmin I, a synaptic vesicle associated protein, was a target site for interaction with *Pb^{2+}* and *Cu^{2+}*

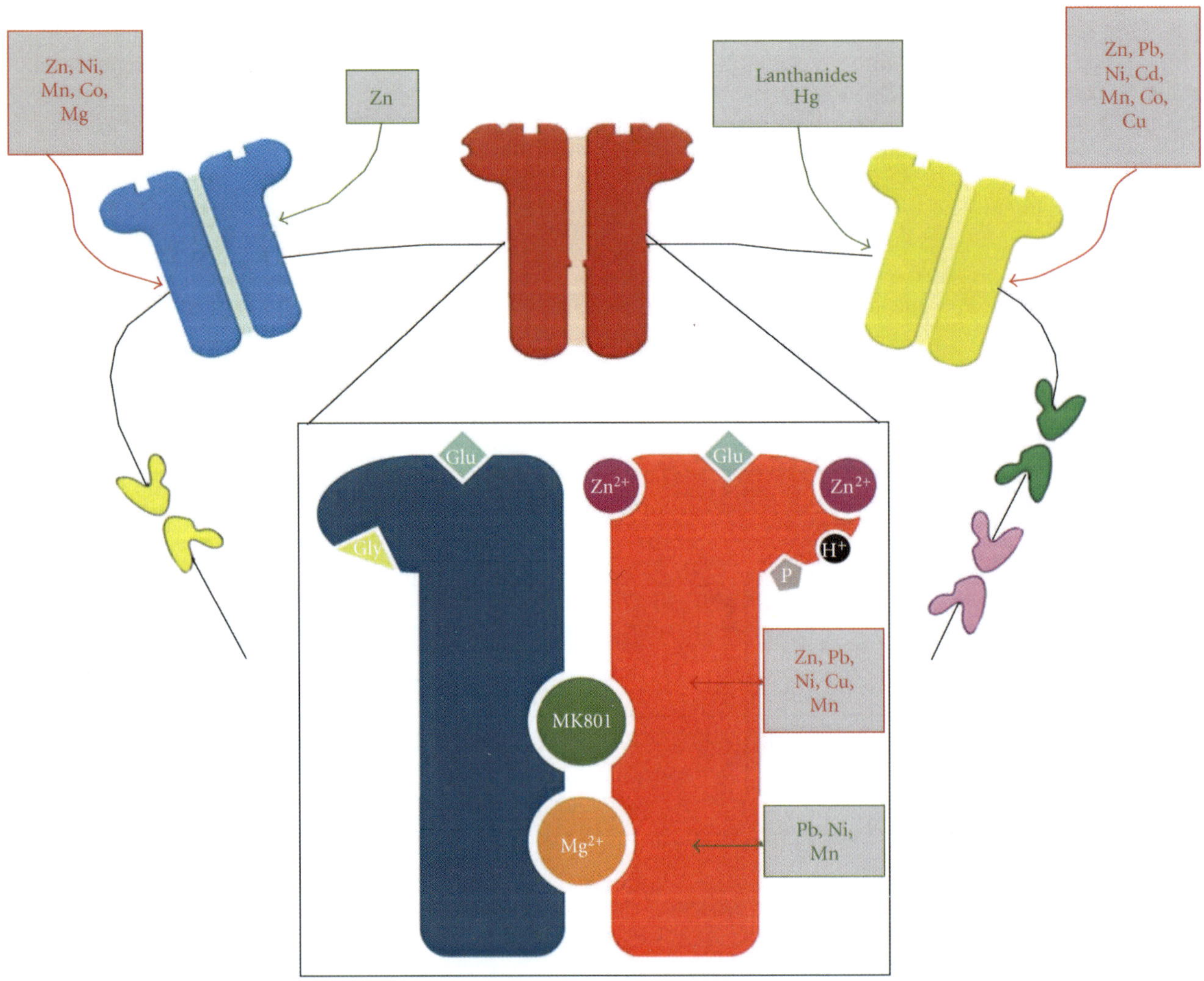

FIGURE 4: Postsynaptic ligand-gated ion channels as targets of neurotoxic metals. The main postsynaptic channels are the AMPA/kainate and NMDA receptors whereas the main inhibitory receptors are the $GABA_A$Rs. Each receptor represents a target for multiple metals. The NMDAR has many modulatory sites identified as it is more extensively studied. NMDAR is composed of a heteromer made of NR1 and NR2, each having multiple subtypes. In the diagram blue arm represents NR1 while the red arm represents NR2, the main modulatory subunit. Most metals have been shown to have effects on NR2 subunit (for values regarding the specific subtypes refer to Section 3.1 and Table 5).

[101–103]. Neurotransmitter release was possibly affected through interaction with many of the targets above as well as through interaction with synthesis and degradation of neurotransmitters and enzymes in the metabolic pathway, which resulted in modulation of neurotransmitter release by metals such as *copper, manganese,* and *tin* [101–103]. The mRNA expression of neurofilaments was affected by *arsenic* [113]. Often contradictory results were obtained regarding the effects of metals, which may indicate that metals had different effects on targets depending on the state of the metal, its concentration, the medium, the area of the brain, and whether the experiment was *in vivo* or *in vitro*.

3. Postsynaptic Targets

The activation of ligand-gated receptor channels is vital for controlling nerve cell inhibition or excitation and, therefore, fashioning the response of individual neurons, neuronal networks, and, ultimately, the entire brain. Consequently the resulting currents through the associated channels will either depolarize or hyperpolarize the postsynaptic terminal under different physiological conditions. The major *excitatory* neurotransmitter in the brain is L-glutamate. There are three classes of ionotropic glutamate receptors named according to their potent excitatory amino acids: α-amino-3-hydroxy-5-methyl-4-isoxazolepropionic acid (AMPA), kainate, and *N*-methyl-D-aspartate (NMDA). The AMPA and kainite-activated channels are designated non-NMDA receptor-channels and will be further discussed in Section 3.2 while metal actions at the NMDA/receptor channel complex are analyzed in the upcoming Section 3.1.

The most abundant *inhibitory* neurotransmitter in the brain is γ-aminobutyric acid (GABA), which acts on its own class of ligand-gated channels. However, these receptors are subject to modulation by other compounds and ions, including metals [118] (Figure 4). As mentioned in the introduction, biological systems utilize metals because of their catalytic versatility, but the high affinity of these metals to specific binding sites could possibly severely impair synaptic transmission and, therefore, cause a malfunction of neuronal networks which might result in changes in perception, learning and memory, and finally change behavior, even at very low and environmentally relevant concentrations.

3.1. The NMDA-Receptor/Channel-Complex. The *N*-methyl-D-aspartate receptor (NMDAR) is a subtype of glutamate ionotropic receptors. The most widely distributed and studied NMDARs are tetrameric assemblies composed of two NR1 subunits and two of the four different NR2 types (named A, B, C, and D), of which NR2A and NR2B are most common [119, 120]. The physiological and pharmacological properties of these receptors are dependent on the NR2 subunit, although different NR1 splice variants may also influence channel performance [121, 122]. NMDAR subunits have a characteristic modular architecture consisting of two extracellular domains, the regulatory amino terminal domain (ATD) and the agonist-binding domain (ABD), and three membrane-spanning segments (M1, M3, and M4) and a reentrant hairpin-like pore loop, M2 [123].

The associated NMDAR channel requires simultaneous binding of two agonists, glutamate (Glu) and glycine (Gly), for opening (for review, [124]). Gly has its binding site in the ABD region of NR1 whereas NR2 ABD binds Glu [120]. The receptor-channel complex has unique properties such as a high Ca^{2+} permeability. Also, the functional activation of NMDAR channels is linked to a voltage-dependent *magnesium-* (*Mg*-) mediated block [125, 126]. Extracellular Mg^{2+} inhibits NMDA responses at membrane potentials close to the resting membrane potential [127]. Studies of the site of action of Mg^{2+} reveal that the N and N+1 site on NR2 subunit are important for the Mg^{2+} block [128]. When the membrane potential is sufficiently depolarized, Mg^{2+} leaves its binding site and even potentiates NMDA responses in low glycine concentrations. This potentiation is shown to be due to increased NMDAR affinity to glycine, in all neurons [129]. However, there was also glycine-independent potentiating effect of Mg^{2+}, which appeared to be largely voltage-independent and subunit specific, being seen only with NR2B-containing receptors. This potentiation has an EC_{50} of ~2 mM [130].

All of these effects reveal the complicated modulation by Mg^{2+} on NMDAR currents. Some data suggest that Mg^{2+} and spermine may completely or partially share a common binding site; similar observations are obtained using spermine [130, 131]. Three different steps in the action of these two substances could be distinguished: (1) increase in glycine affinity, seen in all neurons; (2) voltage-dependent block, also seen in all neurons; and (3) glycine-independent potentiation that was subunit specific [132, 133].

NMDARs contain a number of distinct recognition sites for other endogenous and exogenous ligands, which modulate their functions, such as divalent metal cations, as explored in the later sections (Figure 4).

Zinc is the second most prevalent trace element in the body. Most of the *zinc ions* (Zn^{2+}) are trapped within proteins, but some of it is loosely bound (chelatable zinc) [134]. In the mammalian brain, chelatable *zinc* is distributed mainly in the forebrain and localized almost exclusively within synaptic vesicles of a subset of glutamatergic axon terminals [135]. Since it is accumulated in synaptic vesicles, it has been assumed that *zinc* is released, with glutamate, during neuronal activity. Many studies have showed evidence of quantal corelease of *zinc* and glutamate (for review, [134]).

NMDARs are the best characterized synaptic zinc targets. At low micromolar concentrations, Zn^{2+} selectively inhibited NMDAR-mediated responses. The major effect was through voltage-independent, noncompetitive inhibition seen as a decrease in the opening probability of the channel [136–138]. However, at concentrations higher than 20 μM, Zn^{2+} could also produce voltage-dependent inhibition, probably by binding inside the pore at the Mg^{2+} blocking site [139]. It had been proposed that *zinc* is an endogenous ligand controlling NMDARs functions [140].

An important consideration in NMDAR function and pharmacology is that the Zn^{2+} binding to NR2A and NR2B subunits is associated with discrete subunit selectivity [141]. NMDARs containing the NR2A subunit had a very high sensitivity to extracellular Zn^{2+} (IC_{50} ~15 nM) [133, 142]; however, this inhibition never exceeded 60–80% [142]. The mechanisms of this inhibition occurred in different steps [143]: in the first step Zn^{2+} bound in the interlobe cleft of the NR2A-NTD promoting its closure, which would exert tension on the linkers connecting NTDs to ABDs. This effect would secondarily cause a disruption of the ABD dimer interface. In turn, this disruption relieved the strain on the transmembrane segments, and with proton binding, it allows the closure of the channel gate [133]. This mechanism of enhancement of proton inhibition was supported by subsequent work [144].

Zinc has a much lower affinity to the NR2B subunit, compared to NR2A, with voltage-independent inhibition (IC_{50} ~ 1 μM) [122, 145]. It was suggested that the mechanism of inhibition might be similar to the mechanism described for NR2A receptors. However, *zinc* inhibition of NR2B receptors appeared to not be dependent on pH [122], suggesting that this inhibition might occur through a different mechanism [133]. Studies showed that Zn^{2+} bound with high affinity to a site in NR2A ATD region [146] and with a lower affinity to a site in the same region of the NR2B [145]. The affinities of NR2C and NR2D to Zn^{2+} described to be even higher (IC_{50} > 10 μM) [134].

Lead (Pb^{2+}) is an exogenous heavy metal, which has been a public health concern due to its widespread contamination and its multiple toxic effects. Effects of acute exposure to Pb^{2+} in the micromolar range were originally described in cultured and acutely dissociated neurons as a reversible inhibition of the NMDAR current [19, 147–150]. These studies outlined several features of the effects of Pb^{2+} (for details, see review [151]). First, the inhibition was specific for NMDA channels, which were significantly more sensitive

Table 5: Effects of metals on postsynaptic ligand-gated ion channels (↑—activation/upregulation, ↓—inhibition/downregulation).

Target		NMDA	AMPA/kainate	GABA-A
Lead	Effect	(1) ↓ open channel probability (2) 60% ↓ in current (reversible) (3) >80% block (4) ↓ (5) ↓ (6) ↓ receptor binding (7) ↓		(1) ↓ (35%)
	Conc	(1) 1–10 (2) 50 (3) 100 (4) IC_{50} = 1.52–8.19 (5) IC_{50} = 8.78 (in 0 Zn); IC_{50} = 1.26 (10 Zn) at high site, 94 at low site (6) IC_{50} = 300 (adult); 60 (neonatal) (7) IC_{50} (free) = 0.55		(1) 1m M
	Ref	(1) [16] (2-3) [14] (4) [20] (5) [9] (6) [12] (7) [5]		(1) [10]
Zinc	Effect	(1) ↓ open channel probability	(1) ↑	(1) ↓ ↓ current in voltage independent, noncompetitive manner
		(2) Channel block	(2) ↓	
		(3) NR2A block	(3) ↑	
		(4) NR2B block	(4) ↓	
		(5) ↓	(5) ↑ (16% to kainate, 15% to glu peak and steady state)	
		(6) ↓ receptor binding (76%)	(6) ↓	
		(7) ↓	(7) ↑ AMPA response	
		(8) ↓	(8) ↑ desensitized Kainate responses	

TABLE 5: Continued.

Target		NMDA	AMPA/kainate	GABA-A
			(9) ↓ AMPA and kainate responses	
	Conc	(1) 1–10 μM (2) >20 (3) nM (4) μM (5) High affinity: IC_{50} = 0.77; low affinity: IC_{50} = 153 (6) 1 mM (7) IC_{50} (free) = 1.3 (8) IC_{50} = 42.9	(1) 50 (2) 1 mM (3) <300 (4) >500 (5) 10 (6) IC_{50} = 700 (7) EC_{50} = 30 (8) EC_{50} = 13 (9) IC_{50} = 1.2-1.3 mM	(1) 100 (dose dependent) (2) IC_{50} = 19
	Ref	(1-2) [11] (3) [17, 21] (4) [17] (5) [9] (6) [12] (7) [5] (8) [22]	(1-2) [17] (3-4) [7, 25] (5-6) [15] (7-9) [22]	(1) [13] (2) [10]
Magnesium	Effect	(1) ↑ NMDA-R affinity to glycine in all receptors (2) ↓ elementary current at +ve potentials(+20 to +80) (3) ↑ glycine and voltage-independent and subunit specific (4) external channel block, voltage dependent	(1) ↓ (27%)	
	Conc	(1) 10 mM (2) 10 mM (3) 2 mM (4) IC_{50} (−100 mV) = 2–15	(1) 20 mM	
	Ref	(1–3) [6] (4) [2]	(1) [15]	

Table 5: Continued.

Target		NMDA	AMPA/kainate	GABA-A
Manganese	Effect	(1) ↓ (activity dependent, channel blocker)	(1) ↓ (46%)	(1) Little or no effect
	Conc	(1) Ki = 35.9 (presence of glu and gly); Ki = 157 (no glu nor gly)	(1) 25 mM	(1) 1 mM
	Ref	(1) [8]	(1) [15]	(1) [10]
Copper	Effect	(1) ↓ (2) ↓ receptor binding (54%) (3) ↓ (channel block) (4) ↓ (5) ↓ voltage independent, noncompetitive	(1) ↓ (2) ↓ kainite-induced current (3) ↓ efficacy of kainate	(1) ↓ (voltage independent)
	Conc	(1) ND (2) 1 mM (3) Ki = 195 (no coagonists); two sites (9.4, 248) with glu and gly (4) IC_{50} = 15 (5) IC_{50} (free) = 0.27	(1) (2) IC50 = 4.3 (3) 30	(1) IC_{50} = 5
	Ref	(1) [17, 23] (2) [12] (3) [8] (4) [30] (5) [28]	(1) [17] (2-3) [30]	(1) [10]
Cobalt	Effect	(1) ↓	(1) ↓ (2) ↓	(1) ↓ (2) ↓ (29%)
	Conc	(1) 2 mM	(1) 2 mM (2) IC_{50} = 6.1 mM	(1) 2 mM (2) 1 mM
	Ref	(1) [3]	(1) [3] (2) [15]	(1) [3] (2) [10]

Table 5: Continued.

Target		NMDA	AMPA/kainate	GABA-A
Nickel	Effect	(1) NR2A: ↓, NR2B: ↑ (2) NR2A ↓ (100% at +ve potentials) (3) NR2B ↓ (4) NR2B ↑ (voltage independent)	(1) ↓ (kainite-induced current) (2) ↓ (glu-induced current)	(1) ↓(20%)
	Conc	(1) 30 (2) IC_{50} = 36 at −60 mV and 81 at +40 mV (3) IC_{50} 138 at −60 mV and 442 at +40 mV (4) 3	(1) IC_{50} = 420 (2) IC_{50} = 2.6 mM	(1) 1 mM
	Ref	(1) [16] (2–4) [21]	(1-2) [15]	(1) [10]
Mercuric chloride	Effect			(1) ↑ 130% (2) ↑ (270%)
	Conc			(1) 1 (2) 100
	Ref			(1) [1] (2) [19]
Methyl mercury	Effect	(1) ↓ receptor binding		(1) ↓ amplitude to 82.4%
	Conc	(1) IC_{50} = 0.95 (neonatal); 70 (adult)		(1) 100
	Ref	(1) [12]		(1) [55]
Cadmium	Effect	(1) ↓ receptor binding (58%) (2) ↓ (39% of control) (3) ↓ (4% of control)	(1) ↑ (kainate to 108% and QA to 115%) (2) ↓ (kainate to 79% and QA to 60%)	(1) ↓ (18%)
	Conc	(1) 1 mM (2) 50	(1) 50 (2) 1 mM	(1) 1 mM

Table 5: Continued.

Target		NMDA	AMPA/kainate	GABA-A
		(3) 1 mM		
	Ref	(1) [12] (2-3) [18]	(1-2) [18]	(1) [10]
Lanthanide	Effect	(1) ↓ NMDA response in a voltage-independent manner	(1) ↑ (2) ↓	(1) ↑ (300% max) and ↑ as the potential more −ve
	Conc	(1)) IC_{50} = 2	(1) 1–100 (2) >100	(1) EC_{50} = 231
	Ref	(1) [27]	(1-2) [27]	(1) [10]
Trimethyl-tin (TMT)	Effect	(1) ↓ (35%) reversible	(1) ↓ (20%) irreversible	(1) ↓ (30%) irreversible
	Conc	(1) 100	(1) 100	(1) 100
	Ref	(1) [4]	(1) [4]	(1) [4]

to Pb^{2+} inhibition than other glutamate channels. Secondly, the channel block was independent of voltage [148–150], and therefore the interaction site was likely to be located away from the electric field, or outside the conducting pore. Thirdly, the effect was noncompetitive since increasing the glutamate or glycine concentration could not overcome the block of the current [148, 152]. Biochemical studies suggested that the inhibitory effects of Pb^{2+} on NMDA receptors were age- and brain-region specific [152–154]. One important observation in Pb^{2+} neurotoxicity was that the hippocampus appears to be more sensitive than other brain regions [153, 155, 156].

The effect of Pb^{2+} on glutamate and NMDA-evoked currents depended on the subunit composition of the receptor-channel complex. Concentration-dependent Pb^{2+} inhibited the currents activated by either Glu or NMDA in oocytes expressing NR1-2A or NR1-2B (Table 1, [157]). Yamada and colleagues [158], however, showed that higher concentrations were needed than mentioned before, although, there were methodological differences between the two studies, which could account for the different results (for details, [157]).

Also, Pb^{2+} at low concentrations (<1 μM) acted as a positive modulator of agonist action on NR1-2AB and NR1-2AC receptors whereas at higher concentration *lead* inhibited NR1-2AB and NR1-2AC receptors, but with less potency compared to NR1-2A or NR1-2B [157, 159].

There is incongruity whether *lead* acts via the *zinc* binding site or through a different site. A set of experiments demonstrated that in the presence of increasing amounts of Pb^{2+}, there was a concentration-dependent downward shift of the Zn^{2+} inhibition curve; also, the values of IC_{50} for Zn^{2+} inhibition decreased as a function of increasing Pb^{2+} concentrations. The effects of Zn^{2+} on Pb^{2+} curve and IC_{50} were analogous [160]. These findings suggested that the two metals act via independent binding sites, which is in line with the observation that increasing concentrations of Pb^{2+} did not affect the Zn^{2+} IC_{50} [154]. However, these results were in contrast with other findings which report that the two cations compete for the same binding site [161, 162].

Nickel (Ni^{2+}) is a trace element, which is essential for many biological organisms, but could also induce toxicity. The effects of Ni^{2+} on NMDA channel activity were described as a voltage-dependent and "Mg^{2+}-like" inhibition [127]. Later work showed a potentiation of homomeric NR1a channels [121] and an inhibition of NR1-2A channels [13, 146]. In more recent studies, it is suggested that, besides the voltage-dependent Mg^{2+}-like inhibition, Ni^{2+} causes a potentiation of NR2B-containing channels and a voltage-independent inhibition (Zn^{2+}-like inhibition) in those neurons containing NR2A [163].

Nickel also caused a reduction of single channel current amplitude at negative voltages while the dependence on membrane voltage was slightly steeper for NR2A than NR2B [13]. Several analogies with Mg^{2+}-like inhibition indicated that it might interact with either the N or N+1 site in the pore-forming region of the NR2 subunit [13].

Support for the above theory came from an experiment showing that a single mutation in the NR2B site at the N+1 site would completely abolish the voltage-dependent block Ni^{2+} [123]. The N+1 residue had been shown to be a critical binding site for Mg^{2+} block in NR2A subunit [128]. Moreover, at positive potentials the effects of Ni^{2+} were highly subunit dependent. NR2A-containing channels were blocked in a voltage-independent manner whereas NR2B containing channels were facilitated [13] (see Abbreviation section). However, at higher concentrations (IC_{50}= 442 μM), a voltage-independent inhibition was also present in NR1-2B channels [123]. The voltage-independent inhibition site of Zn^{2+} was investigated as a potential site for Ni^{2+} inhibition, but this did not seem to be the case. Besides the difference in blocking affinity, Zn^{2+} inhibition was pH dependent [122, 164] while Ni^{2+} inhibition was not [163]. Also, Zn^{2+} inhibition was never more than 60–80% (as described in section 3.2.1), while Ni^{2+} inhibition approached 100% at positive potentials [123]. Other results also showed that mutations that affect the inhibition of Zn^{2+} did not modify Ni^{2+} sensitivity [146].

The NR2B-selective potentiation was suggested to share the site of action with spermine, as Ni^{2+} partially obscured the effect of spermine when they were applied concurrently [123].

Although the actions of *zinc, lead, and nickel* on NMDARs were intensively investigated, there are also some reports that other metals have an effect on these receptors and channel activity.

Copper (Cu^{2+}) is an endogenous metal in the human brain [165], and it is an established fact that *copper* represents an integral part of neurotransmission [166]. It is released from synaptic vesicles following neuronal depolarization [167]. The concentration of *copper* in the synaptic cleft could reach up to 100 μM [168]; later studies estimated the concentration of *copper* released into the synaptic cleft to be in the range of ~15 μM [169, 170]. However, the topographic distribution showed marked variations between different brain areas [171]; the highest concentration of *copper* has been found to be in the hypothalamus [172].

Cu^{2+} acts on NMDA receptors and reduces the current—induced by 50 μM NMDA—in a concentration-dependent manner with an IC_{50} of 15.9 μM. This block was completely and quickly reversible, even in the absence of antioxidant dithiotreitol, suggesting that the inhibition was not an oxidizing effect [173]. Further studies showed that Cu^{2+} inhibition was characterized by voltage-independent, but use-dependent mechanism of action, as the degree of inhibition was dramatically decreased in the absence of agonists [174].

Another trace metal required for normal brain function is *manganese (Mn^{2+})*. In the human brain, Mn^{2+} is most concentrated in the globus pallidus, caudate, and putamen, but also found in other areas [175]. Mn^{2+} produces a strong voltage-dependent block in response to NMDA [176]. It was, also, a competitive antagonist of MK-801 binding to the NMDAR-channel. Its inhibitory effects were activity-dependent since Mn^{2+} was a more potent inhibitor in the presence of NMDA coagonists (Glu and Gly) than in their absence [177]. Taking these studies together, they indicate that Mn^{2+} is an NMDAR channel blocker. Interestingly, the inhibitory constant for Mn^{2+}, in the absence of Glu and Gly, was significantly different in neuronal membranes from the cerebellum relative to other brain regions; however, in the presence of the agonists, Mn^{2+} was equally potent in inhibiting NMDARs in different brain regions [177].

3.1.1. The Glycine-Binding Site of the NMDA-Receptor/Channel Complex. The NMDAR glycine-binding site was susceptible to modulation by divalent cations, especially when the glycine site was not saturated. Low, extracellular concentrations of Mg^{2+} potentiated NMDAR currents. The potentiation was the result of an increase in the affinity of NMDAR for glycine [129, 130, 178]. The mean glycine EC_{50} value was 100–133 nM in control conditions and was reduced to 60–62 nM in the presence of 10 μM Mg^{2+} [178]. This increase in affinity was also demonstrated by decreasing the inhibitory potency of NMDAR glycine-site antagonists upon the addition of potentiating concentrations of Mg^{2+}[129, 178, 179]. Ca^{2+} had the same effect as Mg^{2+} [129, 178, 179].

Concentrations of Pb^{2+} and Zn^{2+} higher than 10 μM inhibited NMDAR potentiation by Ca^{2+} and Mg^{2+} [178]. These findings were supported by other studies, which showed that increasing concentrations of Ca^{2+} diminished the inhibition of NMDAR currents by Zn^{2+} [136], or Pb^{2+} [180]. It is suggested that these divalent cations act on the same site, and Ca^{2+} and Mg^{2+} have opposite effects on glycine binding compared to Pb^{2+} and Zn^{2+} [178].

Even the presence or absence of glycine modulated the effects of some of the cations: for example, Cu^{2+} and Mn^{2+} are both potent NMDAR channel inhibitors (as shown above), but in the presence of glycine and glutamate, Cu^{2+} was more potent than Mn^{2+}, and in the absence of glycine, Mn^{2+} was slightly more potent [177].

3.2. AMPA and Kainate Receptors. The two classes of ionotropic glutamate receptor-channels, which are designated non-NMDA channels, are AMPA (α-amino-3-hydroxy-5-methyl-4-isoxazolepropionic acid) and kainate receptors, named after their most potent excitatory amino acids. The AMPAR channel is also activated by kainate (for review, [181]). Also, AMPARs mediate the fast excitatory synaptic transmission in the CNS [182].

AMPA/kainate receptor-gated channels are permeable to Na^+ and K^+ and more or less impermeable to Ca^{2+}; however, there is a subpopulation of central neurons, which contain AMPA/kainate receptors with enhanced Ca^{2+}-permeability [183, 184]. This Ca^{2+} conductance triggered by the AMPA/kainate receptors seemed to be dependent on the absence of the GluR2 subunit [119, 182, 185].

Extracellular calcium ions produced rapid and reversible voltage-independent inhibition of AMPARs, with both Ca^{2+} permeable and Ca^{2+} impermeable AMPAR being equally sensitive [186]. The Ca^{2+} effects were agonist dependent, more prominent in the case of AMPA compared to Glu or kainate. These data suggested that Ca^{2+} enhances desensitization, as two well-known antidesensitization agents prevented Ca^{2+} inhibition through Ca^{2+} binding to a modulatory site in the AMPAR [186].

Effects of *zinc* on AMPA/kainate receptors have also been explored. Zn^{2+} appeared to have a dual effect on AMPAR: at micromolar concentrations, it enhances AMPA receptor responses whereas at millimolar concentrations, it inhibits them [136, 187]. These effects of Zn^{2+} appear to be subunit specific as well. Experiments using cloned AMPAR expressed in oocytes demonstrate that, in normal calcium-containing solution, *zinc* could potentiate current from homomeric GluR3 receptors over a narrow range of 4–7.5 μM Zn^{2+} while homomeric GluR1 receptors could not be potentiated, but are inhibited by 10 μM Zn^{2+} [188]. Additionally, in calcium-free solution, the inhibition caused by Zn^{2+} on GluR1 shifted to $\geq$1 mM and potentiation was attainable reaching a maximum of ~200% at 50 μM Zn^{2+}. Also, GluR3 showed maximum potentiation not significantly different from GluR1 potentiation. The presence of GluR2 subunit in heteromeric expression of GluR2/GluR3 prevented the potentiation by Zn^{2+}, but also allowed inhibition (with 500 μM Zn^{2+}, current was 39% of control). The presence of GluR2 rendered the effects of Zn^{2+} independent of Ca^{2+} levels (for details, [189]).

The effects of other divalent metals effects were explored on these channels but less extensively compared to NMDARs. Various metals caused inhibition of Ca^{2+} impermeable AMPAR with the following rank order of inhibition: $Ni^{2+} > Zn^{2+} > Co^{2+} > Ca^{2+} > Mn^{2+} > Mg^{2+}$ (for values, refer to Table 5) [190]. The proposed mechanism of action is that complexes of divalent cations and AMPAR agonists compete with the free agonists rather than the cations themselves. This mechanism fits the data in which a competitive type of inhibition is observed; in addition, an increase in agonist concentration reduce the inhibitory effects of divalent metals less than that of DNQX (the classical competitive AMPAR antagonist) [190].

3.3. GABA Receptor. γ-Aminobutyric acid (GABA) is the major inhibitory neurotransmitter in the mammalian central nervous system. The synaptic transmission mediated by $GABA_A$ receptor-channel complex leads to a hyperpolarization of the cell membrane due to the fast activation of postsynaptic chloride channels upon the exposure to GABA [191]. The $GABA_AR$ is comprised of pentameric combination of α1–6, β1–4, γ1–3, δ 1, and/or ε1 subunit subtypes that form an intrinsic chloride ion channel, and each subunit comprises four domains. $GABA_ARs$ have some recognized allosteric binding sites such as barbiturates, benzodiazepines, and picrotoxin [192, 193]. The properties of the allosteric binding sites were influenced by the subunit subtype composition of $GABA_AR$ (for review [194]).

3.3.1. Inhibitory Effects of Metal Ions. The $GABA_AR$ response to GABA-evoked currents was modulated by a number of divalent metal cations. *Zinc, cadmium, nickel, manganese, cobalt, lead,* and *copper* inhibited the response to GABA. The inhibition by divalent metals has consistently been shown to be reversible with no or little voltage dependence [14].

Zn^{2+} had the potential to directly interact with the $GABA_AR$ to influence inhibitory postsynaptic currents (IPSC) amplitudes and kinetics [118]. Zn^{2+} suppressed the GABA-induced chloride current with a K_d of 19 μM in a noncompetitive, voltage-independent manner, and without interference with any of the allosteric sites on the GABA-R [195]. Using cultured hippocampal neurons, studies showed that Zn^{2+} reduced the amplitude, slowed the rise time, and accelerated the decay of mIPSCs. Evidence indicated that inhibition of mIPSCs by Zn^{2+} was attributed to an allosteric modulatory site located on the extracellular domain of $GABA_A$ receptors [196, 197]. In accordance with the previous hypothesis, single-channel studies have also shown that Zn^{2+} reduced the opening frequency with no evidence of flickering [198–200].

From another perspective, the effects of Zn^{2+} were subtype-specific. The *zinc*-sensitivity of the channels seemed to be dependent on the absence of γ subunits, as its presence in any combination with other subunits led to the formation of $GABA_A$ receptors almost insensitive to Zn^{2+} [201, 202]. Furthermore, the presence of a δ subunit enhanced *zinc* sensitivity [202, 203]. The exchange of a particular subunit with other members of the same subunit family (α1 versus α3, β1 versus β2, and γ1 versus γ2) did not alter the large difference in Zn^{2+} sensitivity between $GABA_AR$ containing or lacking γ subunit [202]. Later studies showed that recombinant $GABA_AR$, which contain α4, α5, and α6 subunits, were more sensitive to *zinc* than those that contain α1 subunits [204–207]. Given that the majority of synaptic $GABA_AR$ are of the α-, β-, γ-isoform [208], together with the above studies, indicate that a likely target of Zn^{2+} modulation is an extrasynaptic α-, β- or δ-receptor [118].

In rats dorsal root ganglion (DRG) neurons, Cu^{2+} at concentration of 15 μM, suppressed the peak amplitude of the GABA-induced current to approximately 50%; the blocking was exerted and reversed quickly, and it was independent of membrane potential [195].

The similar blocking profiles of Cu^{2+} and Zn^{2+} led to the question whether they shared a common binding site. Competition experiments showed that Zn^{2+} suppression of GABA-induced current was decreased with increasing concentrations of Cu^{2+}, suggesting that Zn^{2+} and Cu^{2+} act on the same allosteric site to inhibit $GABA_AR$ [55].

In a later study, the *copper*-induced block of $GABA_AR$ in Purkinje cells developed slowly, was poorly reversible, and decreased with increasing GABA concentrations. The block occurred at low concentrations indicating a high affinity with an IC_{50} ~35 nM [209]. The copper block of $GABA_AR$ in Purkinje cells seemed to have a higher affinity compared to the block in DRG [195] and olfactory bulb neurons [210]. Another difference between these tissues was that Cu^{2+} in DRG cells interacts in a noncompetitive manner while in Purkinje, Cu^{2+} decreased the potency of GABA without affecting the maximal response. A possible explanation for this discrepancy might be different subunit composition of the $GABA_AR$ [210].

The effects of multiple divalent metals (*cadmium, nickel, manganese, zinc,* and *barium*) were shown in a study of GABA responses of embryonic chick spinal cord neurons. The results were suggestive of an allosteric mechanism of inhibition of $GABA_AR$ currents. Through combination experiments they showed that the ions acted at a common site but possessed different intrinsic efficacies with the following rank: *Zn > Cd> Ni> Mn*. *Ba* was thought to bind to the site but lacked efficacy as an inhibitor of the GABA response [14]. The rank of efficacy was supported by other experiments [195].

3.3.2. Excitatory Effects of Metal Ions. *Lanthanides* comprise a series of 15 metals starting with *lanthanum (La)* and ending with *lutetium*. In sub-millimolar concentrations, lanthanum ions modulate GABA-induced currents [55, 191, 211].

La^{3+} increased the affinity of GABA for the receptor in a concentration-dependent manner with an $EC_{50} = 231\,\mu M$ and maximum enhancement to about 300% of control with 1 mM. This potentiation was completely and quickly reversed, but was more enhanced as the potential became more negative (1.6% per 10 mV) [195]. Also, this effect was independent of the presence or absence of barbiturates, benzodiazepines, picrotoxin, or Zn^{2+}/Cu^{2+}, indicating that it was bound to a site different from all of the binding sites of the above substances [55]. La^{3+} did not activate transmembrane currents, it only potentiated GABA-induced currents; also La^{3+} did not affect the amplitude of the maximum response induced by GABA. These data together suggested that La^{3+} increased the affinity of $GABA_AR$ to its agonist [212]. *Other lanthanides* exhibited enhancing actions, and the efficacy increased with increasing the atomic number, such that Lu^{3+} (1 mM) increased the current to 1230% of control [55]. However, previously it was reported that *lanthanides* generate inward currents on their own in the absence of GABA [55]. This controversy might be due to use of different tissues; as La^{3+} did not activate transmembrane currents in CA1 hippocampal pyramidal neurons whereas La^{3+} generated inward currents in DRG neurons.

Additionally, recombinant $GABA_AR$ studies suggested that changing the α-subunit subtype from $\alpha 1$ to $\alpha 6$ alters the effects of *lanthanum* from potentiation to inhibition at comparable concentrations. These studies also suggested that the maximal inhibition of $GABA_AR$ current by La^{3+} in $\alpha 6$-containing receptors is greater in the presence of δ subunit (83%) than in the presence of γ subunit (32%) [213].

Another cation that might affect $GABA_AR$ is *mercury (Hg)*. In its inorganic form, $GABA_AR$ channel complex was strongly stimulated by low concentrations of *Hg* [214]. *Mercuric chloride* (100 μM) increased the GABA-induced current to 270% of control, and increased it to 115% of control with 0.1 μM [55] indicating its high potency.

3.4. Summary of Postsynaptic Effects. The main **postsynaptic targets** are the ligand-gated receptors including, but not limited to, NMDA, AMPA/kainite, and GABA receptors. Of those, NMDAR channels are the most widely studied receptors due to their association with disease status. Relatively fewer studies have been done on other targets, which could lead to underestimation of their roles in metal toxicity.

Two main mechanisms established for metals effects on NMDAR: Mg^{2+}-like inhibition, which is voltage dependent, or Zn^{2+}-like inhibition, which is voltage independent. *Lead* and *copper* were found to inhibit NMDAR in Zn^{2+}-like pattern. However, *copper*-mediated inhibition of NMDAR was use dependent which was also true for *manganese*-mediated inhibition [160–162]. *Nickel* on the other hand, showed an Mg^{2+}-like inhibition at negative potentials. However, it had different effects on NR2B and NR2A containing channels at positive potentials. It caused a potentiation of NR2B-containing channels and a Zn^{2+}-like inhibition in those containing NR2A. However, at high concentrations, NR2B-containing receptors also showed Zn^{2+}-like inhibition at positive potentials [163]. Another major target on the NMDAR was glycine-binding site with multiple metals affecting it. Ca^{2+} and Mg^{2+} potentiated NMDAR currents whereas Pb^{2+} and Zn^{2+} inhibited NMDAR currents. All of these four divalent metals might act on the same binding site with different effects [178]. Also, the presence or absence of glycine affected the potency of Cu^{2+} and Mn^{2+}, such that in the presence of Gly, Cu^{2+} was more potent, whereas in the absence of Gly, Mn^{2+} was slightly more potent [177].

The main inhibitory receptors in the brain, $GABA_A$, are also modulated by a variety of metals. Certain metals suppressed the GABA-induced chloride current while others augmented it. Multiple divalent metals had inhibitory effects on GABA-induced current. Cu^{2+} and Zn^{2+} suppressed $GABA_AR$ in an equipotent manner, and there was some evidence that they act on the same site. Other divalent metals also showed inhibitory effects through an allosteric mechanism of inhibition, and they demonstrated a common site of action but with different intrinsic efficacies with the rank $Zn^{2+} > Cd^{2+} > Ni^{2+} > Mn^{2+}$ [14].

Interestingly, *Lanthanides* exhibited enhancing effects of GABA-induced currents. The effect was completely and quickly reversible. The efficacy increased with increasing atomic number [55]. However, recombinant $GABA_AR$ studies suggested that changing the α-subunit subtype could alter the effects of lanthanum from potentiation to inhibition in a comparable concentration range.

Mercury was another metal, which had inhibitory and excitatory effects. In its inorganic form, $GABA_AR$ channel complex was strongly stimulated by low concentrations of *Hg*. However, *methyl mercury* was a potent inhibitor of GABA-induced current, and this effect was irreversible [55]. This showed how organic metals might behave differently compared to inorganic cations; however, there is less information in the literature about the effects of organic metals. One of the most toxic organic metal is *trimethyl-tin (TMT)*. At a concentration of 100 μM, around 20–30% of AMPAR and $GABA_AR$ currents were inhibited whereas 35% of NMDAR ion currents were blocked [215].

4. Disruption of Synaptic Plasticity

Multiple reports have demonstrated that human exposure to environmentally concentrations of certain metals can result in cognitive deficits.

Arsenic consumption, mainly through contaminated water, has been found to be associated with impairment

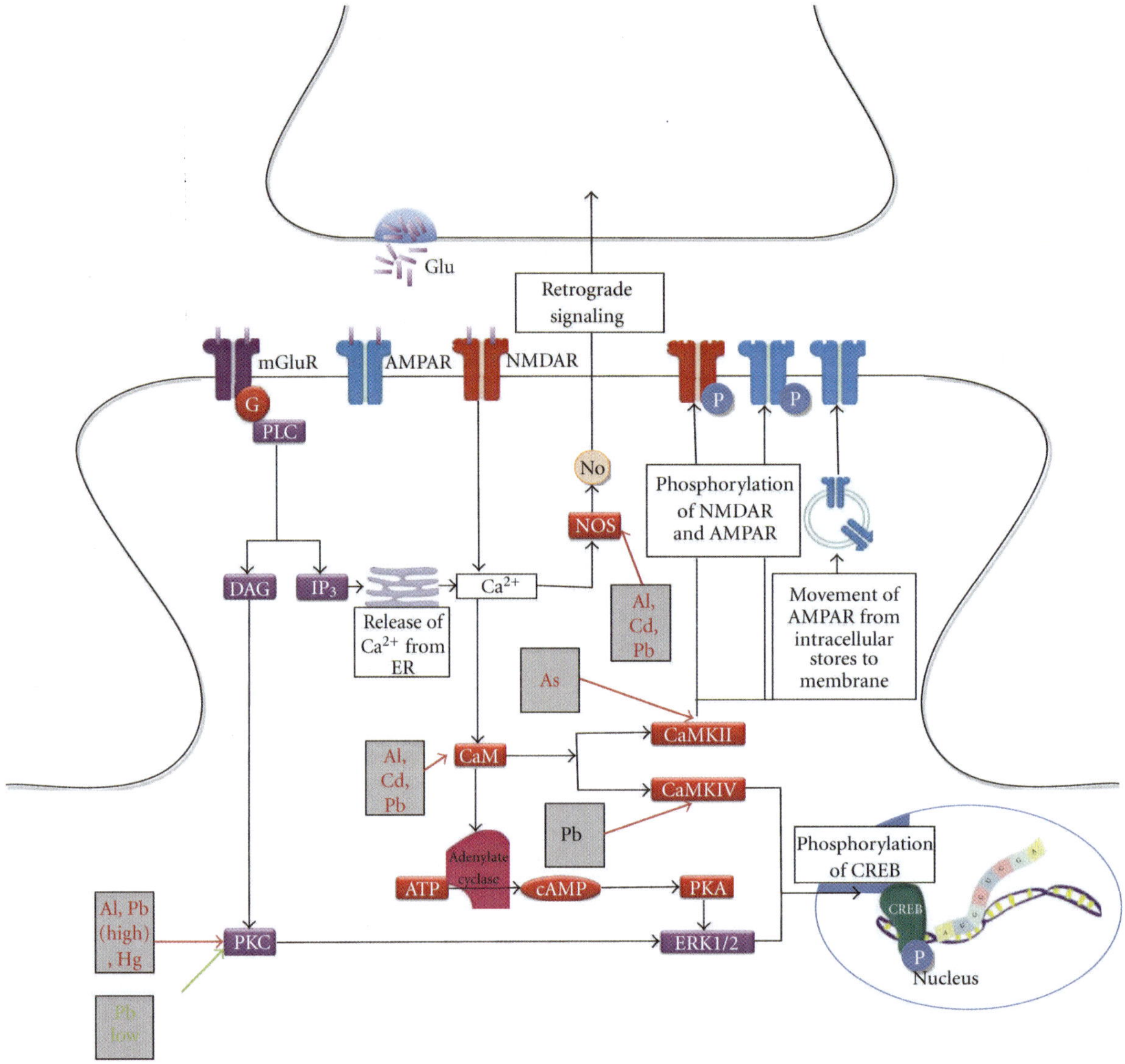

Figure 5: Proteins involved in the formation of long-term potentiation (LTP) and toxic effects of metals. LTP consists of different forms: early-phase LTP (E-LTP), which lasts only a few hours, and late-phase LTP (L-LTP), which lasts for several days. E-LTP includes short-term potentiation (STP), which is dependent on NMDA receptor activation and Ca^{2+}/calmodulin and LTP-1 that involves protein kinase C (PKC) and Ca^{2+}/calmodulin-dependent protein kinase- (CaMK-) dependent phosphorylation. While STP can be formed by activation of NMDA and calmodulin dependent enzymes, LTP-1 requires activation of PKC via DAG that is produced after the activation of mGluRs. PKC and CaMKII then phosphorylate AMPA and NMDA receptors. L-LTP consists of the later phases of LTP, which are LTP-2 and LTP-3. LTP-2 requires synthesis of new proteins and receptors whereas LTP3 requires gene transcription. Activation of adenylate cyclase and cAMP-dependent activation of PKA are required for the formation of the later phases of LTP. LTP-3 depends on the activation of extracellular signal- related kinase 1/2 (ERK1/2) and CaM kinase IV, which in turn phosphorylate CREB and lead to new protein synthesis. Other factors such as p38 mitogen-activated protein kinase (p38 MAPK) leads to the formation of long-term depression (LTD). Several of the molecules required to produce these different forms of LTP have been identified and are targets for metal toxicity, which have been shown (red arrows indicate inhibition whereas green arrows indicate activation by metals. Black arrows indicate activation that occurs during normal formation of LTP).

of long-term memory and a reduction in the verbal IQ of children [216, 217]. *Lead* has been studied extensively for its role in disruption of synaptic plasticity in an attempt to explain the cognitive deficits observed in children with elevated blood lead levels. The CDC currently considers blood Pb^{2+} level of 10 μg/dL to be the threshold for impairment of cognitive function in children [218], although recent studies have observed that cognitive impairment can occur even at blood lead levels <10 μg/dL [219]. There have been reports that *aluminum* also affects synaptic plasticity, which has been implicated in the pathogenesis of Alzheimer's disease, although this topic is highly debated. It has been argued that these detrimental effects on learning, memory, and cognition, which are associated with exposure to metals, may be linked to the disruption of processes that are involved in synaptic plasticity. The formation of long-term potentiation (LTP) is impaired in mice that have inborn low learning capacity indicating the crucial role for synaptic plasticity as the basis of learning and memory. Impairment of LTP has been observed with exposure to *lead* [220]. Moreover, studies have shown that *aluminum* also impaired hippocampal long-term potentiation (LTP) and long-term depression (LTD) in rats both *in vivo* and *in vitro* [221, 222]. Also, multiple metals have been shown to have different concentrations in patients with Parkinson's disease compared to healthy individuals, and the levels of aluminum have been identified as a potential diagnostic marker [223].

To understand how metals and their compounds affect learning and memory, their effects on different stages of LTP and LTD were compared to identify specific sites of interaction for particular metals as well as targets common to more than one metal.

Recently, it has been shown that LTP consists of different succeeding forms: early-phase LTP (E-LTP), which lasts only a few hours, and late-phase LTP (L-LTP), which lasts for several days [224–226]. Several of the molecules required to produce these different forms of LTP have been identified and are targets for metal toxicity [224, 225, 227] (refer to Figure 5 and Table 6).

Early-LTP. it includes short-term potentiation (STP), which is dependent on NMDA receptor activation Ca^{2+}/calmodulin; and LTP-1 that involves protein kinase C (PKC) and Ca^{2+}/calmodulin-dependent protein kinase-(CaMK-) dependent phosphorylation. While STP can be formed by activation of NMDA and calmodulin-dependent enzymes, LTP-1 requires activation of PKC via DAG that is produced after the activation of mGluRs. The activity of mGluR-PKC is important for both increasing activity as well as increasing number of AMPA receptors. PKC and CaMKII then phosphorylate AMPA and NMDA receptors.

Late-LTP. there are two later phases of LTP named LTP-2 and LTP-3. LTP-2 requires synthesis of new proteins and receptors whereas LTP-3 requires gene transcription. Activation of adenylate cyclase and cAMP-dependent activation of PKA are required for the formation of the later phases of LTP. LTP-3 depends on the activation of extracellular signal-related kinase 1/2 (ERK1/2) and CaM kinase IV, which in turn phosphorylate CREB, and this leads to new protein synthesis. p38 mitogen-activated protein kinase (p38 MAPK) is involved in the formation of long-term depression (LTD), and c-JUN-N-terminal kinase (JNK) is thought to participate in LTD [228, 229].

4.1. Disruption of Long-Term Potentiation by Exposure to Metals in Adults

4.1.1. Calmodulin. Calmodulin (CaM) is a regulatory protein that is activated by $[Ca^{2+}]_i$. This protein is found in high concentrations in CNS neurons and is involved in the activation of several other proteins. Some of the CaM-regulated proteins that modulate synaptic plasticity include adenylyl cyclases (AC1 and AC8), protein kinases, calcineurin, calmodulin kinases (CAMK I, II, and IV), nitric oxide synthase, and Ca^{2+} conducting channels. CaM has four Ca^{2+} binding sites. Ca^{2+} binding to CaM leads to a conformational change that exposes a hydrophobic domain which enhances the binding of CaM to other target proteins [226]. It has been hypothesized that in absence of Ca^{2+}, the concentration of free CaM is regulated by neurogranin that binds CaM and releases free CaM in response to PKC and Ca^{2+} [226, 230, 231]. This important molecule has been identified as a target of several neurotoxic metals such as *aluminum, cadmium,* and *lead.*

CaM, when incubated with increasing concentrations of *aluminum* (Al^{3+}) (from 0–1000 μM), showed decreased activity. This decrease in activity, measured by the ability of CaM stimulate activator-deficient cAMP phosphodiesterase was concentration dependent, [20]. Yet, another study showed that an $[Al^{3+}]$: [CaM] ratio of 3 : 1 resulted in 50% decrease in phosphodiesterase activity, and maximal inhibition was observed at a ratio of 4 : 1 [60].

Recently, using highly specific monoclonal antibodies that detect the different conformational states of CaM and monoclonal antibodies against *Al*-CaM complex, researchers found that on dissolving CaM with $AlCl_3 \cdot 6H_2O$ (in increasing concentrations from 0–480 μM), the antibody specific to Ca^{2+} calmodulin conformation (the active form) mAb CAM-1, did not recognize the *Al*-CaM complex (at *Al* concentrations of 240–300 μM) indicating that the CaM was in the inactive conformation. Moreover, the antibodies against the *Al*-calmodulin complex were found to bind to their antigen in the presence of Ca^{2+}. This shows *Al* binds *CaM,* even in the presence of Ca^{2+}, and CaM undergoes a conformational change into an inactive form. Equilibrium dialysis and atomic adsorption studies indicated that Ca^{2+} remained bound to CaM simultaneously with *Al.* When the *Al*-chelator citrate was added to the solution only partial restoration of CaM activity occurred, suggesting that some of the *Al* ions became inaccessible for chelation [62].

The effects of *Cadmium* (Cd^{2+}) were observed *in vivo,* where adult male rats, received 6 mg Cd^{2+}/kg body weight daily for four weeks. Brain CaM activity was determined by measuring the stimulation of phosphodiesterase activity. A

Table 6

Target		Al Effect	Al Concentration	Al Ref	As Effect	As Concentration	As Ref	Cd Effect	Cd Concentration	Cd Ref	Hg Effect	Hg Concentration	Hg Ref	Pb Effect	Pb Concentration	Pb Ref
Pumps	Ca^{2+} ATPase	↓ *in vitro*	10 mg/kg/day Al^{3+}	[1]												
Protein Synthesis	NMDAR NR1													↕ dev.	750 ppm PbAc	[13]
														↑ dev.	750 ppm PbAc	[14]
	NMDAR NR2A													↓ dev.	750 ppm PbAc	[13]
														↓ dev.	750 ppm PbAc	[14]
	NMDAR NR2B													↕ dev.	750ppm PbAc	[13]
														↕ dev.	750 ppm PbAc	[14]
Enzymes	CaM	↓ *in vitro*	10 mg/kg/day Al^{3+}	[1]				↓ *in vivo*	6 mg/kg/day $CdCl_2$	[15]				↑ *in vitro*	30 μM Pb^{2+}	[21]
		↓ *in vitro*	IC_{50} —15 μM $AlCl_3$	[3]				↓ *in vitro*	IC_{50} —0.47 mM $CdCl_2$	[8]						
		↓ *in vitro*	$AlCl_3$— 240 μM	[9]				↓ *in vitro*	10 nM $CdCl_2$	[4]						
	PKC	↓ *in vitro*	10 mg/kg/day Al^{3+}	[1]							↓ *in vitro*	IC_{50}—1.5 μM Hg; IC_{50} — 0.2 2μM CH_3Hg	[2]	↓ dev.	0.1% PbAc	[5]
		↓ *in vivo*	0.3% $AlSO_4$ for 4 months	[18]							↓ *in vitro*	IC_{50}—0.08 μM $HgCl_2$; IC_{50}—1.32 μM CH_3Hg; IC_{50}—0.90 μM $C_6H_5Hg^+$	[7]	↓ *in vitro*	IC_{50} —2.12 μM PbAc	[10]
	NOS													↓ *in vivo*	1500 ppm PbAc	[17]
											↓ *in vivo*	10 mg MeHg/kg	[16]	↑ *in vitro* ↓ *in vitro*	10^{-13} to 4 × 10^{-4} M PbAc > 4 × 10^{-4} M PbAc	[19]
		↓ *in vivo*	2.5% $AlSO_4$ for 3–5 weeks	[20]	↓ *in vivo*	37 ppm $NaAsO_2$	[6]	↓ *in vitro*	100 μM $CdCl_2$	[11]				↓ *in vivo*	125 ppm PbAc	[12]
		↓dev.	3% $AlSO_4$	[27]										↓ dev.	0.2 % PbAc	[22]
														↓ *in vitro*	IC_{50}—0.36 Pb^{2+}	[11]
	CaMK II													↓dev.	1500 ppm PbAc	[25]
	CaMK IV				↓ *in vivo*	4 ppm As_2O_3 for 60 days	[23]									
Transcription factors	P38 MAPK							↑ *in vitro*	5–100 μM $CdCl_2$	[28]				↑ *in vitro*	5 μM Pb^{2+}	[30]
	ERK1/2 phosphorylation							↑ *in vitro*	100–200 μM $CdCl_2$	[28]				↑dev.	2 mg/kg/day PbAc	[30]
														↑ *in vitro*	5 μM Pb^{2+}	[30]
	CREB phosphorylation													↓ dev.	1500 ppm PbAc	[29]

Julka and Gill [20], Nihei and Guilarte [56], Guilarte and McGlothan [57], Vig et al. [58], Sandhir and Gill. [59], Siegel and Haug [60], Cox and Harrison [61], Levi et al. [62], Ohtani-Kaneko et al. [63], Rajanna et al. [64], Xu et al. [65], Inoue et al. [66], Rajanna et al. [64], Saijoh et al. [67], Nihei et al. [68], Johnson et al. [69], Coppi et al. [70], Hermenegildo et al. [71], Zarazua et al. [72], Mittal et al. [73], García-Arenas et al. [74], Chetty et al. [75], Llansola et al. [76], Wang et al. [77], Toscano et al. [78], Rigon et al. [79], Cordova et al. [80], Toscano et al. [81].

significant decrease in the CaM activity was observed after Cd^{2+} treatment. CaM bound to Cd^{2+} was also detected in the brains of rats exposed to $CdCl_2$. It was proposed that, since Cd^{2+} has an ionic radius similar to Ca^{2+}, it might interact with the Ca^{2+}-binding sites on the CaM [58, 61].

Lead was also found to interfere with CaM activity *in vitro* and *in vivo*. *In vitro* incubation of CaM with *lead* (Pb^{2+}) increased the activity of calmodulin in terms of its ability to stimulate cAMP phosphodiesterase and a maximum increase was observed at 30 μM lead concentration whereas at higher concentrations the calmodulin activity was inhibited. CaM-dependent cAMP phosphodiesterase activity increased up to a concentration of 100 μM, following which there was a sharp decline in activity with higher concentrations of *lead*. The involvement of phenomenon of mimicry of calcium by *lead* as a mechanism of toxicity has been proposed. The affinity of *lead* to CaM is stronger than that of calcium and *lead* can displace calcium from calmodulin [59]. An *in vitro* study done on CaM purified from bovine brain showed that Pb^{2+} mimics a natural ligand and raises the maximal activation slightly above the activation by Ca^{2+} [232].

4.1.2. Protein Kinase C (PKC). Protein Kinase C is a Ca^{2+} and phospholipid-dependent serine/threonine kinase that is a receptor for DAG and phorbol esters. There are two classes of PKC. The classical group of PKC consisting of four isozymes: PKC-α, PKC-βI, PKC-βII, and PKC-γ, are Ca^{2+}-dependent and require Ca^{2+} as well as DAG or phorbol ester for their activation. The second group of PKC isoforms consists of five isozymes: PKC-δ, PKC-ε, PKC-η, PKC-θ, and PKC-μ. These do not require Ca^{2+} for their activation by DAG or phorbol ester. Various isozymes of PKC are involved in the formation of LTP. For instance, a null mutation in PKC-γ prevented the induction of LTP [233]. PKC is activated postsynaptically when metabotropic glutamate receptors (mGluR) are activated leading to the formation of DAG and release of intracellular Ca^{2+}, which activates PKC. The mGluR- PKC pathway then increases the number and activity of AMPA receptors [224]. The PKC activity is affected by metal ions such as Al^{3+}, Pb^{2+}, *Hg*, and organic metals such as *methylmercury (MeHg*; refer to Figure 5).

Aluminum (Al^{3+}; 0–100 μM) decreased *in vitro* PKC activity (determined by transfer of ^{32}P from γ-^{32}P-ATP to lysine rich histone in the presence of Ca^{2+} and phosphatidyl serine), and this effect was concentration dependent [20]. *In vivo*, rats fed *aluminum* ($AlSO_4$) orally were found to have more PKC in the particulate fraction of the brain homogenate compared to the soluble fraction. Normally PKC is translocated from the cytosol to the membrane when it is activated. Application of Al^{3+} caused a 70% increase in the total activity of PKC resulting in a greater fraction of it being translocated to the membrane, and hence the presence of greater fraction of PKC in particulate fraction compared to the soluble fraction [69].

Lead acetate upon *in vitro* incubation with PKC from adult rat brains significantly inhibited PKC activity with an IC_{50} of 2.12 μM [64]. However, it was found that while very low concentrations of Pb^{2+} (10^{-13} to 4×10^{-4} M) increased PKC activity, higher Pb^{2+} concentrations ($>4\times10^{-4}$ M) caused an inhibition of PKC activity. When recombinant human PKC iso-enzymes were examined, low concentrations of Pb^{2+} had very little activating effect on PKC-γ but inhibited it at higher concentrations ($>4 \times 10^{-4}$ M) [70]. *In vivo*, on exposure of adult rats to 1500 ppm *lead acetate*, there was a decrease in protein expression of PKCγ by 32% in the cytosol of hippocampal cells and 25% in the membrane fraction [68]. Another study comparing the effects of Pb^{2+} on the PKC in the brain *in vivo* and *in vitro* found a considerable increase in PKC activity *in vitro, but* failed to find a considerable change in PKC activity *in vivo* [234].

In vivo methylmercury chloride administration in rats in five doses of 10 mg/kg body weight leads to a decrease in the enzymatic activity of the cytosolic PKC extracted from the brain, although it did not induce any change in second messenger binding as measured by binding of [^{3}H]PDBu [67].

4.1.3. Ca^{2+}/Calmodulin Kinases. There are two types of Ca^{2+}/calmodulin kinases (CaMK) involved in LTP: CaMKII and CaMKIV. The Ca^{2+}-CaM complex generally activates these kinases. CaMKII is a serine/threonine protein kinase consisting of 12 subunits that are activated when activated calmodulin is associated with them [235]. Studies have shown that CaMKII blockers impede the ability to generate LTP. CaMKII can also be autophosphorylated at Thr^{286} and its activity becomes independent of Ca^{2+}-CaM. This autophosphorylation occurs after the formation of LTP. It is suggested that after activation, CaMKII phosphorylates the AMPA receptor subunit as well as GluR1 and NMDA receptors and therefore enhances their conductance [236, 237].

CaMKIV is also activated similarly but the downstream targets are different for CaMKIV. Experiments have shown that upon activation, CaMKIV can phosphorylate CREB, which in turn mediates the transcriptional control of protein synthesis required for the long-term maintenance of LTP [238].

In vivo, rats exposed to 4 ppm *arsenic trioxide* (As_2O_3) for 60 days showed about a 4-fold decrease in expression of CaMKIV compared to a control group of rats as elucidated by microarray analyses. Western blot analyses reflected similar findings. Moreover, the decrease in expression of the β-subunit of CaMKIV was greater than the decrease in α-subunit expression [77].

4.1.4. Nitric Oxide Synthase. Nitric oxide synthase (NOS) is an enzyme that produces nitric oxide (NO) by oxidizing L-arginine using molecular oxygen and NADPH [239, 240]. There are different kinds of NOS expressed in several cell types. Endothelial cells express constitutive endothelial NOS (eNOS) that is activated by Ca^{2+}. Macrophages express inducible NOS (iNOS), and its expression is inducible by cytokines. Neurons express constitutive Ca^{2+}-activated neuronal NOS (nNOS). Following the activation of NMDA receptors and the influx of Ca^{2+}, it is believed that nNOS

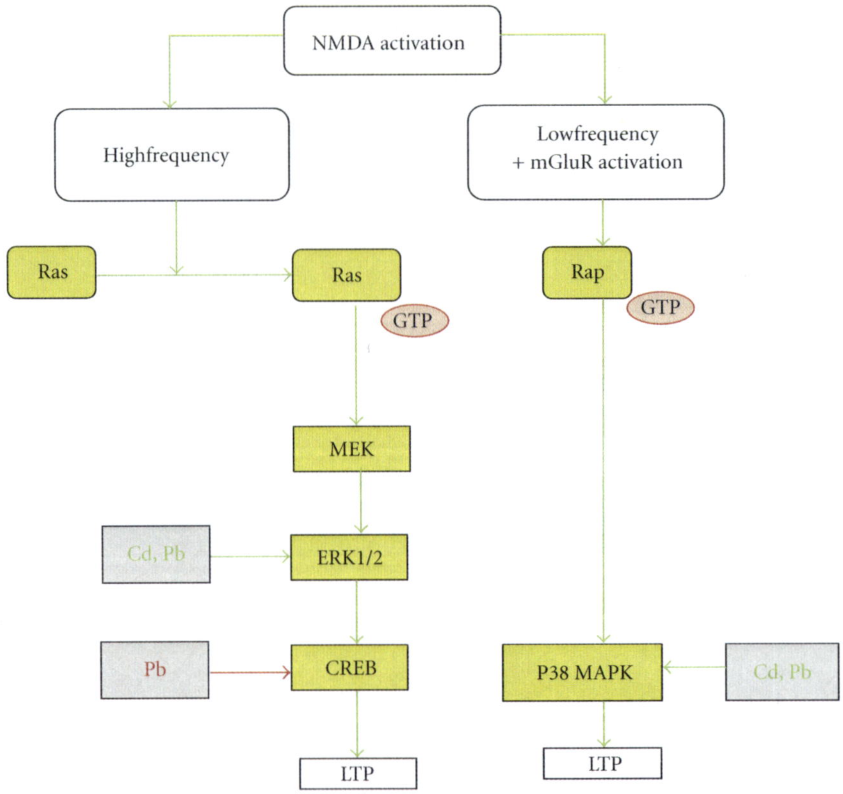

FIGURE 6: Molecules involved in the transcriptional control of LTP and LTD and effects of metals. LTP-3 depends on the activation of ERK1/2 and CaM kinase IV, which in turn phosphorylate CREB, and this leads to new protein synthesis. Other factors such as p38 mitogen-activated protein kinase (p38 MAPK) are involved in the formation of long-term depression (LTD) and c-JUN-N-terminal kinase (JNK) is thought to participate in LTD. A green color indicates an activation or an increase, and a red color indicates an inhibition or a decrease.

produces NO, a retrograde signal, that diffuses into the presynaptic membrane to enhance presynaptic neurotransmitter release by the production of cGMP during the formation of LTP [241, 242].

In vivo, chronic exposure to *aluminum* (Al^{3+}) resulted in the reduced formation of NO after activation of NMDA in the rat cerebellum, as a consequence of decreased calmodulin and NOS [71].

In vivo arsenic exposure to 37 ppm sodium *arsenite* for 10 days, reduced NMDA-induced NOS activity (as measured by sampling of extracellular fluid by means of microdialysis). The maximal NMDA-induced increase of NOS activity (estimated by measuring the changes in extracellular citrulline in the exposed groups) was only 170 ± 24% while under control conditions it reached 278 ± 27% ($P < 0.001$) [72].

In vitro incubation of NOS with 100 μM of *cadmium* (*$CdCl_2$*) resulted in a significant reduction in brain NOS activity as measured by the conversion of radioactive arginine to citrulline. When incubated, the activity of NOS was decreased with an IC_{50} value of 0.22 mM [73].

In vitro incubation of NOS with *lead.* inhibited NOS activity with an IC_{50} of 0.36 mM [73]. *In vivo*, the cNOS activity in the hippocampus and cerebellum (measured by citrulline radioactivity following incubation with radioactive arginine) was decreased in rats that were exposed to 125, 250 and 500 ppm *lead acetate* for 14 days. This decrease was completely reversible by increasing the free Ca^{2+}-concentration. The decrease in NOS activity correlated with blood lead levels [74].

4.1.5. Extracellular Signal-Regulated Kinases (ERK1/2). The extracellular signal-regulated kinases (ERK1/2) are serine threonine kinases that are activated when extracellular signals lead to an increase in intracellular Ras-GTP (GTP-bound form of Ras). Ras-GTP produced by an increase in guanyl nucleotide exchange factors (GEF), a decrease in activity of GTPase-activating proteins (GAPs) or a combination of both then leads to the activation of the enzyme MAPK/ERK kinase (MEK). MEK than activates ERK1 and ERK2 by phosphorylating them. ERK1 and ERK2 (also known as p44 and p42 MAPK) target transcription factors, cytoskeletal proteins, regulatory enzymes, as well as other kinases. In the postsynaptic membrane, calcium influx through the NMDA receptors leads to production of Ras-GTP that can then trigger the cascade leading to phosphorylation of ERK1 and ERK2. CREB maybe one of the targets of the ERK1/2 pathway involved in LTP [229, 243]. CREB, a member of the basic leucine zipper (bZip) family, is a transcription factor that is responsible for initiating new protein synthesis for the maintenance of L-LTP. PKA, CAMK and MAPK can activate CREB by phosphorylation at serine-133. On phosphorylation other proteins such as CREB binding protein are recruited to form a complex, which initiates transcription of CRE containing genes [244–250] (refer to Figure 6).

Exposure of hippocampal slices of rats to Cd^{2+} activates ERK1 and ERK 2 but only at very high concentrations (100–200 μM $CdCl_2$) [79, 229].

On incubation of ERK1/2 with 5 μM Pb^{2+} *in vitro* for 3 hours, there was significant increase in ERK1 and ERK2 phosphorylation in hippocampal homogenates [80].

4.1.6. P38 Mitogen-Activated Protein Kinase (p38 MAPK). Parallel to the ERK1/2 pathway, which is involved in long-term potentiation, another MAPK cascade, which involves p38 MAPK is involved in long-term depression (LTD). Inhibition of p38 MAPK was shown to inhibit a form of hippocampal LTD that involved the activation of mGluR. Inhibition of ERK1/2 by blocking MEK had no effect on this form of synaptic plasticity. The pathways upstream and downstream of p38 MAPK are yet to be elucidated [229, 251] (refer to Figure 6).

Hippocampal slices of postnatal day 14 rats were exposed *to* Cd^{2+} in concentrations between 5–100 μM for 3 hours. A western blot analysis showed that this increased the activity of p38 MAPK, which is involved in the inhibition of LTP [79, 229].

Incubation of ERK1/2 with 5 μM Pb^{2+} for 3 hours resulted in a significant increase in p38 MAPK phosphorylation in hippocampal homogenates [80].

4.2. Disruption of Long-Term Potentiation by Exposure to Metals during Development. Developmental exposure to "neurotoxic" metals differs from exposure in an adult in various ways. The developing brain is more vulnerable than the adult one. The basic circuitry of the brain is laid down during development and any disruption of receptors, neurotransmission, and neurogenesis can prevent the brain from maturing normally. Inappropriate activation of the unspecific receptors in the developing brain can interfere with the normal "tuning." Moreover, the blood-brain barrier is not laid down till approximately six months of age in humans. This absence of blood brain barrier allows toxic agents to enter the brain freely and interfere with its development. Developmental exposure to metals also raises the issue of what Costa et al. labeled as "silent" neurotoxicity. This is when the deleterious effects of various neurotoxic insults do not manifest until several months or years post-partum. For instance, in Guam's disease, unknown neurotoxic agents cause damage to the CNS, which do not become apparent until decades later. Here we discuss developmental exposure of metals and their effects on the molecules involved in the formation of LTP, which are important for the development of memory and learning [252].

N-methyl-D-aspartate receptors (NMDAR) are Ca^{2+} channels, which play an essential role in several forms of synaptic plasticity (see Section 3.1). They have glutamate receptors present which are involved in excitatory synaptic transmission in various parts of the brain. Its unique properties, such as Mg^{2+} block and high permeability to Ca^{2+}, give NMDAR the ability to contribute to the formation of long-term potentiation and long-term depression. Several subunits of NMDA receptors have been identified: NR1 that is ubiquitously expressed; NR2 subunit family that has four distinct types (A, B, C, and D) and two NR3 subunits. The expression of the various subunits is different in different stages of development. For instance, NR2B and NR2D expression is present during the neonatal period and NR2A and NR2C are present in the later stages of development [253]. Due to its many binding sites (especially those for divalent cations), which change in their affinity to their agonists during development, a variety of (toxic non-physiologic) metals might bind to these NMDAR with a high affinity and thereby impair their function.

Lead causes impairment of long-term potentiation in different regions of the hippocampus following chronic *lead* exposure [254, 255]. This has been associated with a disruption in the normal functioning of the NMDA receptors (NMDAR). NMDAR currents decrease after *in vitro* exposure to 5 μM *lead* in hippocampal cells [152]. This can be attributed to the observation that Pb^{2+} alters expression of the different subunits of NMDAR, which has been observed in the hippocampus and cerebral cortex. Additionally, a decrease in expression of NR2A subunit mRNA and proteins in the hippocampus have been seen [56, 57]. Also, the expression of NR1 subunit mRNA in the hippocampus and the cerebral cortex of rats increases [57], but this finding was not supported by another study by Nihei and Guilarte [56], which found no change in the expression of the NR1 subunit protein.

The effects of cadmium (Cd^{2+}) on calmodulin expression were determined in an *in vitro* study done on embryonic rat (ED 15) cerebral cortex, where the cortical slices were incubated with 10 nM *cadmium chloride* for 24 hours. This experiment showed a reduced the amount of calmodulin expression following *cadmium* exposure [63].

Nitric oxide synthase (NOS) was affected by the developmental exposure of rats to *aluminum* (Al^{3+}) and *lead* (Pb^{2+}). Prenatal exposure of developing rats to *aluminum* sulfate (3%) decreased the content of neuronal NOS by 62 ± 12% in the cerebellum [76].

Perinatal exposure to Pb^{2+} decreased NOS activity, as well as NOS expression. Chetty et al., using western blot analysis of nNOS in developing rat brain after perinatal exposure to 0.2% *lead* acetate, found a significant decrease in nNOS protein levels at postnatal day (PND) 21 and 35 in cerebellum, and at PND 21 in hippocampus [75].

Developmental *lead* exposure also affected PKC-γ and CaMKII function. PKC-γ is activated by binding of Ca^{2+} or DAG and on activation, it translocates to the membrane. To determine the effects of Pb^{2+} on PKC-γ and other PKC-subtypes, pregnant rats were exposed to 0.1% *lead acetate*, dissolved in distilled deionized water (DDW) from gestation day 6 to postnatal day 21 (PND). With western blot analysis the expression on PKC-γ was determined. Pb^{2+} reduced PKC-γ mRNA expression significantly in hippocampus and frontal cortex at PND 1, 5, and 10, with greater effect on the membrane PKC-γ than on the cytosolic PKC-γ. Additionally there was a decrease in the activity of PKC-γ following exposure to *lead*. The PKC-γ activity was determined by measuring the amount γ-^{32}P transferred to histone per min per mg protein. In the hippocampus and the frontal cortex, both total and calcium-dependent PKC activities were significantly inhibited [65].

Moreover, rats exposed to 1500 ppm Pb^{2+} during development demonstrated a reduction in the V_{max} of CaMKII (examined by measuring the phosphorylation of a biotinylated substrate for CaMKII) and reduced expression of CaMKII β subunit in the hippocampus, but showed no changes in the sensitivity of calmodulin to CaMKII. In other words, the decrease in CaMKII activity was not due to impairment in its ability to bind CaM [78].

Various metals also inhibited the enzymes related to the transcription of new proteins involved in the formation of LTP. Two such targets are ERK1/2 and CREB.

Prenatal exposure to *aluminum* sulfate (3%) slightly increased the content of ERK [76]. Also, *in vivo* developmental exposure to 2 mg/kg of Pb^{2+} increased both ERK1 and ERK2 phosphorylation in rat hippocampal neurons [80].

On developmental exposure to 1500 ppm of Pb^{2+}, a decrease in the amount of phosphorylated CREB was observed in both the hippocampus (25% decrease) and the cerebral cortex (25% decrease) but there were no significant changes in unphosphorylated CREB levels [81]. Also, significant changes in the binding kinetics of CREB to CRE were observed in the hippocampus. The K_d and B_{max} both were decreased by 38% and 30%, respectively, in the hippocampus but no significant changes in binding kinetics were observed in the cortex [244].

4.3. Summary of Long-Term Effects. Metals affect various mediators of synaptic plasticity. Calmodulin (CaM) activity is affected by *aluminum, cadmium,* and inorganic *lead*. Both *aluminum* and *cadmium* inhibited CaM activity [20, 58, 60–63] whereas inorganic *lead* first increased CaM activity at lower concentrations (possibly by mimicking calcium), but then at higher concentrations it decreased CaM activity [59, 232]. CaM is the central modulator of NMDAR-mediated synaptic plasticity and a majority of the regulators of synaptic plasticity depend on CaM for their activation. Thus, interference with CaM function will indirectly affect the function of numerous LTP- and LTD-related proteins such as adenylyl cyclase, Ca^{2+}/Calmodulin kinases, nitric oxide synthase, and Ca^{2+} channels [226]. Al^{3+}, Pb^{2+}, and *MeHg* affect PKC activity, which is involved in the formation of LTP-1. *In vitro* studies demonstrated that in rat brain, Pb^{2+} inhibited PKC activity at low concentrations but increased PKC activity at higher concentrations. However, when recombinant human PKC-γ was used, an opposite trend was observed [70]. Exposure to Pb^{2+} *in vivo* resulted in a decrease in protein expression whereas *MeHg* decreased the activity of PKC. Al^{3+} inhibited PKC activity *in vitro* but ironically, oral administration lead to increase in PKC activity [20]. *Arsenic trioxide* (As_2O_3) decreases the expression of Ca^{2+}/calmodulin kinase IV (CaMKIV) with a greater decrease in the β-subunit than the α-subunit *in vivo* [77]. Nitric oxide synthase (NOS) activity is decreased by various metals such as Al^{3+}, As^{2+}, Cd^{2+}, and Pb^{2+} [71–73]. The components of the transcription pathway, p38 MAPK and ERK1/2 were phosphorylated more when incubated with Pb^{2+} and Cd^{2+}. As discussed earlier, P38 MAPK is involved in the induction of LTD whereas ERK1/2 is involved in induction of LTP-3 [79, 80, 229].

5. Discussion and Conclusion

Most metals act on multiple modulators of synaptic transmission. Heavy metals such as *mercury, lead,* and *arsenic* interfere with normal functioning of molecules both presynaptically and postsynaptically. They also target molecules involved in synaptic plasticity. As discussed above *in vivo* and *in vitro* studies have shown that metals inappropriately inhibit or activate various molecules involved in synaptic transmission and synaptic plasticity. Even though the current pool of the literature gives us valuable insights into the mechanisms of metal toxicity at the synapse, there are many limitations of the current studies.

Firstly, there is hardly any sufficient information with regard to the effect of metals at ***different stages of development***. Postsynaptically, there is a strong suggestion that the different effects on development are due to different subunit expression. As discussed in Section 3.2, Pb^{2+} was a more potent inhibitor of Glu-activated currents in NMDAR expressing NR2A or NR2B compared to receptors expressing both these subunits [157]. At the same time, Pb^{2+} showed high- and low-affinity components for its inhibition in PN14 and PN21 hippocampal membranes. These data suggested that the high-affinity Pb^{2+}-sensitive site was associated with receptors expressing NR2A or NR2B subunits, while the low-affinity site was associated with receptors expressing both subunits (to see the effects on other brain areas, review [153]). The support to this hypothesis came from studies showing that the developmental pattern of NR2A and NR2B mRNA in the hippocampus was similar to that in the data presented [256].

This developmental aspect is not well studied for most of the metals and also for AMPA/kainate and GABA receptors. The effects of divalent metals on AMPA/kainate receptors seem to be dependent upon the subunit composition as well, particularly the presence of GluR2 subunit which rendered the channel impermeable to Ca^{2+}. Zn^{2+} and Co^{2+} both had dual effects on AMPA-Rs: at micromolar concentrations they enhanced AMPA receptor responses whereas at millimolar concentrations, they had inhibitory actions. Various metals caused inhibition of Ca^{2+} impermeable AMPA-R, the inhibition was fast, reversible, and voltage independent. The rank order of activities was $Ni^{2+} > Zn^{2+} > Co^{2+} > Ca^{2+} > Mn^{2+} > Mg^{2+}$ [190]. The proposed mechanism of action was that complexes of AMPAR agonists and divalent cations compete with the free agonists for the binding sites.

Prenatal exposure to heavy metals also leads to various changes in the LTP machinery in the developing brain as discussed before. *Lead*, for instance, changed the expression pattern for NMDAR subunits, and decreased the expression and activity of PKC-γ, CaMKII β, and nNOS in various areas of the brain. These results could explain why the development exposure to some metals causes cognitive deficits in children.

Moreover, a majority of the studies were done *in vitro*, and the *in vivo* studies were done in rats. In most *in vitro* studies, either brain homogenates or purified target molecules were incubated with a given metal. These studies therefore may not accurately depict the physiologic effects of the metals since they do not undergo the physiological process of absorption from the gut as in the human body, and the alterations that may occur in the blood before the metals reach the target tissue. Also, the solutions used for the preservation of the cells may interfere with the experimental results rendering them inaccurate. Moreover, the contents of the media and the forms of metals used were inconsistent between studies. Consequently properties such as solubility of metals in the media and presence of anions and pH were variable and beyond the scope of this study to discuss. It is definitely a limitation of *in vitro* studies, which makes it difficult to compare the different experiments, even when an identical concentration of the same metals was used. However, the ease of carrying out the experiment and lack of requirement for storage space for animals make them a likely choice for most researchers. *In vivo* studies may be closer to the physiologic processes; however it becomes harder than to vary the concentrations of metals and monitor them at the selected site of interest.

In addition, most of the findings presented in this review both *in vivo* and *in vitro* were based on studies done using rats. Even though it is easy to measure concentrations of metals, levels of proteins and enzymes in rats, elucidating the clinical manifestations in animal models can be challenging. Also, it is hard to find whether the effects in rats are similar to those in humans and if the effects in rats are representative of the effects in humans. Higher cognitive functions in humans might alter the presentation of the toxicity in ways that cannot be adjusted for because much of the mechanisms of the functioning of the human nervous system are not fully understood today.

Another important limitation of the currently available literature is that the majority of studies discussed were on effects of inorganic metals on the brain cells or brain molecules, and very few centered around organic metals which are perhaps even more significant than inorganic metal toxicity since in some cases the organic forms are more toxic than the inorganic forms, as for *mercury* [257]. There is a rapidly growing body of evidence that the majority of metals may actually be methylated to their organic form as the body attempts to detoxify metals. For *arsenic*, in the past it was believed that conversion of arsenic to *monomethyl arsenic* and *dimethyl-arsenic* was a method of detoxification; however, the view has changed since then with the recognition that methylated metabolites of trivalent arsenic are carcinogenic [258]. *Antimony, mercury, lead, tin, and selenium* are known to cause public health problems in their methylated forms. *Cadmium, cobalt, mercury, and nickel* reportedly undergo biomethylation; however, the effects of biomethylation have been studied more in unicellular organisms rather than plants and animals, therefore it has been suggested that although biomethylation does occur in plants and animals, the rates are likely to vary on the basis of the animal and the metal, and its concentration [259].

There are some situations that have not been considered in most experimental designs. One such issue that arises with the study of metals is the problem that most studies are not reflective with regard to the actual exposure in nature where humans are simultaneously exposed to more than one metal. Very few studies have targeted this issue, most likely due to the complicated nature of conducting an experiment with many variables and determining the contribution of each. One study by Platt and Büsselberg who examined the effects of combinations of Pb^{2+}, Zn^{2+}, and Al^{3+}, on voltage-activated calcium channels by simultaneous application of various combinations of two metals determined that regardless of the order in which the metals were added, the actions were in fact additive [260]. Whether this is the case with other metals is not certain and there is not enough data in the literature describing effects of combinations of metals. Another limitation of the study is that some targets may not be as relevant as others in causing the clinical symptoms of metal toxicity; however, it is not possible to know at this stage the exact contribution of each target.

Finally, the most important objective is to put these effects of metals into practical use. This can be done by using the data of the toxic concentrations of metals to make a meaningful decision in regard to their acceptable blood levels. There is evidence to suggest that currently accepted levels for some metals are still not "safe" levels. Even at the currently accepted blood *lead* levels of $10\,\mu g/dL$, it is causative of preterm labor and adverse pregnancy outcome [261]. Therefore, there is a need to reevaluate the accepted blood concentrations of metals in light of the newer evidence as it appears.

Metal neurotoxicity is a field, which is abounding with the literature and excellent research; however, in the current literature some metals are highlighted while for other metals (or metal compounds) hardly any data are available. There is an emphasis on certain metals such as *lead*, whose harmful effects are well known while there is very little known about certain metal groups such as *lanthanides* and *actinides*.

There are certain targets where metal actions have been excessively examined such as voltage-activated calcium channels while there is little known about the effects of metals on parts of signaling pathways such as phosphodiesterases and IP_3. This raises the need to evaluate new targets for metals, which have not been studied before, which may prove to have a groundbreaking effect in the field of neurotoxicity.

To summarize, exposure to different metals occurs due to industrial activities, environmental, and food chain contamination. This paper elucidated the various targets of metals in synaptic transmission and synaptic plasticity. Exposure to metals had varied effects on different synaptic targets, which were dependent on the form of metal, the concentration of metal, route of exposure (*in vitro* or *in vivo*), the medium used, and even the duration of exposure in some cases.

Abbreviations

$[Ca^{2+}]_i$: Intracellular calcium concentration
ABD: Agonist-binding domain
AC: Adenylate cyclase
Ach: Acetylcholine
Al: Aluminum
$AlCl_3$: Aluminum trichloride
AMPA: α-amino-3-hydroxy-5-methyl-4-isoxazolepropionic acid
As: Arsenic
As_2O_3: Arsenic trioxide
ATD: Amino terminal domain
ATP: Adenosine triphosphate
ATPase: Adenosine triphosphatase
Ba: Barium
BAPTA: 1,2-bis(2-aminophenoxy)ethane-N,N,N9,N9-tetracetic acid tetrakis(acetoxymethyl) ester
B_{max}: Maximal binding
Ca: Calcium
CaM: Calmodulin
CaMK: Ca^{2+}/calmodulin-dependent protein kinase
cAMP: Cyclic adenosine monophosphate
Cd: Cadmium
$CdCl_2$: Cadmium chloride
CDDP: *cis-Diammine-dichloroplatin*
CH_3Hg: Methylmercury
CNS: Central nervous system
Co: Cobalt
Cr: Chromium
CRE: cAMP response elements
CREB: Ca^{+2}/cAMP response element-binding protein
Cu: Copper
DAG: Diacylglycerol
DDW: Distilled deionized water
DOC2: Double C2 domain
DOPAC: 3.4-dihydroxyphenylacetic acid
DOPAC: 3.4-dihydroxyphenylacetic acid
DRG: Dorsal root ganglion
E-LTP: Early-phase LTP
ED: Embryonic day
eNOS: Eendothelial NOS
EPP: End-plate potential
ERK1/2: Extracellular signal-related kinase 1/2
Et_3Pb: Triethyl lead
Et_3Sn: Triethyl-tin
Fe: Iron
GABA: γ-Aminobutyric acid
GAP: GTPase-activating protein
GEF: Guanyl nucleotide exchange factors
$G_{i/o}$: Inhibitory Sguanine nucleotide binding protein/other guanine nucleotide-binding protein
Glu: Glutamate
GluR: Glutamate Receptor
Gly: Glycine
GPCR: G-protein-coupled Receptors
Gpp(NH)p: 5′ Guanylylimidodiphosphate
G_s: Stimulatory guanine nucleotide binding protein
GTP: Guanosine-5′-triphosphate
Hg: Mercury
HVA: Homovanillic acid
IC_{50}: Concentration for 50% inhibition
iNOS: Inducible NOS
IP_3: Inositol triphosphate
Inositol triphosphate: Inhibitory postsynaptic currents
IQ: Intelligence quotient
JNK: c-JUN-N-terminal kinase
K: Potassium
KCl: Potassium chloride
K_d: Dissociation constant
L-LTP: Late-phase LTP
La: Lanthanum
Li: Lithium
LTD: Long-term depression
LTP: Long-term potentiation
mAb: Monoclonal antibody
MAPK: Mitogen-activated protein kinase
Me_3Pb: Trimethyl lead
Me_3Sn: Trimethyl-tin
MeHg: Methylmercury
MEK: MAPK/ERK kinase
MEPP: Miniature end-plate potential
Met: Methionine
Mg: Magnesium
mGluR: Metabotropic glutamate receptors
mIPSC: Miniature inhibitory postsynaptic currents
Mn: Manganese
mRNA: Messenger ribo nucleic acid
Na: Sodium
NADPH: Reduced nicotinamide adenine dinucleotide phosphate
Ni: Nickel
NMDA: N-methyl-D-aspartate
NMDAR: N-methyl-D-aspartate receptors
nNOS: Neuronal NOS
NOS: Nitric oxide synthase
NT: Neurotransmitter
Pb: Lead
PKA: Protein kinase A
PLC: Phospholipase C
PND: Postnatal day
Ras: Rat sarcoma family
RBC: Red blood cells
Sn: Tin

SNAP-25: Synaptosome-associated protein 25 kDa
SNARE: SNAP and NSF attachment receptor
$SnCl_2$: Stannous chloride
Sr: Strontium

STP: Short-term potentiation
Thr: Threonine
VGCC: Voltage-gated calcium Channel
V_m: Membrane voltage
Zn: Zinc.

Authors' Contribution

S. Sadiq, Z. Ghazala and A. Chowdhury contributed equally.

References

[1] P. J. Craig, G. Eng, and R. O. Jenkins, "Occurrence and pathways of organometallic compounds in the environment—general considerations," in *Organometallic Compounds in the Environment*, P. J. Craig, Ed., pp. 1–55, John Wiley & Sons, Chichester, UK, 2003.

[2] H. A. Waldron, "Lead poisoning in the ancient world," *Medical History*, vol. 17, no. 4, pp. 391–399, 1973.

[3] D. R. Crapper, S. S. Krishnan, and S. Quittkat, "Aluminium, neurofibrillary degeneration and Alzheimer's disease," *Brain*, vol. 99, no. 1, pp. 67–80, 1976.

[4] B. Michalke, S. Halbach, and V. Nischwitz, "JEM spotlight: metal speciation related to neurotoxicity in humans," *Journal of Environmental Monitoring*, vol. 11, no. 5, pp. 939–954, 2009.

[5] H. Needleman, "Low level lead exposure: history and discovery," *Annals of Epidemiology*, vol. 19, no. 4, pp. 235–238, 2009.

[6] D. Swandulla and C. M. Armstrong, "Calcium channel block by cadmium in chicken sensory neurons," *Proceedings of the National Academy of Sciences of the United States of America*, vol. 86, no. 5, pp. 1736–1740, 1989.

[7] A. M. Florea, E. Dopp, and D. Büsselberg, "Elevated Ca2+i transients induced by trimethyltin chloride in HeLa cells: types and levels of response," *Cell Calcium*, vol. 37, no. 3, pp. 251–258, 2005.

[8] A. Vahidnia, G. B. van der Voet, and F. A. de Wolff, "Arsenic neurotoxicity—a review," *Human and Experimental Toxicology*, vol. 26, no. 10, pp. 823–832, 2007.

[9] P. C. L. Wong, J. C. K. Lai, L. Lim, and A. N. Davison, "Selective inhibition of L-glutamate and gammaaminobutyrate transport in nerve ending particles by aluminium, manganese, and cadmium chloride," *Journal of Inorganic Biochemistry*, vol. 14, no. 3, pp. 253–260, 1981.

[10] A. L. S. Rodrigues, A. Regner, M. A. Rubin, and D. O. Souza, "Effects of lead on adenylate cyclase activity in rat cerebral cortex," *Neurochemical Research*, vol. 24, no. 8, pp. 1037–1042, 1999.

[11] R. H. Chow, "Cadmium block of squid calcium currents. Macroscopic data and a kinetic model," *Journal of General Physiology*, vol. 98, no. 4, pp. 751–770, 1991.

[12] A. Minami, A. Takeda, D. Nishibaba, S. Takefuta, and N. Oku, "Cadmium toxicity in synaptic neurotransmission in the brain," *Brain Research*, vol. 894, no. 2, pp. 336–339, 2001.

[13] C. Marchetti and P. Gavazzo, "NMDA receptors as targets of heavy metal interaction and toxicity," *Neurotoxicity Research*, vol. 8, no. 3-4, pp. 245–258, 2005.

[14] J. J. Celentano, M. Gyenes, T. T. Gibbs, and D. H. Farb, "Negative modulation of the γ-aminobutyric acid response by extracellular zinc," *Molecular Pharmacology*, vol. 40, no. 5, pp. 766–773, 1991.

[15] A. M. Florea and D. Büsselberg, "Occurrence, use and potential toxic effects of metals and metal compounds," *BioMetals*, vol. 19, no. 4, pp. 419–427, 2006.

[16] C. I. Ragan, "Metal ions in neuroscience," *Metal-Based Drugs*, vol. 4, no. 3, pp. 125–132, 1997.

[17] A. Tomaszewski and D. Büsselberg, "Cisplatin modulates voltage gated channel currents of dorsal root ganglion neurons of rats," *NeuroToxicology*, vol. 28, no. 1, pp. 49–58, 2007.

[18] D. Purves et al., "Synaptic transmission," in *Neuroscience*, pp. 85–118, Sinauer Associates, Sunderland, UK, 2008.

[19] D. Busselberg, B. Platt, D. Michael, D. O. Carpenter, and H. L. Haas, "Mammalian voltage-activated calcium channel currents are blocked by Pb2+, Zn2+, and Al3+," *Journal of Neurophysiology*, vol. 71, no. 4, pp. 1491–1497, 1994.

[20] D. Julka and K. D. Gill, "Altered calcium homeostasis: a possible mechanism of aluminium-induced neurotoxicity," *Biochimica et Biophysica Acta*, vol. 1315, no. 1, pp. 47–54, 1996.

[21] V. Kumar and K. D. Gill, "Aluminium neurotoxicity: neurobehavioural and oxidative aspects," *Archives of Toxicology*, vol. 83, no. 11, pp. 965–978, 2009.

[22] A. Welling, "Voltage-dependent calcium channels," *Biotrend Reviews*, pp. 1–2009, 2009.

[23] D. Busselberg, M. L. Evans, H. Rahmann, and D. O. Carpenter, "Lead and zinc block a voltage-activated calcium channel of Aplysia neurons," *Journal of Neurophysiology*, vol. 65, no. 4, pp. 786–795, 1991.

[24] D. Busselberg, M. Pekel, D. Michael, and B. Platt, "Mercury (Hg2+) and zinc (Zn2+): two divalent cations with different actions on voltage-activated calcium channel currents," *Cellular and Molecular Neurobiology*, vol. 14, no. 6, pp. 675–686, 1994.

[25] M. L. Evans, D. Busselberg, and D. O. Carpenter, "Pb2+ blocks calcium currents of cultured dorsal root ganglion cells," *Neuroscience Letters*, vol. 129, no. 1, pp. 103–106, 1991.

[26] R. K. Hajela, S. Q. Peng, and W. D. Atchison, "Comparative effects of methylmercury and Hg2+ on human neuronal N- and R-type high-voltage activated calcium channels transiently expressed in human embryonic kidney 293 cells," *Journal of Pharmacology and Experimental Therapeutics*, vol. 306, no. 3, pp. 1129–1136, 2003.

[27] D. Busselberg, M. L. Evans, H. L. Haas, and D. O. Carpenter, "Blockade of mammalian and invertebrate calcium channels by lead," *NeuroToxicology*, vol. 14, no. 2-3, pp. 249–258, 1993.

[28] G. Audesirk and T. Audesirk, "The effects of inorganic lead on voltage-sensitive calcium channels differ among cell types and among channel subtypes," *NeuroToxicology*, vol. 14, no. 2-3, pp. 259–266, 1993.

[29] E. Reuveny and T. Narahashi, "Potent blocking action of lead on voltage-activated calcium channels in human neuroblastoma cells SH-SY5Y," *Brain Research*, vol. 545, no. 1-2, pp. 312–314, 1991.

[30] G. Audesirk and T. Audesirk, "Effects of inorganic lead on voltage-sensitive calcium channels in N1E-115 neuroblastoma cells," *NeuroToxicology*, vol. 12, no. 3, pp. 519–528, 1991.

[31] D. Busselberg, D. Michael, M. L. Evans, D. O. Carpenter, and H. L. Haas, "Zinc (Zn2+) blocks voltage gated calcium

channels in cultured rat dorsal root ganglion cells," *Brain Research*, vol. 593, no. 1, pp. 77–81, 1992.

[32] L. Schild and E. Moczydlowski, "Competitive binding interaction between Zn2+ and saxitoxin in cardiac Na+ channels. Evidence for a sulfhydryl group in the Zn2+ saxitoxin binding site," *Biophysical Journal*, vol. 59, no. 3, pp. 523–537, 1991.

[33] E. Gawrisch, R. Leonhardt, and D. Büsselberg, "Voltage-activated calcium channel currents of rat dorsal root ganglion cells are reduced by trimethyl lead," *Toxicology Letters*, vol. 92, no. 2, pp. 117–122, 1997.

[34] T. Hattori and H. Maehashi, "Stannous chloride-induced increase in calcium entry into motor nerve terminals of the frog," *European Journal of Pharmacology*, vol. 166, no. 3, pp. 527–530, 1989.

[35] S. P. H. Alexander, A. Mathie, and J. A. Peters, "Ion channels," *British Journal of Pharmacology*, vol. 141, no. S1, pp. S71–S91, 2004.

[36] M. Sue Marty and W. D. Atchison, "Pathways mediating Ca2+ entry in rat cerebellar granule cells following in vitro exposure to methyl mercury," *Toxicology and Applied Pharmacology*, vol. 147, no. 2, pp. 319–330, 1997.

[37] A. L. Goldin, R. L. Barchi, J. H. Caldwell et al., "Nomenclature of voltage-gated sodium channels," *Neuron*, vol. 28, no. 2, pp. 365–368, 2000.

[38] J. E. Sirois and W. D. Atchison, "Methylmercury affects multiple subtypes of calcium channels in rat cerebellar granule cells," *Toxicology and Applied Pharmacology*, vol. 167, no. 1, pp. 1–11, 2000.

[39] T. J. Shafer and W. D. Atchison, "Methylmercury blocks N- and L-type Ca++ channels in nerve growth factor-differentiated pheochromocytoma (PC12) cells," *Journal of Pharmacology and Experimental Therapeutics*, vol. 258, no. 1, pp. 149–157, 1991.

[40] M. Pekel, B. Platt, and D. Busselberg, "Mercury (Hg2+) decreases voltage-gated calcium channels currents in rat DRG and Aplysia neurons," *Brain Research*, vol. 632, no. 1-2, pp. 121–126, 1993.

[41] A. Tomaszewski and D. Büsselberg, "SnCl2 reduces voltage-activated calcium channel currents of dorsal root ganglion neurons of rats," *NeuroToxicology*, vol. 29, no. 6, pp. 958–963, 2008.

[42] C. Frelin, C. Cognard, P. Vigne, and M. Lazdunski, "Tetrodotoxin-sensitive and tetrodotoxin-resistant Na+ channels differ in their sensitivity to Cd2+ and Zn2+," *European Journal of Pharmacology*, vol. 122, no. 2, pp. 245–250, 1986.

[43] J. Györi, O. Platoshyn, D. O. Carpenter, and J. Salánki, "Effect of inorganic and organic tin compounds on ACh- and voltage- activated Na currents," *Cellular and Molecular Neurobiology*, vol. 20, no. 5, pp. 591–604, 2000.

[44] A. Ravindran, L. Schild, and E. Moczydlowski, "Divalent cation selectivity for external block of voltage-dependent Na+ channels prolonged by batrachotoxin. Zn2+ induces discrete substates in crdiac Na+ channels," *Journal of General Physiology*, vol. 97, no. 1, pp. 89–115, 1991.

[45] W. A. Coetzee, Y. Amarillo, J. Chiu et al., "Molecular diversity of K+ channels," *Annals of the New York Academy of Sciences*, vol. 868, no. 1, pp. 233–285, 1999.

[46] R. C. Huang, Y. W. Peng, and K. W. Yau, "Zinc modulation of a transient potassium current and histochemical localization of the metal in neurons of the suprachiasmatic nucleus," *Proceedings of the National Academy of Sciences of the United States of America*, vol. 90, no. 24, pp. 11806–11810, 1993.

[47] C. C. Kuo and F. P. Chen, "Zn2+ modulation of neuronal transient K+ current: fast and selective binding to the deactivated channels," *Biophysical Journal*, vol. 77, no. 5, pp. 2552–2562, 1999.

[48] T. X. Xu, N. Gong, and T. L. Xu, "Divalent cation modulation of A-type potassium channels in acutely dissociated central neurons from wide-type and mutant Drosophila," *Journal of Neurogenetics*, vol. 19, no. 2, pp. 87–107, 2005.

[49] C. S. Watkins and A. Mathie, "Modulation of the gating of the transient outward potassium current of rat isolated cerebellar granule neurons by lanthanum," *Pflugers Archiv: European Journal of Physiology*, vol. 428, no. 3-4, pp. 209–216, 1994.

[50] M. L. Mayer and K. Sugiyama, "A modualtory action of divalent cations on transient outward current in cultured rat sensory neurones," *Journal of Physiology*, vol. 396, pp. 417–433, 1988.

[51] R. Leonhardt, H. Haas, and D. Büsselberg, "Methyl mercury reduces voltage-activated currents of rat dorsal root ganglion neurons," *Naunyn-Schmiedeberg's Archives of Pharmacology*, vol. 354, no. 4, pp. 532–538, 1996.

[52] A. P. de Jong and M. Verhage, "Presynaptic signal transduction pathways that modulate synaptic transmission," *Current Opinion in Neurobiology*, vol. 19, no. 3, pp. 245–253, 2009.

[53] R. Sandhir and K. D. Gill, "Calmodulin and cAMP dependent synaptic vesicle protein phosphorylation in rat cortex following lead exposure," *International Journal of Biochemistry*, vol. 26, no. 12, pp. 1383–1389, 1994.

[54] U. Ewers and R. Erbe, "Effects of lead, cadmium and mercury on brain adenylate cyclase," *Toxicology*, vol. 16, no. 3, pp. 227–237, 1980.

[55] T. Narahashi, J. Y. Ma, O. Arakawa, E. Reuveny, and M. Nakahiro, "GABA receptor-channel complex as a target site of mercury, copper, zinc, and lanthanides," *Cellular and Molecular Neurobiology*, vol. 14, no. 6, pp. 599–621, 1994.

[56] M. K. Nihei and T. R. Guilarte, "NNMDAR-2A subunit protein expression is reduced in the hippocampus of rats exposed to Pb2+ during development," *Molecular Brain Research*, vol. 66, no. 1-2, pp. 42–49, 1999.

[57] T. R. Guilarte and J. L. McGlothan, "Hippocampal NMDA receptor MRNA undergoes subunit specific changes during developmental lead exposure," *Brain Research*, vol. 790, no. 1-2, pp. 98–107, 1998.

[58] P. J. S. Vig, K. Ravi, and R. Nath, "Interaction of metals with brain calmodulin purified from normal and cadmium exposed rats," *Drug and Chemical Toxicology*, vol. 14, no. 1-2, pp. 207–218, 1991.

[59] R. Sandhir and K. D. Gill, "Lead perturbs calmodulin dependent cyclic AMP metabolism in rat central nervous system," *Biochemistry and Molecular Biology International*, vol. 33, no. 4, pp. 729–742, 1994.

[60] N. Siegel and A. Haug, "Aluminum interaction with calmodulin. Evidence for altered structure and function from optical and enzymatic studies," *Biochimica et Biophysica Acta*, vol. 744, no. 1, pp. 36–45, 1983.

[61] J. L. Cox and S. D. Harrison, "Correlation of metal toxicity with in vitro calmodulin inhibition," *Biochemical and Biophysical Research Communications*, vol. 115, no. 1, pp. 106–111, 1983.

[62] R. Levi, T. Wolf, G. Fleminger, and B. Solomon, "Immunodetection of aluminium and aluminium induced conformational changes in calmodulin-implications in Alzheimer's disease," *Molecular and Cellular Biochemistry*, vol. 189, no. 1-2, pp. 41–46, 1998.

[63] R. Ohtani-Kaneko, H. Tazawa, M. Yokosuka, M. Yoshida, M. Satoh, and C. Watanabe, "Suppressive effects of cadmium on neurons and affected proteins in cultured developing cortical cells," *Toxicology*, vol. 253, no. 1-3, pp. 110–116, 2008.

[64] B. Rajanna, C. S. Chetty, S. Rajanna, E. Hall, S. Fail, and P. R. Yallapragada, "Modulation of protein kinase C by heavy metals," *Toxicology Letters*, vol. 81, no. 2-3, pp. 197–203, 1995.

[65] S. Z. Xu, L. Bullock, C. J. Shan, K. Cornelius, and B. Rajanna, "PKC isoforms were reduced by lead in the developing rat brain," *International Journal of Developmental Neuroscience*, vol. 23, no. 1, pp. 53–64, 2005.

[66] Y. Inoue, K. Saijoh, and K. Sumino, "Action of mercurials on activity of partially purified soluble protein kinase C from mice brain," *Pharmacology and Toxicology*, vol. 62, no. 5, pp. 278–281, 1988.

[67] K. Saijoh, T. Fukunaga, H. Katsuyama, Myeong Jin Lee, and K. Sumino, "Effects of methylmercury on protein kinase A and protein kinase C in the mouse brain," *Environmental Research*, vol. 63, no. 2, pp. 264–273, 1993.

[68] M. K. Nihei, J. L. McGlothan, C. D. Toscano, and T. R. Guilarte, "Low level Pb2+ exposure affects hippocampal protein kinase Cγ gene and protein expression in rats," *Neuroscience Letters*, vol. 298, no. 3, pp. 212–216, 2001.

[69] G. V. W. Johnson, K. W. Cogdill, and R. S. Jope, "Oral alumimum alters in vitro protein phosphorylation and kinase activities in rat brain," *Neurobiology of Aging*, vol. 11, no. 3, pp. 209–216, 1990.

[70] A. A. Coppi, J. Lesniak, D. Zieba, and F. A. X. Schanne, "The effects of lead on PKC isoforms," *Annals of the New York Academy of Sciences*, vol. 919, pp. 304–306, 2000.

[71] C. Hermenegildo, R. Sáez, C. Minoia, L. Manzo, and V. Felipo, "Chronic exposure to aluminium impairs the glutamate-nitric oxide-cyclic GMP pathway in the rat in vivo," *Neurochemistry International*, vol. 34, no. 3, pp. 245–253, 1999.

[72] S. Zarazúa, F. Pérez-Severiano, J. M. Delgado, L. M. Martínez, D. Ortiz-Pérez, and M. E. Jiménez-Capdeville, "Decreased nitric oxide production in the rat brain after chronic arsenic exposure," *Neurochemical Research*, vol. 31, no. 8, pp. 1069–1077, 2006.

[73] C. K. Mittal, W. B. Harrell, and C. S. Mehta, "Interaction of heavy metal toxicants with brain constitutive nitric oxide synthase," *Molecular and Cellular Biochemistry*, vol. 149-150, pp. 263–265, 1995.

[74] G. García-Arenas, V. Ramírez-Amaya, I. Balderas et al., "Cognitive deficits in adult rats by lead intoxication are related with regional specific inhibition of cNOS," *Behavioural Brain Research*, vol. 149, no. 1, pp. 49–59, 2004.

[75] C. S. Chetty, G. R. Reddy, K. S. Murthy, J. Johnson, K. Sajwan, and D. Desaiah, "Perinatal lead exposure alters the expression of neuronal nitric oxide synthase in rat brain," *International Journal of Toxicology*, vol. 20, no. 3, pp. 113–120, 2001.

[76] M. Llansola, M. D. Miñana, C. Montoliu et al., "Prenatal exposure to aluminum reduces expression of neuronal nitric oxide synthase and of soluble guanylate cyclase and impairs glutamatergic neurotransmission in rat cerebellum," *Journal of Neurochemistry*, vol. 73, no. 2, pp. 712–718, 1999.

[77] Y. Wang, S. Li, F. Piao, Y. Hong, P. Liu, and Y. Zhao, "Arsenic down-regulates the expression of Camk4, an important gene related to cerebellar LTD in mice," *Neurotoxicology and Teratology*, vol. 31, no. 5, pp. 318–322, 2009.

[78] C. D. Toscano, J. P. O'Callaghan, and T. R. Guilarte, "Calcium/calmodulin-dependent protein kinase II activity and expression are altered in the hippocampus of Pb2+-exposed rats," *Brain Research*, vol. 1044, no. 1, pp. 51–58, 2005.

[79] A. P. Rigon, F. M. Cordova, C. S. Oliveira et al., "Neurotoxicity of cadmium on immature hippocampus and a neuroprotective role for p38MAPK," *NeuroToxicology*, vol. 29, no. 4, pp. 727–734, 2008.

[80] F. M. Cordova, A. L. S. Rodrigues, M. B. O. Giacomelli et al., "Lead stimulates ERK1/2 and p38MAPK phosphorylation in the hippocampus of immature rats," *Brain Research*, vol. 998, no. 1, pp. 65–72, 2004.

[81] C. D. Toscano, H. Hashemzadeh-Gargari, J. L. McGlothan, and T. R. Guilarte, "Developmental Pb2+ exposure alters NMDAR subtypes and reduces CREB phosphorylation in the rat brain," *Developmental Brain Research*, vol. 139, no. 2, pp. 217–226, 2002.

[82] C. Klein, R. K. Sunahara, T. Y. Hudson, T. Heyduk, and A. C. Howlett, "Zinc inhibition of cAMP signaling," *Journal of Biological Chemistry*, vol. 277, no. 14, pp. 11859–11865, 2002.

[83] C. Klein, T. Heyduk, and R. K. Sunahara, "Zinc inhibition of adenylyl cyclase correlates with conformational changes in the enzyme," *Cellular Signalling*, vol. 16, no. 10, pp. 1177–1185, 2004.

[84] N. E. Ziv and C. C. Garner, "Cellular and molecular mechanisms of presynaptic assembly," *Nature Reviews Neuroscience*, vol. 5, no. 5, pp. 385–399, 2004.

[85] J. B. Suszkiw, "Presynaptic disruption of transmitter release by lead," *NeuroToxicology*, vol. 25, no. 4, pp. 599–604, 2004.

[86] T. A. Slotkin and F. J. Seidler, "Protein kinase C is a target for diverse developmental neurotoxicants: transcriptional responses to chlorpyrifos, diazinon, dieldrin and divalent nickel in PC12 cells," *Brain Research*, vol. 1263, no. C, pp. 23–32, 2009.

[87] J. Rizo and T. C. Südhof, "Snares and munc18 in synaptic vesicle fusion," *Nature Reviews Neuroscience*, vol. 3, no. 8, pp. 641–653, 2002.

[88] F. Splettstoesser, A. M. Florea, and D. Büsselberg, "IP3 receptor antagonist, 2-APB, attenuates cisplatin induced Ca2+-influx in HeLa-S3 cells and prevents activation of calpain and induction of apoptosis," *British Journal of Pharmacology*, vol. 151, no. 8, pp. 1176–1186, 2007.

[89] T. A. Sarafian, "Methyl mercury increases intracellular Ca2+ and inositol phosphate levels in cultured cerebellar granule neurons," *Journal of Neurochemistry*, vol. 61, no. 2, pp. 648–657, 1993.

[90] S. K. Aggarwal, "A histochemical approach to the mechanism of action of cisplatin and its analogues," *Journal of Histochemistry and Cytochemistry*, vol. 41, no. 7, pp. 1053–1073, 1993.

[91] M. Gemba, E. Nakatani, M. Teramoto, and S. Nakano, "Effect of cisplatin on calcium uptake by rat kidney cortical mitochondria," *Toxicology Letters*, vol. 38, no. 3, pp. 291–297, 1987.

[92] M. Sue Marty and W. D. Atchison, "Elevations of intracellular Ca2+ as a probable contributor to decreased viability in cerebellar granule cells following acute exposure to methylmercury," *Toxicology and Applied Pharmacology*, vol. 150, no. 1, pp. 98–105, 1998.

[93] R. J. DeLorenzo, "The calmodulin hypothesis of neurotransmission," *Cell Calcium*, vol. 2, no. 4, pp. 365–385, 1981.

[94] C. R. Angle and M. S. McIntire, "Red cell lead, whole blood lead, and red cell enzymes," *Environmental Health Perspectives*, vol. 7, pp. 133–137, 1974.

[95] M. Aschner and J. L. Aschner, "Mercury neurotoxicity: mechanisms of blood-brain barrier transport," *Neuroscience and Biobehavioral Reviews*, vol. 14, no. 2, pp. 169–176, 1990.

[96] M. T. Antonio, L. Corredor, and M. L. Leret, "Study of the activity of several brain enzymes like markers of the neurotoxicity induced by perinatal exposure to lead and/or cadmium," *Toxicology Letters*, vol. 143, no. 3, pp. 331–340, 2003.

[97] M. Aschner and J. L. Aschner, "Cellular and molecular effects of trimethyltin and triethyltin: relevance to organotin neurotoxicity," *Neuroscience and Biobehavioral Reviews*, vol. 16, no. 4, pp. 427–435, 1992.

[98] E. W. Haeffner, H. P. Zimmermann, and C. J. K. Hoffmann, "Influence of triethyl lead on the activity of enzymes of the ascites tumor cell plasma membrane and its microviscosity," *Toxicology Letters*, vol. 23, no. 2, pp. 183–188, 1984.

[99] K. E. Stine, L. W. Reiter, and J. J. Lemasters, "Alkyltin inhibition of ATPase activities in tissue homogenates and subcellular fractions from adults and neonatal rats," *Toxicology and Applied Pharmacology*, vol. 94, no. 3, pp. 394–406, 1988.

[100] T. C. Südhof and J. Rizo, "Synaptotagmins: C2-domain proteins that regulate membrane traffic," *Neuron*, vol. 17, no. 3, pp. 379–388, 1996.

[101] C. M. L. S. Bouton, L. P. Frelin, C. E. Forde, H. A. Godwin, and J. Pevsner, "Synaptotagmin I is a molecular target for lead," *Journal of Neurochemistry*, vol. 76, no. 6, pp. 1724–1735, 2001.

[102] D. Rajalingam, T. K. S. Kumar, and C. Yu, "The C2A domain of synaptotagmin exhibits a high binding affinity for copper: implications in the formation of the multiprotein FGF release complex," *Biochemistry*, vol. 44, no. 44, pp. 14431–14442, 2005.

[103] K. M. Kathir, L. Gao, D. Rajalingam et al., "NMR characterization of copper and lipid interactions of the C2B domain of synaptotagmin I-relevance to the non-classical secretion of the human acidic fibroblast growth factor (hFGF-1)," *Biochimica et Biophysica Acta*, vol. 1798, no. 2, pp. 297–302, 2010.

[104] T. O. Brock and J. P. O'Callaghan, "Quantitative changes in the synaptic vesicle proteins synapsin I and p38 and the astrocyte-specific protein glial fibrillary acidic protein are associated with chemical-induced injury to the rat central nervous system," *Journal of Neuroscience*, vol. 7, no. 4, pp. 931–942, 1987.

[105] J. Wang, M. F. Rahman, H. M. Duhart et al., "Expression changes of dopaminergic system-related genes in PC12 cells induced by manganese, silver, or copper nanoparticles," *NeuroToxicology*, vol. 30, no. 6, pp. 926–933, 2009.

[106] S. V. Verstraeten, L. Aimo, and P. I. Oteiza, "Aluminium and lead: molecular mechanisms of brain toxicity," *Archives of Toxicology*, vol. 82, no. 11, pp. 789–802, 2008.

[107] R. B. Mailman, M. R. Krigman, G. D. Frye, and I. Hanin, "Effects of postnatal trimethyltin or triethyltin treatment on CNS catecholamine, GABA, and acetylcholine systems in the rat," *Journal of Neurochemistry*, vol. 40, no. 5, pp. 1423–1429, 1983.

[108] T. Hattori and H. Maehashi, "Acceleration by stannous ion of the evoked release of transmitter from motor nerve endings in the frog," *Brain Research*, vol. 473, no. 1, pp. 157–160, 1988.

[109] M. F. M. Braga, E. F. R. Pereira, M. Marchioro, and E. X. Albuquerque, "Lead increases tetrodotoxin-insensitive spontaneous release of glutamate and GABA from hippocampal neurons," *Brain Research*, vol. 826, no. 1, pp. 10–21, 1999.

[110] S. V. Doctor, L. G. Costa, D. A. Kendall, and S. D. Murphy, "Trimethyltin inhibits uptake of neurotransmitters into mouse forebrain synaptosomes," *Toxicology*, vol. 25, no. 2-3, pp. 213–221, 1982.

[111] B. C. Seidman and M. A. Verity, "Selective inhibition of synaptosomal γ-aminobutyric acid uptake by triethyllead: role of energy transduction and chloride ion," *Journal of Neurochemistry*, vol. 48, no. 4, pp. 1142–1149, 1987.

[112] D. N. Skilleter, "The decrease of mitochondrial substrate uptake caused by trialkyltin and trialkyl lead compounds in chloride media and its relevance to inhibition of oxidative phosphorylation," *Biochemical Journal*, vol. 146, no. 2, pp. 465–471, 1975.

[113] A. Vahidnia, F. Romijn, M. Tiller, G. B. Van Der Voet, and F. A. De Wolff, "Arsenic-induced toxicity: effect on protein composition in sciatic nerve," *Human and Experimental Toxicology*, vol. 25, no. 11, pp. 667–674, 2006.

[114] H. P. Zimmermann, K. H. Doenges, and G. Roderer, "Interaction of triethyl lead chloride with microtubules in vitro and in mammalian cells," *Experimental Cell Research*, vol. 156, no. 1, pp. 140–152, 1985.

[115] H. Faulstich, C. Stournaras, K. H. Doenges, and H. P. Zimmermann, "The molecular mechanism of interaction of Et3Pb+ with tubulin," *FEBS Letters*, vol. 174, no. 1, pp. 128–131, 1984.

[116] C. Stournaras, G. Weber, and H. P. Zimmermann, "High cytotoxicity and membrane permeability of Et3Pb+ in mammalian and plant cells," *Cell Biochemistry and Function*, vol. 2, no. 4, pp. 213–216, 1984.

[117] H. P. Zimmermann, U. Plagens, and P. Traub, "Influence of triethyl lead on neurofilaments in vivo and in vitro," *NeuroToxicology*, vol. 8, no. 4, pp. 569–578, 1987.

[118] T. G. Smart, A. M. Hosie, and P. S. Miller, "Zn2+ ions: modulators of excitatory and inhibitory synaptic activity," *Neuroscientist*, vol. 10, no. 5, pp. 432–442, 2004.

[119] R. Dingledine, K. Borges, D. Bowie, and S. F. Traynelis, "The glutamate receptor ion channels," *Pharmacological Reviews*, vol. 51, no. 1, pp. 7–61, 1999.

[120] P. Paoletti and J. Neyton, "NMDA receptor subunits: function and pharmacology," *Current Opinion in Pharmacology*, vol. 7, no. 1, pp. 39–47, 2007.

[121] M. Hollmann, J. Boulter, C. Maron et al., "Zinc potentiates agonist-induced currents at certain splice variants of the NMDA receptor," *Neuron*, vol. 10, no. 5, pp. 943–954, 1993.

[122] S. F. Traynelis, M. F. Burgess, F. Zheng, P. Lyuboslavsky, and J. L. Powers, "Control of voltage-independent Zinc inhibition of NMDA receptors by the NR1 subunit," *Journal of Neuroscience*, vol. 18, no. 16, pp. 6163–6175, 1998.

[123] P. Gavazzo, P. Guida, I. Zanardi, and C. Marchetti, "Molecular determinants of multiple effects of nickel on NMDA receptor channels," *Neurotoxicity Research*, vol. 15, no. 1, pp. 38–48, 2009.

[124] R. Schoepfer, H. Monyer, B. Sommr et al., "Molecular biology of glutamate receptors," *Progress in Neurobiology*, vol. 42, no. 2, pp. 353–357, 1994.

[125] M. L. Mayer, G. L. Westbrook, and P. B. Buthrie, "Voltage-dependent block by Mg2+ of NMDA responses in spinal cord neurones," *Nature*, vol. 309, no. 5965, pp. 261–263, 1984.

[126] L. Nowak, P. Bregestovski, and P. Ascher, "Magnesium gates glutamate-activated channels in mouse central neurones," *Nature*, vol. 307, no. 5950, pp. 462–465, 1984.

[127] B. Ault, R. H. Evans, A. A. Francis, D. J. Oakes, and J. C. Watkins, "Selective depression of excitatory amino acid induced depolarizations by magnesium ions in isolated

spinal cord preparations," *Journal of Physiology*, vol. 307, pp. 413–428, 1980.

[128] L. P. Wollmuth, T. Kuner, and B. Sakmann, "Adjacent asparagines in the NR2-subunit of the NMDA receptor channel control the voltage-dependent block by extracellular Mg2+," *Journal of Physiology*, vol. 506, no. 1, pp. 13–32, 1998.

[129] L. Y. Wang and J. F. MacDonald, "Modulation by magnesium of the affinity of NMDA receptors for glycine in murine hippocampal neurones," *Journal of Physiology*, vol. 486, no. 1, pp. 83–95, 1995.

[130] P. Paoletti, J. Neyton, and P. Ascher, "Glycine-independent and subunit-specific potentiation of NMDA responses by extracellular Mg2+," *Neuron*, vol. 15, no. 5, pp. 1109–1120, 1995.

[131] E. Kumamoto, "Neuromodulation by Mg2+ and polyamines of excitatory amino acid currents in rodent neurones in culture," *Magnesium Research*, vol. 9, no. 4, pp. 317–327, 1996.

[132] M. Benveniste and M. L. Mayer, "Multiple effects of spermine on N-methyl-D-aspartic acid receptor responses of rat cultured hippocampal neurones," *Journal of Physiology*, vol. 464, pp. 131–163, 1993.

[133] L. Mony, J. N. C. Kew, M. J. Gunthorpe, and P. Paoletti, "Allosteric modulators of NR2B-containing NMDA receptors: molecular mechanisms and therapeutic potential," *British Journal of Pharmacology*, vol. 157, no. 8, pp. 1301–1317, 2009.

[134] P. Paoletti, A. M. Vergnano, B. Barbour, and M. Casado, "Zinc at glutamatergic synapses," *Neuroscience*, vol. 158, no. 1, pp. 126–136, 2009.

[135] C. J. Frederickson, S. W. Suh, D. Silva, C. J. Frederickson, and R. B. Thompson, "Importance of zinc in the central nervous system: the zinc-containing neuron," *Journal of Nutrition*, vol. 130, no. 5, pp. 1471S–1483S, 2000.

[136] M. L. Mayer, L. Vyklicky, and G. L. Westbrook, "Modulation of excitatory amino acid receptors by group IIB metal cations in cultured mouse hippocampal neurones," *Journal of Physiology*, vol. 415, pp. 329–350, 1989.

[137] G. L. Westbrook and M. L. Mayer, "Micromolar concentrations of Zn2+ antagonize NMDA and GABA responses of hippocampal neurons," *Nature*, vol. 328, no. 6131, pp. 640–643, 1987.

[138] C. W. Christine and D. W. Choi, "Effect of zinc on NMDA receptor-mediated channel currents in cortical neurons," *Journal of Neuroscience*, vol. 10, no. 1, pp. 108–116, 1990.

[139] P. Legendre and G. L. Westbrook, "The inhibition of single N-methyl-D-aspartate-activated channels by zinc ions on cultured rat neurones," *Journal of Physiology*, vol. 429, pp. 429–449, 1990.

[140] P. Paoletti, F. Perin-Dureau, A. Fayyazuddin, A. Le Goff, I. Callebaut, and J. Neyton, "Molecular organization of a zinc binding N-terminal modulatory domain in a NMDA receptor subunit," *Neuron*, vol. 28, no. 3, pp. 911–925, 2000.

[141] G. A. Herin and E. Aizenman, "Amino terminal domain regulation of NMDA receptor function," *European Journal of Pharmacology*, vol. 500, no. 1–3, pp. 101–111, 2004.

[142] P. Paoletti, P. Ascher, and J. Neyton, "High-affinity zinc inhibition of NMDA NR1-NR2A receptors," *Journal of Neuroscience*, vol. 17, no. 15, pp. 5711–5725, 1997.

[143] M. Gielen, A. Le Goff, D. Stroebel, J. W. Johnson, J. Neyton, and P. Paoletti, "Structural rearrangements of NR1/NR2A NMDA receptors during allosteric inhibition," *Neuron*, vol. 57, no. 1, pp. 80–93, 2008.

[144] K. Erreger and S. F. Traynelis, "Zinc inhibition of rat NR1/NR2A N-methyl-d-aspartate receptors," *Journal of Physiology*, vol. 586, no. 3, pp. 763–778, 2008.

[145] J. Rachline, F. Perin-Dureau, A. Le Goff, J. Neyton, and P. Paoletti, "The micromolar zinc-binding domain on the NMDA receptor subunit NR2B," *Journal of Neuroscience*, vol. 25, no. 2, pp. 308–317, 2005.

[146] A. Fayyazuddin, A. Villarroel, A. Le Goff, J. Lerma, and J. Neyton, "Four residues of the extracellular N-terminal domain of the NR2A subunit control high-affinity Zn2+ binding to NMDA receptors," *Neuron*, vol. 25, no. 3, pp. 683–694, 2000.

[147] D. Busselberg, D. Michael, and B. Platt, "Pb2+ reduces voltage- and N-methyl-D-aspartate (NMDA)-activated calcium channel currents," *Cellular and Molecular Neurobiology*, vol. 14, no. 6, pp. 711–722, 1994.

[148] M. Alkondon, A. C. S. Costa, V. Radhakrishnan, R. S. Aronstam, and E. X. Albuquerque, "Selective blockade of NMDA-activated channel currents may be implicated in learning deficits caused by lead," *FEBS Letters*, vol. 261, no. 1, pp. 124–130, 1990.

[149] K. Ishihara, M. Alkondon, J. G. Montes, and E. X. Albuquerque, "Ontogenically related properties of N-methyl-D-aspartate receptors in rat hippocampal neurons and the age-specific sensitivity of developing neurons to lead," *Journal of Pharmacology and Experimental Therapeutics*, vol. 273, no. 3, pp. 1459–1470, 1995.

[150] H. Ujihara and E. X. Albuquerque, "Developmental change of the inhibition by lead of NMDA-activated currents in cultured hippocampal neurons," *Journal of Pharmacology and Experimental Therapeutics*, vol. 263, no. 2, pp. 868–875, 1992.

[151] C. Marchetti, "Molecular targets of lead in brain neurotoxicity," *Neurotoxicity Research*, vol. 5, no. 3, pp. 221–235, 2003.

[152] T. R. Guilarte and R. C. Miceli, "Age-dependent effects of lead on [3H]MK-801 binding to the NMDA receptor-gated ionophore: In vitro and in vivo studies," *Neuroscience Letters*, vol. 148, no. 1-2, pp. 27–30, 1992.

[153] T. R. Guilarte, "Pb2+ inhibits NMDA receptor function at high and low affinity sites: developmental and regional brain expression," *NeuroToxicology*, vol. 18, no. 1, pp. 43–52, 1997.

[154] T. R. Guilarte, R. C. Miceli, and D. A. Jett, "Biochemical evidence of an interaction of lead at the zinc allosteric sites of the NMDA receptor complex: effects of neuronal development," *NeuroToxicology*, vol. 16, no. 1, pp. 63–71, 1995.

[155] D. P. Alfano and T. L. Petit, "Neonatal lead exposure alters the dendritic development of hippocampal dentate granule cells," *Experimental Neurology*, vol. 75, no. 2, pp. 275–288, 1982.

[156] T. L. Petit, D. P. Alfano, and J. C. LeBoutillier, "Early lead exposure and the hippocampus: a review and recent advances," *NeuroToxicology*, vol. 4, no. 1, pp. 79–94, 1983.

[157] I. A. Omelchenko, C. S. Nelson, J. L. Marino, and C. N. Allen, "The sensitivity of N-methyl-D-aspartate receptors to lead inhibition is dependent on the receptor subunit composition," *Journal of Pharmacology and Experimental Therapeutics*, vol. 278, no. 1, pp. 15–20, 1996.

[158] Y. Yamada, H. Ujihara, H. Sada, and T. Ban, "Pb2+ reduces the current from NMDA receptors expressed in Xenopus oocytes," *FEBS Letters*, vol. 377, no. 3, pp. 390–392, 1995.

[159] I. A. Omelchenko, C. S. Nelson, and C. N. Allen, "Lead inhibition of N-methyl-D-aspartate receptors containing NR2A, NR2C and NR2D subunits," *Journal of Pharmacology*

and Experimental Therapeutics, vol. 282, no. 3, pp. 1458–1464, 1997.

[160] S. M. Lasley and M. E. Gilbert, "Lead inhibits the rat N-methyl-D-aspartate receptor channel by binding to a site distinct from the zinc allosteric site," *Toxicology and Applied Pharmacology*, vol. 159, no. 3, pp. 224–233, 1999.

[161] T. R. Guilarte, R. C. Miceli, and D. A. Jett, "Neurochemical aspects of hippocampal and cortical Pb2+ neurotoxicity," *NeuroToxicology*, vol. 15, no. 3, pp. 459–466, 1994.

[162] S. Schulte, W. E. Muller, and K. D. Friedberg, "In vitro and in vivo effects of lead on specific 3H-MK-801 binding to NMDA-receptors in the brain of mice," *NeuroToxicology*, vol. 16, no. 2, pp. 309–318, 1995.

[163] C. Marchetti and P. Gavazzo, "Subunit-dependent effects of nickel on NMDA receptor channels," *Molecular Brain Research*, vol. 117, no. 2, pp. 139–144, 2003.

[164] C. M. Low, F. Zheng, P. Lyuboslavsky, and S. F. Traynelis, "Molecular determinants of coordinated proton and zinc inhibition of N-methyl-D-aspartate NR1/NR2A receptors," *Proceedings of the National Academy of Sciences of the United States of America*, vol. 97, no. 20, pp. 11062–11067, 2000.

[165] Y. H. Hung, A. I. Bush, and R. A. Cherny, "Copper in the brain and Alzheimer's disease," *Journal of Biological Inorganic Chemistry*, vol. 15, no. 1, pp. 61–76, 2010.

[166] A. I. Bush and R. E. Tanzi, "Therapeutics for Alzheimer's disease based on the metal hypothesis," *Neurotherapeutics*, vol. 5, no. 3, pp. 421–432, 2008.

[167] A. Barnea, D. E. Hartter, G. Cho, K. R. Bhasker, B. M. Katz, and M. D. Edwards, "Further characterization of the process of in vitro uptake of radiolabeled copper by the rat brain," *Journal of Inorganic Biochemistry*, vol. 40, no. 2, pp. 103–110, 1990.

[168] J. Kardos, I. Kovacs, F. Hajos, M. Kalman, and M. Simonyi, "Nerve endings from rat brain tissue release copper upon depolarization. A possible role in regulating neuronal excitability," *Neuroscience Letters*, vol. 103, no. 2, pp. 139–144, 1989.

[169] A. Hopt, S. Korte, H. Fink et al., "Methods for studying synaptosomal copper release," *Journal of Neuroscience Methods*, vol. 128, no. 1-2, pp. 159–172, 2003.

[170] D. E. Hartter and A. Barnea, "Evidence for release of copper in the brain: depolarization-induced release of newly taken-up 67copper," *Synapse*, vol. 2, no. 4, pp. 412–415, 1988.

[171] P. Y. Wong and K. Fritze, "Determination by neutron activation of copper, manganese, and zinc in the pineal body and other areas of brain tissue," *Journal of Neurochemistry*, vol. 16, no. 8, pp. 1231–1234, 1969.

[172] J. Donaldson, T. S. Pierre, J. L. Minnich, and A. Barbeau, "Determination of Na+, K+, Mg2+, Cu2+, Zn2+ , and Mn2+ in rat brain regions," *Canadian Journal of Biochemistry*, vol. 51, no. 1, pp. 87–92, 1973.

[173] T. Weiser and M. Wienrich, "The effects of copper ions on glutamate receptors in cultured rat cortical neurons," *Brain Research*, vol. 742, no. 1-2, pp. 211–218, 1996.

[174] V. Vlachová, "Copper modulation of NMDA responses in mouse and rat cultured hippocampal neurons," *European Journal of Neuroscience*, vol. 8, no. 11, pp. 2257–2264, 1996.

[175] N. A. Larsen, H. Pakkenberg, E. Damsgaard, and K. Heydorn, "Topographical distribution of arsenic, manganese, and selenium in the normal human brain," *Journal of Neurosurgical Sciences*, vol. 42, no. 3, pp. 407–416, 1979.

[176] M. L. Mayer and G. L. Westbrook, "Permeation and block of N-methyl-D-aspartic acid receptor channels by divalent cations in mouse cultured central neurones," *Journal of Physiology*, vol. 394, pp. 501–527, 1987.

[177] T. R. Guilarte and M. K. Chen, "Manganese inhibits NMDA receptor channel function: implications to psychiatric and cognitive effects," *NeuroToxicology*, vol. 28, no. 6, pp. 1147–1152, 2007.

[178] H. Hashemzadeh-Gargari and T. R. Guilarte, "Divalent cations modulate N-methyl-D-aspartate receptor function at the glycine site," *Journal of Pharmacology and Experimental Therapeutics*, vol. 290, no. 3, pp. 1356–1362, 1999.

[179] Y. Gu and L. Y. M. Huang, "Modulation of glycine affinity for NMDA receptors by extracellular Ca2+ in trigeminal neurons," *Journal of Neuroscience*, vol. 14, no. 7, pp. 4561–4570, 1994.

[180] M. Marchioro, K. L. Swanson, Y. Aracava, and E. X. Albuquerque, "Glycine- and calcium-dependent effects of lead on N-methyl-D-aspartate receptor function in rat hippocampal neurons," *Journal of Pharmacology and Experimental Therapeutics*, vol. 279, no. 1, pp. 143–153, 1996.

[181] M. Hollmann and S. Heinemann, "Cloned glutamate receptors," *Annual Review of Neuroscience*, vol. 17, pp. 31–108, 1994.

[182] S. R. Platt, "The role of glutamate in central nervous system health and disease—a review," *Veterinary Journal*, vol. 173, no. 2, pp. 278–286, 2007.

[183] R. M. Pruss, R. L. Akeson, M. M. Racke, and J. L. Wilburn, "Agonist-activated cobalt uptake identifies divalent cation-permeable kainate receptors on neurons and glial cells," *Neuron*, vol. 7, no. 3, pp. 509–518, 1991.

[184] M. Iino, S. Ozawa, and K. Tsuzuki, "Permeation of calcium through excitatory amino acid receptor channels in cultured rat hippocampal neurones," *Journal of Physiology*, vol. 424, pp. 151–165, 1990.

[185] B. S. Meldrum, "Glutamate as a neurotransmitter in the brain: review of physiology and pathology," *Journal of Nutrition*, vol. 130, no. 4, pp. 1007S–1015S, 2000.

[186] S. L. Buldakova, K. V. Bolshakov, D. B. Tikhonov, and L. G. Magazanik, "Ca2+-dependent desensitization of AMPA receptors," *NeuroReport*, vol. 11, no. 13, pp. 2937–2941, 2000.

[187] F. A. Rassendren, P. Lory, J. P. Pin, and J. Nargeot, "Zinc has opposite effects on NMDA and non-NMDA receptors expressed in Xenopus oocytes," *Neuron*, vol. 4, no. 5, pp. 733–740, 1990.

[188] J. C. Dreixler and J. P. Leonard, "Subunit-specific enhancement of glutamate receptor responses by zinc," *Molecular Brain Research*, vol. 22, no. 1–4, pp. 144–150, 1994.

[189] J. C. Dreixler and J. P. Leonard, "Effects of external calcium on zinc modulation of AMPA receptors," *Brain Research*, vol. 752, no. 1-2, pp. 170–174, 1997.

[190] N. A. Dorofeeva, D. B. Tikhonov, O. I. Barygin, T. B. Tikhonova, Y. I. Salnikov, and L. Magazanik, "Action of extracellular divalent cations on native α-amino-3-hydroxy-5-methylisoxazole-4-propionate (AMPA) receptors," *Journal of Neurochemistry*, vol. 95, no. 6, pp. 1704–1712, 2005.

[191] W. J. Zhu, J. F. Wang, L. Corsi, and S. Vicini, "Lanthanum-mediated modification of GABA(A) receptor deactivation, desensitization and inhibitory synaptic currents in rat cerebellar neurons," *Journal of Physiology*, vol. 511, no. 3, pp. 647–661, 1998.

[192] R. W. Olsen and A. J. Tobin, "Molecular biology of GABA(A) receptors," *FASEB Journal*, vol. 4, no. 5, pp. 1469–1480, 1990.

[193] R. D. Schwartz, "The GABA(A) receptor-gated ion channel: biochemical and pharmacological studies of structure and

function," *Biochemical Pharmacology*, vol. 37, no. 18, pp. 3369–3375, 1988.

[194] W. Sieghart, "Structure and pharmacology of γ-aminobutyric acid(A) receptor subtypes," *Pharmacological Reviews*, vol. 47, no. 2, pp. 181–234, 1995.

[195] J. Y. Ma and T. Narahashi, "Differential modulation of GABA(A) receptor-channel complex by polyvalent cations in rat dorsal root ganglion neurons," *Brain Research*, vol. 607, no. 1-2, pp. 222–232, 1993.

[196] A. Barberis, E. Cherubini, and J. W. Mozrzymas, "Zinc inhibits miniature GABAergic currents by allosteric modulation of GABA(A) receptor gating," *Journal of Neuroscience*, vol. 20, no. 23, pp. 8618–8627, 2000.

[197] E. H. Buhl, T. S. Otis, and I. Mody, "Zinc-induced collapse of augmented inhibition by GABA in a temporal lobe epilepsy model," *Science*, vol. 271, no. 5247, pp. 369–373, 1996.

[198] P. Legendre and G. L. Westbrook, "Noncompetitive inhibition of γ-aminobutyric acid(A) channels by Zn," *Molecular Pharmacology*, vol. 39, no. 3, pp. 267–274, 1991.

[199] T. G. Smart, "A novel modulatory binding site for zinc on the GABA(A) receptor complex in cultured rat neurones," *Journal of Physiology*, vol. 447, pp. 587–625, 1992.

[200] G. Kilic, O. Moran, and E. Cherubini, "Currents activated by GABA and their modulation by Zn2+ in cerebellar granule cells in culture," *European Journal of Neuroscience*, vol. 5, no. 1, pp. 65–72, 1993.

[201] W. Sieghart, "GABA(A) receptors: ligand-gated Cl- ion channels modulated by multiple drug-binding sites," *Trends in Pharmacological Sciences*, vol. 13, no. 12, pp. 446–450, 1992.

[202] A. Draguhn, T. A. Verdorn, M. Ewert, P. H. Seeburg, and B. Sakmann, "Functional and molecular distinction between recombinant rat GABA(A) receptor subtypes by Zn2+," *Neuron*, vol. 5, no. 6, pp. 781–788, 1990.

[203] N. C. Saxena and R. L. Macdonald, "Assembly of GABA(A) receptor subunits: role of the δ subunit," *Journal of Neuroscience*, vol. 14, no. 11, pp. 7077–7086, 1994.

[204] J. L. Fisher and R. L. Macdonald, "The role of an α subtype M2-M3 his in regulating inhibition of GABA(A) receptor current by zinc and other divalent cations," *Journal of Neuroscience*, vol. 18, no. 8, pp. 2944–2953, 1998.

[205] N. C. Saxena and R. L. Macdonald, "Properties of putative cerebellar γ-aminobutyric acidA receptor isoforms," *Molecular Pharmacology*, vol. 49, no. 3, pp. 567–579, 1996.

[206] F. Knoflach, D. Benke, Y. Wang et al., "Pharmacological modulation of the diazepam-insensitive recombinant γ-aminobutyric acid(A) receptors $\alpha4\beta2\gamma2$ and $\alpha6\beta2\gamma2$," *Molecular Pharmacology*, vol. 50, no. 5, pp. 1253–1261, 1996.

[207] G. White and D. A. Gurley, "α subunits influence Zn block of γ2 containing GABA(A) receptor currents," *NeuroReport*, vol. 6, no. 3, pp. 461–464, 1995.

[208] S. J. Moss and T. G. Smart, "Constructing inhibitory synapses," *Nature Reviews Neuroscience*, vol. 2, no. 4, pp. 240–250, 2001.

[209] I. N. Sharonova, V. S. Vorobjev, and H. L. Haas, "High-affinity copper block of GABAA receptor-mediated currents in acutely isolated cerebellar Purkinje cells of the rat," *European Journal of Neuroscience*, vol. 10, no. 2, pp. 522–528, 1998.

[210] P. Q. Trombley and G. M. Shepherd, "Differential modulation by zinc and copper of amino acid receptors from rat olfactory bulb neurons," *Journal of Neurophysiology*, vol. 76, no. 4, pp. 2536–2546, 1996.

[211] B. Barilà, A. Cupello, and M. Robello, "Modulation by lanthanum ions of γ-aminobutyric acidA receptors of rat cerebellum granule cells in culture: clues on their subunit composition," *Neuroscience Letters*, vol. 298, no. 1, pp. 13–16, 2001.

[212] A. A. Boldyreva, "Lanthanum potentiates GABA-activated currents in rat pyramidal neurons of CA1 hippocampal field," *Bulletin of Experimental Biology and Medicine*, vol. 140, no. 4, pp. 403–405, 2005.

[213] N. C. Saxena, T. R. Neelands, and R. L. Macdonald, "Contrasting actions of lanthanum on different recombinant γ-aminobutyric acid receptor isoforms expressed in l929 fibroblasts," *Molecular Pharmacology*, vol. 51, no. 2, pp. 328–335, 1997.

[214] O. Arakawa, M. Nakahiro, and T. Narahashi, "Mercury modulation of GABA-activated chloride channels and non-specific cation channels in rat dorsal root ganglion neurons," *Brain Research*, vol. 551, no. 1-2, pp. 58–63, 1991.

[215] K. Krüger, V. Diepgrond, M. Ahnefeld et al., "Blockade of glutamatergic and GABAergic receptor channels by trimethyltin chloride," *British Journal of Pharmacology*, vol. 144, no. 2, pp. 283–292, 2005.

[216] G. A. Wasserman, X. Liu, F. Parvez et al., "Water arsenic exposure and children's intellectual function in Araihazar, Bangladesh," *Environmental Health Perspectives*, vol. 112, no. 13, pp. 1329–1333, 2004.

[217] J. Calderón, M. E. Navarro, M. E. Jimenez-Capdeville et al., "Exposure to arsenic and lead and neuropsychological development in Mexican children," *Environmental Research*, vol. 85, no. 2, pp. 69–76, 2001.

[218] S. G. Gilbert and B. Weiss, "A rationale for lowering the blood lead action level from 10 to 2 μg/dL," *NeuroToxicology*, vol. 27, no. 5, pp. 693–701, 2006.

[219] M. M. Téllez-Rojo, D. C. Bellinger, C. Arroyo-Quiroz et al., "Longitudinal associations between blood lead concentrations lower than 10 μg/dL and neurobehavioral development in environmentally exposed children in Mexico City," *Pediatrics*, vol. 118, no. 2, pp. e323–e330, 2006.

[220] D. O. Carpenter, "Effects of metals on the nervous system of humans and animals," *International Journal of Occupational Medicine and Environmental Health*, vol. 14, no. 3, pp. 209–218, 2001.

[221] B. Platt, D. O. Carpenter, D. Busselberg, K. G. Reymann, and G. Riedel, "Aluminum impairs hippocampal long-term potentiation in rats in vitro and in vivo," *Experimental Neurology*, vol. 134, no. 1, pp. 73–86, 1995.

[222] J. Chen, M. Wang, D. Ruan, and J. She, "Early chronic aluminium exposure impairs long-term potentiation and depression to the rat dentate gyrus in vivo," *Neuroscience*, vol. 112, no. 4, pp. 879–887, 2002.

[223] S. S. Ahmed and W. Santosh, "Metallomic profiling and linkage map analysis of early Parkinson's disease: a new insight to aluminum marker for the possible diagnosis," *PloS One*, vol. 5, no. 6, Article ID e11252, 2010.

[224] C. R. Raymond, "LTP forms 1, 2 and 3: different mechanisms for the 'long' in long-term potentiation," *Trends in Neurosciences*, vol. 30, no. 4, pp. 167–175, 2007.

[225] K. G. Reymann and J. U. Frey, "The late maintenance of hippocampal LTP: requirements, phases, 'synaptic tagging', 'late-associativity' and implications," *Neuropharmacology*, vol. 52, no. 1, pp. 24–40, 2007.

[226] Z. Xia and D. R. Storm, "The role of calmodulin as a signal integrator for synaptic plasticity," *Nature Reviews Neuroscience*, vol. 6, no. 4, pp. 267–276, 2005.

[227] E. Miyamoto, "Molecular mechanism of neuronal plasticity: induction and maintenance of long-term potentiation in the hippocampus," *Journal of Pharmacological Sciences*, vol. 100, no. 5, pp. 433–442, 2006.

[228] Y. Izumi, K. Tokuda, and C. F. Zorumski, "Long-term potentiation inhibition by low-level N-methyl-D-aspartate receptor activation involves calcineurin, nitric oxide, and p38 mitogen-activated protein kinase," *Hippocampus*, vol. 18, no. 3, pp. 258–265, 2008.

[229] G. M. Thomas and R. L. Huganir, "MAPK cascade signalling and synaptic plasticity," *Nature Reviews Neuroscience*, vol. 5, no. 3, pp. 173–183, 2004.

[230] L. Prichard, J. C. Deloulme, and D. R. Storm, "Interactions between neurogranin and calmodulin in vivo," *Journal of Biological Chemistry*, vol. 274, no. 12, pp. 7689–7694, 1999.

[231] J. Baudier, J. C. Deloulme, A. Van Dorsselaer, D. Black, and H. W. D. Matthes, "Purification and characterization of a brain-specific protein kinase C substrate, neurogranin (p17). Identification of a consensus amino acid sequence between neurogranin and neuromodulin (GAP43) that corresponds to the protein kinase C phosphorylation site and the calmodulin-binding domain," *Journal of Biological Chemistry*, vol. 266, no. 1, pp. 229–237, 1991.

[232] E. Habermann, K. Crowell, and P. Janicki, "Lead and other metals can substitute for Ca2+ in calmodulin," *Archives of Toxicology*, vol. 54, no. 1, pp. 61–70, 1983.

[233] G. M. J. Ramakers, P. Pasinelli, J. J. H. Hens, W. H. Gispen, and P. N. E. De Graan, "Protein kinase C in synaptic plasticity: changes in the in situ phosphorylation state of identified pre- and postsynaptic substrates," *Progress in Neuro-Psychopharmacology and Biological Psychiatry*, vol. 21, no. 3, pp. 455–486, 1997.

[234] J. D. Cremin Jr. and D. R. Smith, "In vitro vs in vivo Pb effects on brain protein kinase C activity," *Environmental Research*, vol. 90, no. 3, pp. 191–199, 2002.

[235] S. J. R. Lee, Y. Escobedo-Lozoya, E. M. Szatmari, and R. Yasuda, "Activation of CaMKII in single dendritic spines during long-term potentiation," *Nature*, vol. 458, no. 7236, pp. 299–304, 2009.

[236] R. V. Omkumar, M. J. Kiely, A. J. Rosenstein, K. T. Min, and M. B. Kennedy, "Identification of a phosphorylation site for calcium/calmodulin- dependent protein kinase II in the NR2B subunit of the N-methyl-D-aspartate receptor," *Journal of Biological Chemistry*, vol. 271, no. 49, pp. 31670–31678, 1996.

[237] R. C. Malenka and R. A. Nicoll, "Long-term potentiation—a decade of progress?" *Science*, vol. 285, no. 5435, pp. 1870–1874, 1999.

[238] K. A. Anderson and C. D. Kane, "Ca2+/calmodulin-dependent protein kinase IV and calcium signaling," *BioMetals*, vol. 11, no. 4, pp. 331–343, 1998.

[239] B. Mayer, M. John, B. Heinzel et al., "Brain nitric oxide synthase is a biopterin- and flavin-containing multi-functional oxido-reductase," *FEBS Letters*, vol. 288, no. 1-2, pp. 187–191, 1991.

[240] M. J. Lohse, U. Forstermann, and H. H. H. W. Schmidt, "Pharmacology of NO: cGMP signal transduction," *Naunyn-Schmiedeberg's Archives of Pharmacology*, vol. 358, no. 1, pp. 111–112, 1998.

[241] H. Prast and A. Philippu, "Nitric oxide as modulator of neuronal function," *Progress in Neurobiology*, vol. 64, no. 1, pp. 51–68, 2001.

[242] Y. F. Lu, E. R. Kandel, and R. D. Hawkins, "Nitric oxide signaling contributes to late-phase LTP and CREB phosphorylation in the hippocampus," *Journal of Neuroscience*, vol. 19, no. 23, pp. 10250–10261, 1999.

[243] Y. Keshet and R. Seger, "The MAP kinase signaling cascades: a system of hundreds of components regulates a diverse array of physiological functions," *Methods in Molecular Biology*, vol. 661, pp. 3–38, 2010.

[244] C. D. Toscano, J. L. McGlothan, and T. R. Guilarte, "Lead exposure alters cyclic-AMP response element binding protein phosphorylation and binding activity in the developing rat brain," *Developmental Brain Research*, vol. 145, no. 2, pp. 219–228, 2003.

[245] B. E. Lonze and D. D. Ginty, "Function and regulation of CREB family transcription factors in the nervous system," *Neuron*, vol. 35, no. 4, pp. 605–623, 2002.

[246] J. C. Chrivia, R. P. S. Kwok, N. Lamb, M. Hagiwara, M. R. Montminy, and R. H. Goodman, "Phosphorylated CREB binds specifically to the nuclear protein CBP," *Nature*, vol. 365, no. 6449, pp. 855–859, 1993.

[247] K. Deisseroth, H. Bito, and R. W. Tsien, "Signaling from synapse to nucleus: postsynaptic CREB phosphorylation during multiple forms of hippocampal synaptic plasticity," *Neuron*, vol. 16, no. 1, pp. 89–101, 1996.

[248] G. E. Hardingham and H. Bading, "The Yin and Yang of NMDA receptor signalling," *Trends in Neurosciences*, vol. 26, no. 2, pp. 81–89, 2003.

[249] M. R. Montminy and L. M. Bilezikjian, "Binding of a nuclear protein to the cyclic-AMP response element of the somatostatin gene," *Nature*, vol. 328, no. 6126, pp. 175–178, 1987.

[250] A. J. Silva, J. H. Kogan, P. W. Frankland, and S. Kida, "CREB and memory," *Annual Review of Neuroscience*, vol. 21, pp. 127–148, 1998.

[251] V. Y. Bolshakov, L. Carboni, M. H. Cobb, S. A. Siegelbaum, and F. Belardetti, "Dual MAP kinase pathways mediate opposing forms of long-term plasticity at CA3-CA1 synapses," *Nature Neuroscience*, vol. 3, no. 11, pp. 1107–1112, 2000.

[252] L. G. Costa, M. Aschner, A. Vitalone, T. Syversen, and O. P. Soldin, "Developmental neuropathology of environmental agents," *Annual Review of Pharmacology and Toxicology*, vol. 44, pp. 87–110, 2004.

[253] S. Cull-Candy, S. Brickley, and M. Farrant, "NMDA receptor subunits: diversity, development and disease," *Current Opinion in Neurobiology*, vol. 11, no. 3, pp. 327–335, 2001.

[254] Y. Z. Xu, D. Y. Ruan, Y. Wu et al., "Nitric oxide affects LTP in area CA1 and CA3 of hippocampus in low-level lead-exposed rat," *Neurotoxicology and Teratology*, vol. 20, no. 1, pp. 69–73, 1998.

[255] L. Altmann, F. Weinsberg, K. Sveinsson, H. Lilienthal, H. Wiegand, and G. Winneke, "Impairment of long-term potentiation and learning following chronic lead exposure," *Toxicology Letters*, vol. 66, no. 1, pp. 105–112, 1993.

[256] J. Zhong, D. P. Carrozza, K. Williams, D. B. Pritchett, and P. B. Molinoff, "Expression of mRNAs encoding subunits of the NMDA receptor in developing rat brain," *Journal of Neurochemistry*, vol. 64, no. 2, pp. 531–539, 1995.

[257] L. R.F. Faro, R. Durán, J. L.M. Do Nascimento, M. Alfonso, and C. W. Picanço-Diniz, "Effects of methyl mercury on the in vivo release of dopamine and its acidic metabolites DOPAC and HVA from striatum of rats," *Ecotoxicology and Environmental Safety*, vol. 38, no. 2, pp. 95–98, 1997.

[258] M. Stýblo, Z. Drobná, I. Jaspers, S. Lin, and D. J. Thomas, "The role of biomethylation in toxicity and carcinogenicity

of arsenic: a research update," *Environmental Health Perspectives*, vol. 110, supplement 5, pp. 767–771, 2002.
[259] J. S. Thayer, "Biological methylation of less-studied elements," *Applied Organometallic Chemistry*, vol. 16, no. 12, pp. 677–691, 2002.
[260] B. Platt and D. Busselberg, "Combined actions of Pb2+, Zn2+, and Al3+ on voltage-activated calcium channel currents," *Cellular and Molecular Neurobiology*, vol. 14, no. 6, pp. 831–840, 1994.
[261] M. Vigeh, K. Yokoyama, Z. Seyedaghamiri et al., "Blood lead at currently acceptable levels may cause preterm labour," *Occupational and Environmental Medicine*, vol. 68, no. 3, pp. 231–234, 2011.

4

Nervous System of *Periplaneta americana* Cockroach as a Model in Toxinological Studies: A Short Historical and Actual View

Maria Stankiewicz,[1] Marcin Dąbrowski,[1] and Maria Elena de Lima[2]

[1] *Biophysics Laboratory, Institute of General and Molecular Biology, N. Copernicus University, 87-100 Torun, Poland*
[2] *Departamento de Bioquímica e Imunologia, Instituto de Ciências Biológicas, Universidade Federal de Minas Gerais, Belo Horizonte, 31270-901 MG, Brazil*

Correspondence should be addressed to Maria Stankiewicz, stankiew@umk.pl

Academic Editor: Yonghua Ji

Nervous system of *Periplaneta americana* cockroach is used in a wide range of pharmacological studies, including electrophysiological techniques. This paper presents its role as a preparation in the development of toxinological studies in the following electrophysiological methods: double-oil-gap technique on isolated giant axon, patch-clamp on DUM (dorsal unpaired median) neurons, microelectrode technique *in situ* conditions on axon in connective and DUM neurons in ganglion, and single-fiber oil-gap technique on last abdominal ganglion synapse. At the end the application of cockroach synaptosomal preparation is mentioned.

1. Introduction

The cockroach, especially the *Periplaneta americana* species, is recognized as a very useful model in neurobiological studies [1]. The field of toxinology owes much to the use of various nervous preparations obtained from this insect. *Periplaneta americana* represents an excellent model applied in different pharmacological methods, especially in electrophysiology, which plays a vital part in most of research activity in toxinology. It may be based on using natural and "artificial" preparations, as for example the transfected *Xenopus* oocytes. A wide range of nervous functions have been described on the basis of studies on various parts of cockroach nervous system (Figure 1(a)) and the experiments can be performed on natural models. Biophysical principles of the nervous system function in insects are much the same as in mammals. In both groups of animals similar neurotransmitters can be found, although their distribution varies. Thus the observations made on the cockroach can nearly be applied in vertebrates. On the other hand, some arthropod neurotoxins show high selectivity to insect nervous system and they are considered as potent bioinsecticides. Cockroach model has been largely used for the description of their mode of action. In the following paragraphs, various electrophysiological methods using cockroach preparations will be presented, along with their contribution to the development of toxinology.

2. Giant Axon and Single-Fiber Double-Oil-Gap Method

Cell body and the dendritic tree of the *P. americana* giant interneurons, located in the last abdominal ganglion, have been well identified for a long time. They possess unmyelinated, very long (1.5–2 cm), large diameter (up to 50 μm) axons. The axons, being surrounded by glial Schwann cells, can be isolated manually (Figure 1(b)) under microscope, and their activity can be observed using the double-oil-gap method—a refined electrophysiological technique—Figure 2(a) [2–5]. Such axonal preparation exhibits simple bioelectrical properties; one type of voltage-dependent sodium and potassium (Kdr) channels can be found; they are responsible for generating short (0.5 ms) action potentials. Double-oil-gap technique permits, in current-clamp, to evoke large (up to 100 mV) axonal action potentials (Figure 2(b)(A)), to follow their evolution and to control the resting potential as well as the level of local response. Passive characteristics

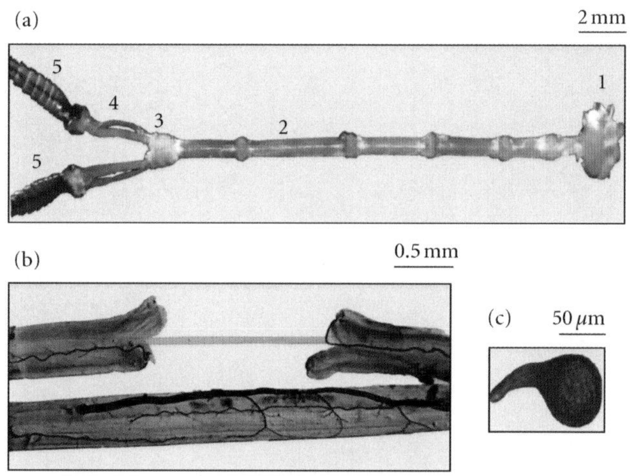

FIGURE 1: Cockroach (*Periplaneta americana*) nervous system. (a) Isolated abdominal nerve cord with last thoracic (1) ganglion and cercal nerves (4) linked to cerci (5). Giant axon is isolated from one connective between the 4th and the 5th ganglion (2). DUM neurons and cercal nerve-giant interneuron synapses are located in last abdominal ganglion (3). (b) Isolated giant axon dissected from one connective, accompanied by the second connective which protects the axon when the preparation is transferred to experimental chamber; axon diameter ~50 μm. (c) Isolated DUM neuron.

of axonal membrane (resistance and capacitance) can be analyzed using longer (e.g., 5 ms) hyperpolarizing pulses (Figure 2(b)(B)); the application of long depolarizing pulses allows to observe delayed rectification (Figure 2(b)(B)).

In voltage-clamp configuration, depolarizing voltage pulses induce a short, inwardly directed, tetrodotoxin-sensitive sodium current and delayed, noninactivating outward potassium current (Figure 2(d)), most sensitive to 3,4 diaminopyridine′ [6]; hyperpolarizing pulses are used to record the leak current. At holding potential of −60 mV, about 50% of sodium current is inactivated; this inactivation is completely removed when the HP reaches −80 mV and, in these conditions, a larger current can be observed, similarly to what has been reported by Pichon [2] (Figure 2(e)). Double-oil-gap method has several advantages: (1) the recordings are stable and long-lasting (up to 1 hour), (2) various experimental protocols in current-clamp as well in voltage-clamp can be applied, (3) the quantity of the tested molecules can be very small (e.g., 0.2 mL 10^{-7} M in the case of a highly active substance), (4) it is inexpensive. However, the preparation of an isolated axon is a sophisticated procedure and requires much experience.

The activity of giant axon can also be recorded in *in situ* conditions in the whole nerve cord [7]. In such case, axon is left on its place in nervous chain, stays in contact with others axons and its microenvironment is much less changed compared to isolated axon. After one connective is desheathed, the giant axons become accessible for microelectrodes. Introducing them allows to record the exact axonal resting potential in its *semi*-physiological microenvironment. Extracellular stimulation, even performed from some mm distance, evokes action potentials similar in size and amplitude to action potential recorded from the isolated axon (Figure 2(c)), however, long-pulse stimulation can only accelerate the generation of action potential. The accessibility of the axon *in situ* to the tested molecules is much more limited, however, their effect can be considered more physiological in such conditions.

Double-oil-gap method has been used in toxinological studies for many years. The long history of anti-insect scorpion toxins started with this technique, when in the 1970–80s the toxins purified from North African scorpions (*Androctonus australis* Hector—AaH IT and *Buthus judaicus*—Bj IT) by Professor Eliahu Zlotkin and collaborators from the Hebrew University of Jerusalem, Israel, and Faculté de Médecine, Marseille, France [8], were tested for the first time on cockroach isolated giant axon by electrophysiologist Professor Marcel Pelhate, at Angers University, France [9, 10]. Toxicity tests and biochemical studies, especially by means of binding assays, established the specificity of this toxin, which has been confirmed by electrophysiological experiments. In the subsequent years, the story developed with the application of more and more modern methods and presently many details of arthropod toxins' selectivity to insects are known [11–13]. Their applicability as bioinsecticides is now under consideration [12, 14, 15].

Scorpion toxins, active on sodium channels, are divided into two large groups: *alpha* and *beta* toxins, modifying mainly the channels' inactivation and activation, respectively [12, 13, 16, 17]. Among *alpha* toxins, an *alpha*-like subgroup has been established [18, 19]. The insect-selective toxins, depressant and excitatory, are *beta* toxins. Several toxins related to these groups were tested and their mode of action was determined using the single-fiber oil-gap method. It helped to discriminate between excitatory and depressant groups of toxins. The most distinctive features of axonal bioelectric activity modification induced by excitatory toxins (AaH IT1 from *Androctonus australis* Hector, Bj IT1 from *Buthotus judaicus*—[9, 10, 20]; Bm 32-VI and Bm 33-I from *Buthus martensi*—[21]; are a slight depolarization, a decrease in threshold for action potential generation (Figure 3(a)(A) and (B)), and the repetitive activity instead of a single

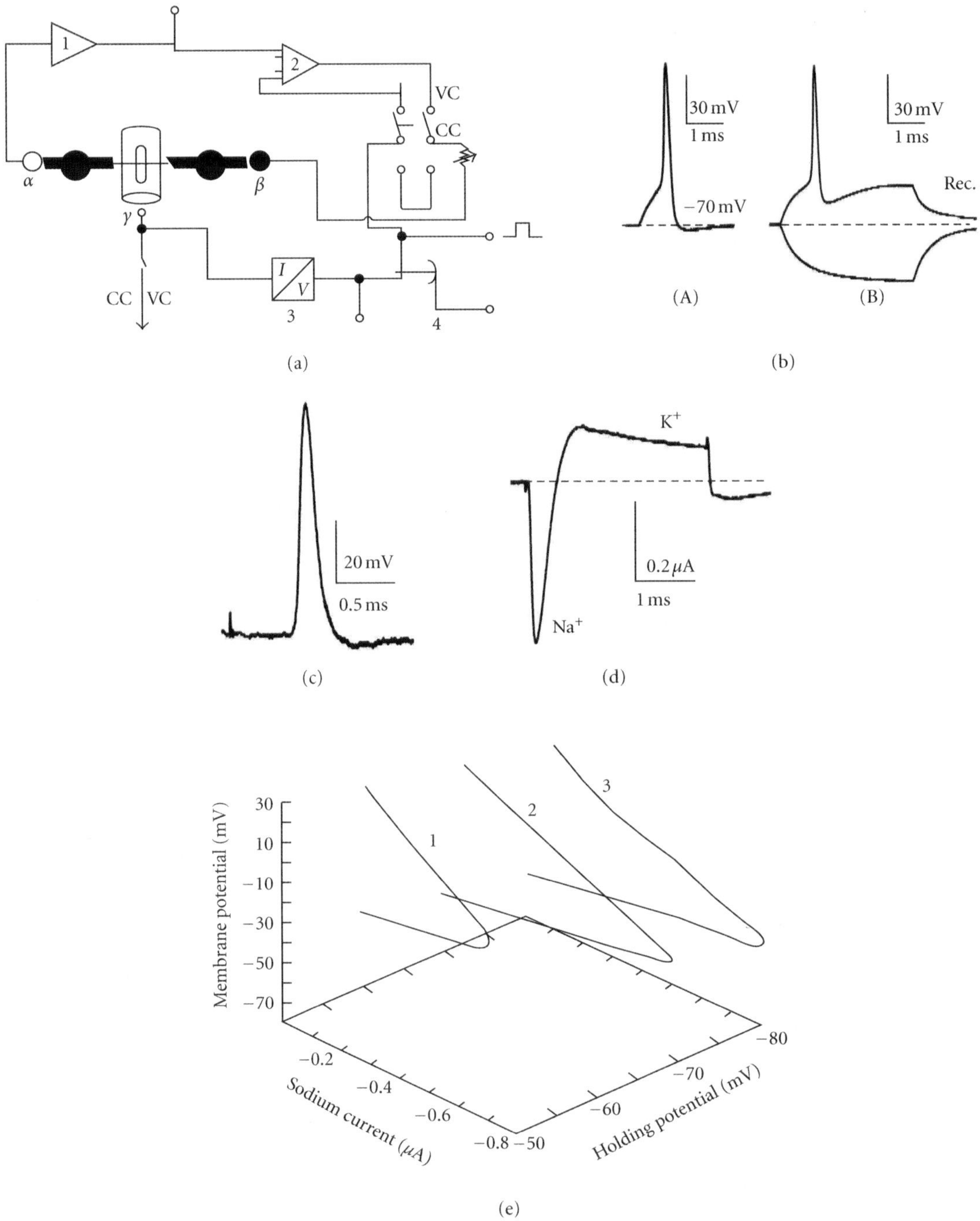

FIGURE 2: Single-fiber double-oil-gap method on isolated giant axon. (a) Electronic arrangement of technique for current- and voltage-clamp recordings (CC and VC, resp.)—according to [4]. α and β are the lateral (recording and stimulating) electrodes immersed in 180 mM KCl—they have contact with the cut ends of axons in connective and represent intracellular electrodes; γ electrode is plunged in physiological saline (with the tested substances)—it has contact with the extracellular side of the isolated axon. Amplifier 1 is a high-input impedance, negative capacitance amplifier, 2—high-gain differential amplifier, 3—current-to-voltage converter; 4—analogue compensator for leakage and fast and slow capacitive currents. In CC γ electrode is grounded and resistor = 3 MΩ. (b)(A) Action potential evoked by a 0.5 ms depolarizing current pulse. (b)(B) The effect of long symmetrical current pulses: the hyperpolarizing one—used to estimate the passive axonal membrane properties and the depolarizing one—used to observe the membrane rectification (Rec.). (c) Action potential recorded from *in situ* giant axon using microelectrode. (d) Total current recorded under voltage pulse from holding potential −70 mV to −10 mV; K^+—potassium component, Na^+—sodium component. (e) Voltage-dependence of sodium current recorded at various holding potentials: −1 : −60, 2 : −70 and 3 : −80 mV. The points (not shown) for curves are mean values from 5 experiments performed in control conditions. Note that at holding potential of −60 mV, about 50% of Na current is inactivated.

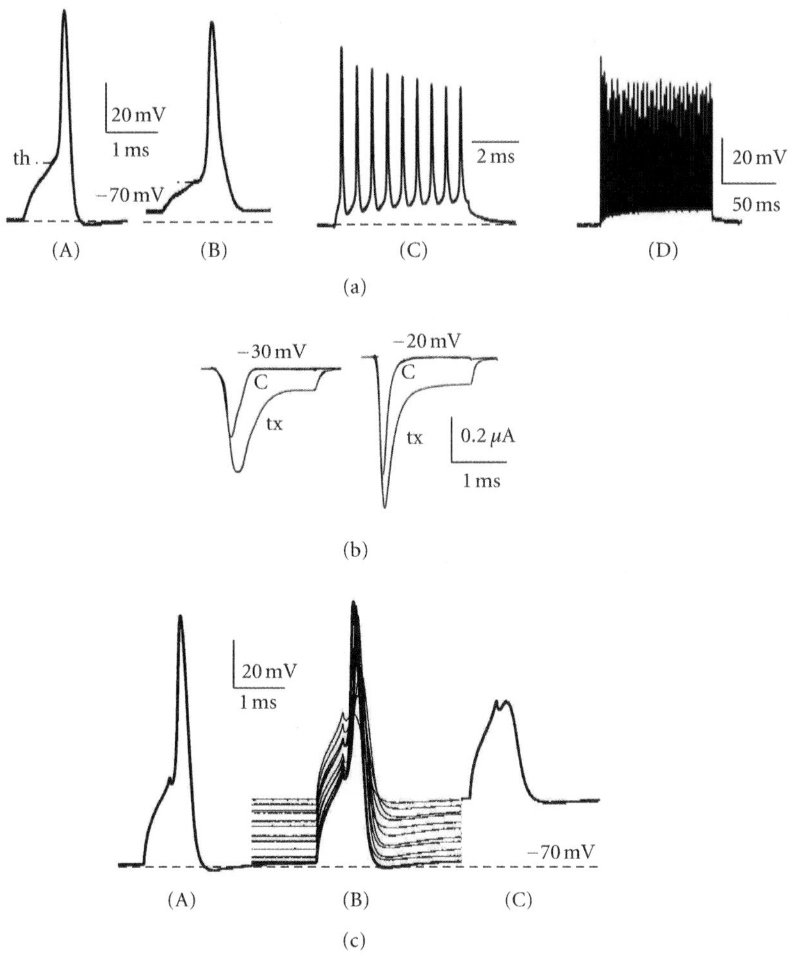

Figure 3: The effects of beta group of scorpion toxins on axonal bioelectrical activity. (a) The effect of Bj-xtrIT—a recombinant excitatory anti-insect toxin from *Buthus judaicus* scorpion: (A) control action potential; (B) action potential recorded from the same axon in 10 min of toxin action (10^{-7} M)—note much lower threshold (th) for action potential generation and a slight membrane depolarization; (C) repetitive activity evoked after artificial repolarization of axonal membrane and stimulation with single, short (0.5 ms) current pulse; (D) long duration, high frequency repetitive activity observed after the artificial membrane hyperpolarization to −80 mV—activity was evoked by a single, short stimulation. (b) Bigger and prolonged sodium current recorded after 10 min of Bj-xtrIT presence (tx, 10^{-7} M) compared to control (c); currents were elicited with voltage pulses from HP = −70 mV to −30 and −20 mV. (c) Axonal activity modified by Lqh IT2 (10^{-6} M)—anti-insect depressant toxin. (A) control action potential and (B) the progressive decrease of its amplitude together with the membrane depolarization induced by toxin; (C) block of action potential generation observed after 15 min of toxin action.

response to current stimulation (Figure 3(a)(C)). The ability of the axon to generate such bursting discharges manifested itself especially when it was artificially repolarized or hyperpolarized (Figure 3(a)(D)). Exalted axonal excitability resulted from the increase in sodium current amplitude at negative membrane potentials and its prolongation observed under voltage pulse (Figure 3(b)). The analysis of sodium current voltage dependence revealed a shift in sodium current voltage dependence towards more negative membrane potentials [20]. In toxicity tests, these toxins caused an immediate contraction paralysis of fly larvae and a quick excitatory "knock-down" effect on locusts [8, 10], which remains consistent with the observations done in electrophysiological experiments.

The name "depressant toxins" comes from the flaccid paralysis they cause in fly larvae. The toxins within this group (Bj IT2—[10]; toxin from *Scorpio maurus palmatus* venom—[22]; Bot IT3 and BoT IT4 from *Buthus occitanus tunetanus*—[23, 24]; BmK ITa and BmK ITb from *Buthus martensi* Karsch—[23]; Lqh IT2—[25] evidently increase sodium permeability at resting potential, inducing relatively fast depolarization and distinct decrease in action potential amplitude (Figure 3(c)(A) and (B)), eventually blocking the conduction (Figure 3(c)(C)). In voltage-clamp experiments, the lowering of peak sodium current was observed, however, along with a development of a constant current, at holding potential equal to axonal resting potential, that is, −60 mV.

There have also been cases of finding toxins of which the effects on axonal electrophysiological activity appear intermediate between those of excitatory and depressant groups, for instance: BcTx1 from East African scorpion *Babycurus centrurimorphus* [26] or BoT IT2, which, moreover, induced a new, unusual current with slow activation/deactivation kinetics [23, 24, 27]. Bot IT2 is insect-selective; its binding site is similar to that one of AaH IT1 excitatory toxin, but amino acid sequence resembles the ones found in depressant toxins [23, 24]. Similar modification of axonal bioelectrical activity by Bot IT2 has been evidenced using a toxin from the venom of ant, *Paraponera clavata*, also tested on the cockroach isolated axon [28].

The comparative analysis of electrophysiological effects of several excitatory and depressant toxins suggests that the discrimination between these two groups of toxins is not always easy and certainly not possible only on the basis of bioelectrical activity modifications. Parallel biochemical and structural studies are absolutely required. As mentioned above, these two groups of toxins belong to one very large group of *beta* toxins that bind to receptor 4 on sodium channel [13, 14, 17].

Toxin VII from South American scorpion, *Tityus serrulatus*, is a typical *beta* toxin with no selectivity to any group of organisms [29, 30]. Its effect on cockroach axon can also be described as intermediate between those of excitatory and depressant toxins. In the presence of the toxin, resting depolarization was observed jointly with a tendency to repetitive discharges. Sodium current was activated at more negative potential than normally; it was prolonged, but holding current development was slower than in the case of depressant toxins [31].

Scorpion *alpha* toxins bind to the receptor site 3 on sodium channel and inhibit the channel's inactivation [12]. In voltage-clamp experiments, short sodium current is prolonged during depolarizing voltage pulse (Figure 4(b)); potassium current is not modified. In current-clamp, short action potentials are extended and transformed into *plateau* action potentials (Figure 4(a)). Such effects were observed when the first anti-insect toxin LqhαIT from *Leiurus quinquestriatus hebraeus* scorpion venom was tested on cockroach isolated axon [32, 33]. Later, several new anti-insect toxins with similar Lqh*a*IT characteristics were described, as for example BoT IT1 [23, 24].

Alpha toxin (LqhαIT) was also tested on cockroach giant axon in *in situ* conditions. The first observed effect, after the toxin's application, was a repetitive generation of slightly prolonged action potentials in response to short stimulation—such effect has never been observed in the experiments on isolated giant axon (Figure 4(c)). Later on, *plateau* action potential sometimes appeared (Figure 4(d)), but it was never as long in duration as in the case of isolated axon, even after a prolonged application of high toxin concentration. The influence of axonal microenvironment created by glial cells and other axons is a very likely factor in this matter. And it is necessary to consider the fact that the experimental conditions may vary from the physiological ones in a very diverse degree, which in turn may affect significantly the effects of the tested molecules.

Electrophysiological experiments performed on the cockroach axon helped to define a new group of scorpion neurotoxins: the *alpha*-like toxins. Receptor site of these molecules overlaps with receptor site 3 on sodium channel, where *alpha* toxins bind [18, 19]. *Alpha*-like toxins do not express selectivity toward insect or mammalian sodium channels. Pharmacological characteristics of *alpha*-like toxins are similar but not identical with those of *alpha* neurotoxins. They induce *plateau* potentials, but in addition, they depolarize progressively the axonal membrane. They inhibit the inactivation of sodium current, but to a lesser degree than in the case of LqhαIT. Moreover, a tail current appears, which increases when depolarizing pulses are applied repeatedly (every 5 s) and at the same time, the peak sodium current decreases [18, 19].

Along with the science progressing, modern techniques in molecular biology were applied and a "new era" in scorpion anti-insect toxins launched. One of the most noteworthy approaches towards this issue so far have been presented by Professor Michael Gurevitz and Dr. Dalia Gordon from the Department of Molecular Biology and Ecology of Plants, Tel Aviv University, Israel. They and their collaborators isolated the genetic material responsible for the synthesis of toxins from the scorpion venom, they defined the cDNA sequence and developed artificial expression systems [33–36]. New, recombinant toxins LqhαITr [36], Lqh IT2 [37] and Bj-xtrIT [38], tested on the cockroach isolated giant axon, showed much resemblance in their mode of action to the native counterparts. Such studies provided an extremely valuable conclusion: the activity of properly prepared recombinant toxins is the same as that of the native ones. This was a huge step in the field of toxinology. Nowadays, the recombinant toxins are accessible in a greater number than the native molecules and the advent of further mutations is feasible. It is pivotal now to study the molecular basis of anti-insect selectivity, as well as anti-mammalian specificity.

Toxicity tests, binding studies and electrophysiological recordings along with the molecular modeling, gene cloning and the site-directed mutagenesis create an opportunity to investigate the molecular basis of toxins' activity. The experiments performed on *alpha*-like toxins from *Buthus martensi* Karsch using cockroach axon showed that mutation of a single amino acid can change completely the toxin mode of action [39]. A phrase: "a story of one amino acid" may well summarize the long history of multiapproach studies on depressant toxins from *Leiurus quinquestriatus hebraeus.* In the experiments on the isolated axon of the cockroach, it has been shown that the replacement of the amino acid in position 58 from Asn to Asp is able to change completely the toxin's mode of action. At the same time, its affinity to sodium channel target and its toxicity decreased. Conclusion from these studies was as follows: Asn in position 58 plays the mandatory role in the activity of depressant toxins [13, 40].

The isolated axon of the cockroach was also used in the tests on the toxins obtained from the spider venom. In most cases they prolonged the duration of action potential, however, *plateau* action potential could only be generated in the presence of a potassium channel blocker. Sodium current inactivation was inhibited in the presence of the toxin, but never to such a degree as in the case of scorpion *alpha* toxins [41–43]. Postapplication of LqhαIT increased the late sodium current recorded during depolarizing pulse (Stankiewicz, personal observations).

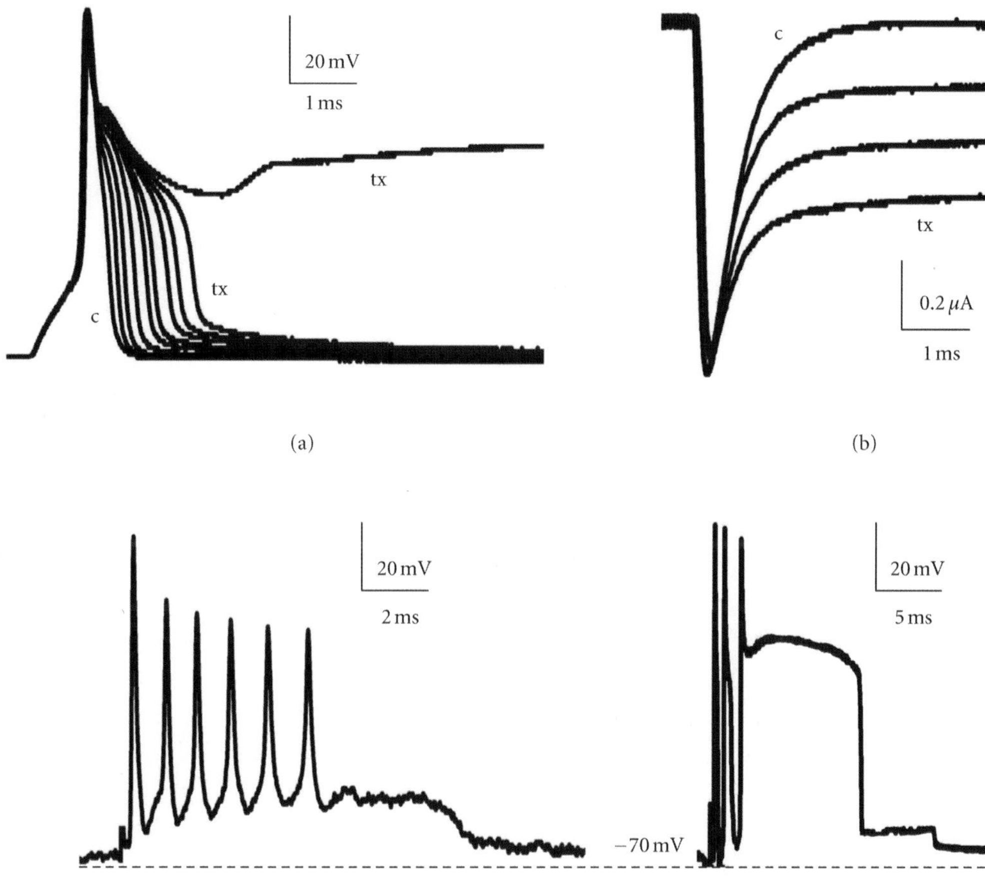

Figure 4: (a) The effect of LqhαIT (10^{-7} M)—recombinant anti-insect *alpha* toxin from *Leiurus quinquestriatus hebraeus* venom on axonal action potential; c—control action potential, tx—progressive increase of action potential duration until *plateau* action potential under toxin. (b) sodium current prolonged until the end of depolarizing pulse in toxin presence (tx). (c) Repetitive discharges induced by LqhαIT (5×10^{-6} M) recorded from the axon in connective (*in situ*), using microelectrode technique; connective was stimulated by extracellular silver electrodes through an isolated unit. (d) *Plateau* action potential generated sometimes by axon *in situ* in toxin presence.

3. DUM Neurons in Patch-Clamp and Microelectrode Techniques

In 1989 and 1990 two articles describing the application of patch-clamp technique in the study on the activity of neurosecretory dorsal unpaired median (DUM—Figure 1(c)) neurons from terminal ganglion of *Periplaneta americana* nerve cord were published [44, 45]. The technique of single DUM cell isolation and patch-clamp recording on it have been developed in Laboratory of Neurophysiology at Angers University in France by Professor Bruno Lapied. DUM neurons possess an endogenous pacemaker activity which depends on a wide range of ionic membrane conductances [46]. Various types of receptors provide a very precise regulation of the neurons' spontaneous activity and neurosecretory function. DUM neurons represent an outstanding model for studies on intracellular processes [47–49] as well as for pharmacological tests [50, 51]. They have also been used in toxinological experiments.

There were several experiments on DUM cells performed simultaneously with observations on an isolated axon. Although DUM neurons represent a much more complex model of bioelectrical activity than the axon, the observations were similar and the conclusions-compatible [25, 52]. Background sodium channels (bNa) in DUM neurons were examined using the patch-clamp cell-attached technique [53]. They appeared to be a new target for LqhαIT toxin, even more sensitive than the classical voltage-dependent Na channels in this preparation. The activity of bNa is limited at membrane potential −50 mV (DUM neuron resting potential) and can be "liberated" under LqhαIT action or at very negative (−90 mV) membrane potential. In the presence of the toxin (10^{-8} M), unclustered, brief single channel openings in control (at −50 mV) were transformed into large, multistep amplitude bursting activity, separated by periods of silence. Open probability of the channels increased by about 20-fold. Such channel activity was well corresponding to the transformation observed in DUM neurons: from regular beating, spontaneous activity to rhythmic bursting [53, 54].

Background sodium channels in DUM neurons are also the target for *beta* toxin (VII) from Brazilian scorpion,

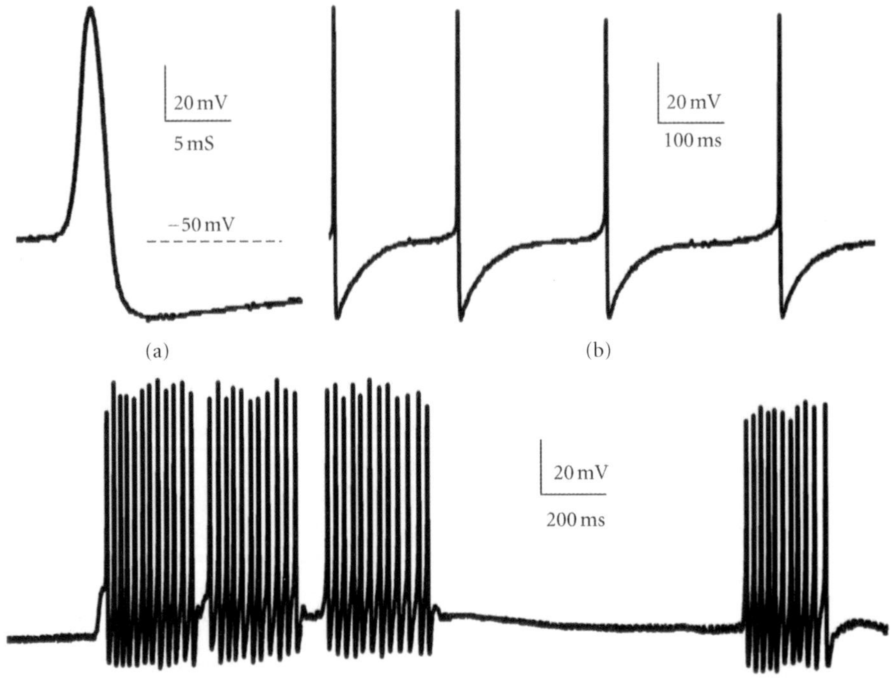

FIGURE 5: Activity of dorsal unpaired median (DUM) neurons from terminal abdominal ganglion, examined with the microelectrode technique. (a) Single action potential and (b) regular spontaneous activity recorded from the neuron in the ganglion—in *in situ* conditions, in control. (c) Radical change of neuron regular beating discharges into bursting activity in LqhαIT (10^{-6} M) presence.

Tityus serrulatus, venom [55]. In the toxin's presence, single-amplitude openings of the channels were replaced by events with several distinct subconductance current levels. Channel open probability rose by about 50-fold and similarly did the open-time duration; additionally, very long duration events emerged. Classical voltage-dependent sodium channels were also modified in a manner typical for *beta* toxin. The experiments performed with calcium imaging demonstrated the rise in the intracellular calcium concentration in the presence of toxin VII. A very complex study of this phenomenon evidenced the participation of high-voltage activated N-type calcium channels and the activation of noncapacitative calcium entry (NCCE). An important conclusion has been drawn from these studies that the reduction of the activity of NCCE may prove a useful strategy in the development of a drug for antienvenoming therapy [55].

The activity of DUM neurons can also be observed in *in situ* conditions using the microelectrode technique. Terminal abdominal ganglion is separated from the nerve cord, desheated and fixed. Neurons remain in their place in ganglion surrounded by glial cells and other neurons. DUM neurons are recognized by spontaneous action potentials when the microelectrode enters the cell. The pattern of neuronal activity is similar to the recordings obtained on isolated cells, however, the effect of toxins is not exactly the same. The application of *alpha* toxin (LqhαIT, 10^{-5} and 10^{-4} M) never induced *plateau* action potential *in situ*; only transformation from regular firing into bursting activity was observed and the bursts were generated from a level of slight depolarization (Figure 5(c)). In the ganglion, DUM cells are mainly under the influence of glial cells, as well as other neurons; thus, the ionic microenvironment remains partially undisturbed. In order to investigate the toxin's mechanism of action, isolated neurons should be used by all means, however, *in situ* experiments may in some cases reveal more on physiological effect of toxic molecules. The interactions between two neurotoxins observed on isolated and *in situ* DUM cells are also different (Stankiewicz et al., in preparation).

4. Cercal Nerve—Giant Interneuron Synapse and Single-Fiber Oil-Gap Technique

The information about mechanical stimulation arising in the cockroach cercal sensory neurons is transmitted to giant interneurons. Cercal nerves X and XI are connected with giant interneurone dendritic tree by inhibitory and excitatory synapses, respectively, located in the last abdominal ganglion. The activity of these synapses can be observed using the single-fiber oil-gap technique (Figure 6(a)), developed by Professor Jean-Jacques Callec in Rennes University [56, 57], later improved and applied for several years by Professor Bernard Hue from Laboratory of Neurophysiology at Angers University, France [58–60]. This method allows the extracellular recording of spontaneous and evoked excitatory postsynaptic potentials (EPSP) as well as inhibitory postsynaptic potentials (IPSP) [57, 60, 61]. Nerve XI is classified as excitatory and its fibers activate nicotinic receptors at

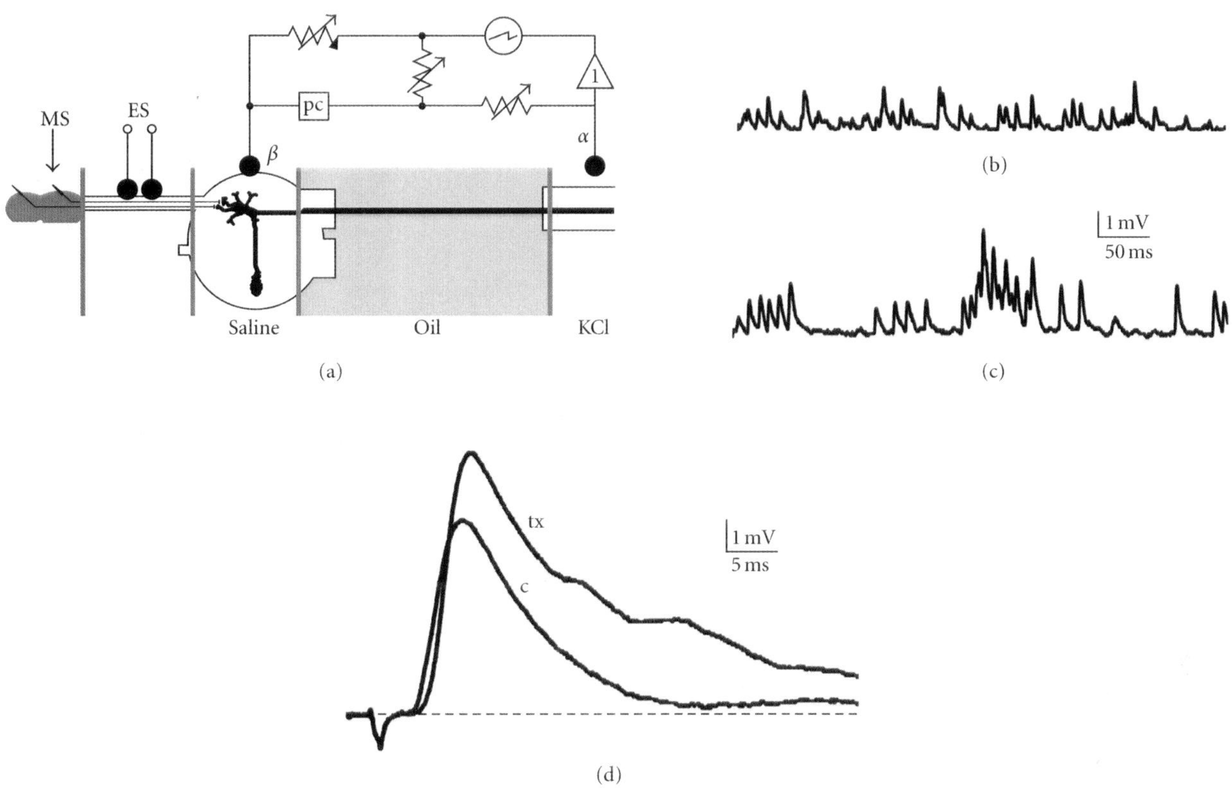

Figure 6: Single-fiber oil-gap method applied for studying synaptic transmission between cercal nerve and giant interneurone. (a) The scheme of electronic circuit used to record postsynaptic events. Recording electrode (α) bathed in isotonic KCl solution is connected with high-input impedance, negative capacitance amplifier (1); extracellular electrode β is in contact with last abdominal ganglion. Wheatstone bridge is connected to recording circuit and it is used to apply polarizing current (pc) through postsynaptic membrane. The desheated ganglion is superfused with saline or test solution. The dissected axon is bathed in paraffin-oil. MS—mechanical stimulation, ES—electrical stimulation applied to cercal nerve (according to [59, 60]). (b) Control conditions—unitary excitatory postsynaptic potentials (uEPSP) recorded as spontaneous activity of preparation and (d) c—control excitatory compound postsynaptic potential (cEPSP) observed as the effect of cercal nerve electrical stimulation. (c) The increased spontaneous activity (uEPSPs) and (d) tx—cEPSPs observed 10 min after LqhαIT (10^{-6} M) application using pneumatic injection in synapse vicinity.

postsynaptic membrane. Unitary excitatory postsynaptic potentials (uEPSP) result from the stimulation of single hair mechanoreceptors covering the cercus; composed postsynaptic potentials (cEPSP) are the effect of cercal nerve XI electrical stimulation. At the presynaptic face of such synapses, muscarinic receptors are present, the role of which is to regulate the acetylcholine releasing by negative feedback [62]. Muscarinic receptors were also found on postsynaptic membrane [63]. Stimulation of nerve X evokes inhibitory postsynaptic potentials (IPSP) via activation of GABA receptors [61]. Single-fiber oil-gap method allows to perform long-term experiments (even up to 12 hours) and well-adjusted perfusion of the ganglion enables to obtain reliable dose-response curves. Using the iontophoretic application of acetylcholine or carbachol to postsynaptic mem-brane vicinity permits to discriminate between pre- and postsynaptic action of the tested drugs. Synaptic preparation from the cockroach represents a remarkably useful model for pharmacological studies, however, obtaining a high-quality stable preparation requires much experience.

Cockroach synaptic model allowed to test the toxins which are active on cholinergic receptors. Snake venom is a well-known source for them. *Alpha*-bungarotoxins and k-bungarotoxins completely blocked uEPSP and cEPSP at concentration of 10^{-7} M. All performed experimental protocols indicated that the toxins block neuronal postsynaptic nicotinic receptors and α-bungarotoxin was more effective [64, 65]. Scorpion *alpha* toxin LqhαIT induced a substantial increase in the postsynaptic spontaneous activity, that is, in the frequency and the amplitude of uEPSP (Figures 6(b) and 6(c)), as well as in the amplitude and duration of cEPSP (Figure 6(d)). Higher presynaptic activity results in the increased releasing of acetylcholine, however, it activates the negative feedback via presynaptic muscarinic receptors in turn and after several minutes of the toxin's action, a decrease in postsynaptic events can be observed (Stankiewicz, personal observations).

The experiments performed using the single-fiber oil-gap method with the scolopendra, *Scolopendra* sp., venom determined its components which induced the depolarization of the cockroach postsynaptic membrane and the decrease in EPSP amplitude. Such effect was limited after pretreatment with atropine. Along with the studies performed on *Drosophila* muscarinic receptors (Dm1) expressed in *Xenopus* oocytes, it was evidenced that the venom of scolopendra comprises a component acting as agonist on insect muscarinic receptors [66].

Lastly, the experiments performed on cockroach synaptic preparation contributed to studies which allowed to explain the mechanism of synergistic interaction between chemical neurotoxins: pyrethroids (permethrin) and carbamates (propoxur) [67]. The conclusions from these studies are important for practical implementation in the field of crop protection.

5. Synaptosomal Preparation from Cockroach Nerve Cord

The nerve cords of cockroach (*Periplaneta americana*) have also been used to prepare synaptosomes, which are functional vesicles containing the nervous terminals. The synaptosomal preparation is easy to obtain and has been applied in several pharmacological tests. As illustration, binding assays of many radiolabeled toxins have been successfully characterized with synaptosomes [24, 42, 43, 68]. In addition, studies of photoaffinity labeling using ^{125}I TsVII as a ligand in synaptosomes of nerve cord from cockroach indicated for the first time the molecular weight of the scorpion toxin receptor from the insect nervous system which was suggested to be associated with voltage sensitive Na^+ channels [68]. More recently this preparation was also successful applied in binding studies involving radiolabelled spider toxins acting in sodium channels (De Lima, in preparation). Results obtained from electrophysiological experiments are often completed using synaptosomal preparation coming from cockroach nervous system.

6. Summary

Nervous system of the cockroach (*Periplaneta americana*) can be recognized as a remarkably useful model preparation in multiple electrophysiological techniques, which allows to perform pharmacological tests on diverse levels of nervous system organization. Confronting the results obtained reveals that a toxin may affect the activity of the same nervous structure with diverse effects, depending on the experimental conditions and this conclusion should be taken into account prior to any definite statement concerning the mode of action of any toxin.

Acknowledgments

Work was supported by the Ministry of Science and Higher Education of Poland; Grant no. N N303 320637. M. de Lima has been supported by FAPEMIG, CAPES, CNPq, and INCT-TOX Grants in Brazil. M. Dąbrowski is a beneficiary of Ph. D. grant within the Project "Enhancing Educational Potential of Nicolaus Copernicus University in the Disciplines of Mathematical and Natural Sciences; (Project no. POKL.04.01.01-00-081/10)," Poland. Maria Stankiewicz expresses great gratitude to Professor Marcel Pelhate, Professor Bernard Hue, and Professor Bruno Lapied from Laboratoire de Neurophysiologie (at present Recepteurs et Canaux Ioniques Membranaires) at Angers University, France, for teaching her all the techniques on the cockroach described in the paper and for their generous placing at her disposal all the facilities in their laboratory during many years. Many thanks also to all collaborators, especially to Dr. Dalia Gordon and Professor Michael Gurevitz from Tel Aviv University, Israel.

References

[1] I. Huber, E. P. Masler, and B. R. Rao, Eds., *Cockroaches as Models for Neurobiology: Applications in Biomedical Research*, CRC Press, Boca Raton, Fla, USA, 1990.

[2] Y. Pichon, *Aspects electriques et ioniques du fonctionnement nerveux chez les insectes. Cas particulier de la chaine nerveuse abdominale d'une blatte* Periplaneta americana *L.*, dissertation, These d'Etat, Rennes, France, 1969.

[3] Y. Pichon and J. Boistel, "Current-voltage relations in the isolated giant axon of the cockroach under voltage-clamp conditions," *Journal of Experimental Biology*, vol. 47, no. 2, pp. 343–355, 1967.

[4] M. Pelhate and D. B. Sattelle, "Pharmacological properties of insect axons: a review," *Journal of Insect Physiology*, vol. 28, no. 11, pp. 889–903, 1982.

[5] M. Pelhate, Y. Pichon, and D. J. Beadle, "Cockroach axons and cell bodies: electrical activity," in *Cockroaches as Models for Neurobiology: Applications in Biomedical Research*, I. Huber, E. P. Masler, and B. R. Rao, Eds., pp. 131–148, CRC Press , Boca Raton, Fla, USA, 1990.

[6] M. Pelhate and Y. Pichon, "Selective inhibition of potassium current in the giant axon of the cockroach," *The Journal of Physiology*, vol. 343, pp. 90–91P, 1974.

[7] Y. Pichon and J. Boistel, "Microelectrode study of the resting and action potentials of the cockroach giant axon with special reference to the role played by the nerve sheath," *Journal of Experimental Biology*, vol. 47, no. 2, pp. 357–373, 1967.

[8] E. Zlotkin, H. Rochat, Kopeyan, F. Miranda, and S. Lissitzky, "Purification and properties of the insect toxin from the venom of the scorpion *Androctonus australis* Hector," *Biochimie*, vol. 53, no. 10, pp. 1073–1078, 1971.

[9] M. Pelhate and E. Zlotkin, "Actions of insect toxin and other toxins derived from the venom of the scorpion *Androctonus australis* on isolated giant axons of the cockroach (*Periplaneta americana*)," *Journal of Experimental Biology*, vol. 97, pp. 67–77, 1982.

[10] D. Lester, P. Lazarovici, M. Pelhate, and E. Zlotkin, "Purification, characterization and action of two insect toxins from the venom of the scorpion *Buthus judaicus*," *Biochimica et Biophysica Acta*, vol. 701, pp. 370–381, 1982.

[11] I. Karbat, F. Frolow, O. Froy et al., "Molecular basis of the high insecticidal potency of scorpion α-toxins," *Journal of Biological Chemistry*, vol. 279, no. 30, pp. 31679–31686, 2004.

[12] D. Gordon, I. Karbat, N. Ilan et al., "The differential preference of scorpion α-toxins for insect or mammalian sodium channels: implications for improved insect control," *Toxicon*, vol. 49, no. 4, pp. 452–472, 2007.

[13] M. Gurevitz, I. Karbat, L. Cohen et al., "The insecticidal potential of scorpion β-toxins," *Toxicon*, vol. 49, no. 4, pp. 473–489, 2007.

[14] D. Gordon, "Sodium channels as targets for neurotoxins. Mode of action and interaction of neurotoxins with receptor

sites on sodium channels," in *Toxins and Signal Transduction*, Y. Gutman and P. Lazarovici, Eds., pp. 119–153, Harwood, The Netherlands, 1997.

[15] N. Gilles, M. Gurevitz, and D. Gordon, "Allosteric interactions among pyrethroid, brevetoxin, and scorpion toxin receptors on insect sodium channels raise an alternative approach for insect control," *FEBS Letters*, vol. 540, no. 1-3, pp. 81–85, 2003.

[16] F. Couraud, E. Jover, J. M. Dubois, and H. Rochat, "Two types of scorpion toxin receptor sites, one related to the activation, the other to the inactivation of the action potential sodium channel," *Toxicon*, vol. 20, no. 1, pp. 9–16, 1982.

[17] M. Gurevitz, O. Froy, N. Zilberberg et al., "Sodium channel modifiers from scorpion venom: structure-activity relationship, mode of action and application," *Toxicon*, vol. 36, no. 11, pp. 1671–1682, 1998.

[18] I. Krimm, N. Gilles, P. Sautière et al., "Nmr structures and activity of a novel α-like toxin from the scorpion *Leiurus quinquestriatus hebraeus*," *Journal of Molecular Biology*, vol. 285, no. 4, pp. 1749–1763, 1999.

[19] S. Cestèle, M. Stankiewicz, P. Mansuelle et al., "Scorpion alpha-like toxins, toxic to both mammals and insects, differentially interact with receptor site 3 on voltage-gated sodium channels in mammals and insects," *European Journal of Neuroscience*, vol. 11, pp. 975–985, 1999.

[20] M. Pelhate, M. Stankiewicz, and R. Ben Khalifa, "Anti-insect scorpion toxins: historical account, activities and prospects," *Comptes Rendus Des Séances De La Société De Biologie Et De Ses Filiales*, vol. 192, no. 3, pp. 463–484, 1998.

[21] P. Escoubas, M. Stankiewicz, T. Takaoka et al., "Sequence and electrophysiological characterization of two insect-selective excitatory toxins from the venom of the chinese scorpion *Buthus martensi*," *FEBS Letters*, vol. 483, no. 2-3, pp. 175–180, 2000.

[22] P. Lazarovici, P. Yanai, M. Pelhate, and E. Zlotkin, "Insect toxic components from the venom of a chactoid scorpion, *Scorpio maurus palmatus* (scorpionidae)," *Journal of Biological Chemistry*, vol. 257, no. 14, pp. 8397–8404, 1982.

[23] L. Borchani, P. Mansuelle, M. Stankiewicz et al., "A new scorpion venom toxin paralytic to insects that affects Na^+ channel activation. purification, structure, antigenicity and mode of action," *European Journal of Biochemistry*, vol. 241, no. 2, pp. 525–532, 1996.

[24] L. Borchani, M. Stankiewicz, C. Kopeyan et al., "Purification, structure and activity of three insect toxins from *Buthus occitanus tunetanus* venom," *Toxicon*, vol. 35, no. 3, pp. 365–382, 1997.

[25] R. Benkhalifa, M. Stankiewicz, B. Lapied et al., "Refined electrophysiological analysis suggests that a depressant toxin is a sodium channel opener rather than a blocker," *Life Sciences*, vol. 61, no. 8, pp. 819–830, 1997.

[26] R. B. Khalifa, M. Stankiewicz, M. Pelhate et al., "Action of babycurus-toxin 1 from the east african scorpion *Babycurus centrurimorphus* on the isolated cockroach giant axon," *Toxicon*, vol. 35, no. 7, pp. 1069–1080, 1997.

[27] M. Stankiewicz, F. Grolleau, B. Lapied, L. Borchani, M. El Ayeb, and M. Pelhate, "Bot it2, a toxin paralytic to insects from the *Buthus occitanus tunetanus* venom modifying the activity of insect sodium channels," *Journal of Insect Physiology*, vol. 42, no. 4, pp. 397–405, 1996.

[28] T. Piek, A. Duval, B. Hue et al., "Poneratoxin, a novel peptide neurotoxin from the venom of the ant, *Paraponera clavata*," *Comparative Biochemistry and Physiology. C*, vol. 99, no. 3, pp. 487–495, 1991.

[29] M. E. DeLima, M. F. Martin, C. R. Diniz, and H. Rochat, "*Tityus serrulatus* toxin VII bears pharmacological properties of both beta-toxin and insect toxin from scorpion venoms," *Biochemical and Biophysical Research Communications*, vol. 139, pp. 296–302, 1986.

[30] B. Becerril, S. Marangoni, and L. D. Possani, "Toxins and genes isolated from scorpions of the genus *Tityus*," *Toxicon*, vol. 35, no. 6, pp. 821–835, 1997.

[31] M. Stankiewicz, R. BenKhalifa, M. E. DeLima, and M. Pelhate, "Action of a typical beta scorpion toxin, *Tityus* toxin VII on the cockroach axonal membrane," *Toxicon*, vol. 37, article 310, 1999.

[32] M. Eitan, E. Fowler, R. Herrmann, A. Duval, M. Pelhate, and E. Zlotkin, "A scorpion venom neurotoxin paralytic to insects that affects sodium current inactivation: purification, primary structure, and mode of action," *Biochemistry*, vol. 29, no. 25, pp. 5941–5947, 1990.

[33] M. Gurevitz, D. Urbach, E. Zlotkin, and N. Zilberberg, "Nucleotide sequence and structure analysis of a cDNA encoding an alpha insect toxin from the scorpion *Leiurus quinquestriatus hebraeus*," *Toxicon*, vol. 29, no. 10, pp. 1270–1272, 1991.

[34] M. Gurevitz, E. Zlotkin, and N. Zilberberg, "Characterization of the transcript for a depressant insect selective neurotoxin gene with an isolated cDNA clone from the scorpion *Buthotus judaicus*," *FEBS Letters*, vol. 269, no. 1, pp. 229–232, 1990.

[35] N. Zilberberg, E. Zlotkin, and M. Gurevitz, "The cDNA sequence of a depressant insect selective neurotoxin from the scorpion *Buthotus judaicus*," *Toxicon*, vol. 29, no. 9, pp. 1155–1158, 1991.

[36] N. Zilberberg, D. Gordon, M. Pelhate et al., "Functional expression and genetic alteration of an alpha scorpion neurotoxin," *Biochemistry*, vol. 35, no. 31, pp. 10215–10222, 1996.

[37] M. Turkov, S. Rashi, Z. Noam et al., "*In vitro* folding and functional analysis of an anti-insect selective scorpion depressant neurotoxin produced in *Escherichia coli*," *Protein Expression and Purification*, vol. 10, no. 1, pp. 123–131, 1997.

[38] O. Froy, N. Zilberberg, D. Gordon et al., "The putative bioactive surface of insect-selective scorpion excitatory neurotoxins," *Journal of Biological Chemistry*, vol. 274, no. 9, pp. 5769–5776, 1999.

[39] C. G. Wang, M. H. Ling, C. W. Chi, D. C. Wang, M. Stankiewicz, and M. Pelhate, "Purification of two depressant insect neurotoxins and their gene cloning from the scorpion *Buthus martensi* karsch," *Journal of Peptide Research*, vol. 61, no. 1, pp. 7–16, 2003.

[40] D. Strugatsky, N. Zilberberg, M. Stankiewicz et al., "Genetic polymorphism and expression of a highly potent scorpion depressant toxin enable refinement of the effects on insect Na channels and lluminate the key role of Asn-58," *Biochemistry*, vol. 44, no. 25, pp. 9179–9187, 2005.

[41] G. Corzo, P. Escoubas, M. Stankiewicz, M. Pelhate, C. P. Kristensen, and T. Nakajima, "Isolation, synthesis and pharmacological characterization of δ-palutoxins IT, novel insecticidal toxins from the spider *Paracoelotes luctuosus* (amaurobiidae)," *European Journal of Biochemistry*, vol. 267, no. 18, pp. 5783–5795, 2000.

[42] M. E. De Lima, M. Stankiewicz, A. Hamon et al., "The toxin tx4(6-1) from the spider *Phoneutria nigriventer* slows down Na(+) current inactivation in insect CNS via binding to receptor site 3," *Journal of Insect Physiology*, vol. 48, no. 1, pp. 53–61, 2002.

[43] M. E. De Lima, S. G. Figueiredo, A. M. Pimenta et al., "Peptides of arachnid venoms with insecticidal activity targeting

sodium channels," *Comparative Biochemistry and Physiology. Toxicology & Pharmacology*, vol. 146, pp. 264–279, 2007.

[44] B. Lapied, C. O. Malecot, and M. Pelhate, "Ionic species involved in the electrical activity of single aminergic neurons isolated from the sixth abdominal ganglion of the cockroach *Periplaneta americana*," *The Journal of Experimental Biology*, vol. 144, pp. 535–549, 1989.

[45] B. Lapied, C. O. Malecot, and M. Pelhate, "Patch-clamp study of the properties of the sodium current in cockroach single isolated adult aminergic neurones," *Journal of Experimental Biology*, vol. 151, pp. 387–403, 1990.

[46] F. Grolleau and B. Lapied, "Dorsal unpaired median neurones in the insect central nervous system: towards a better understanding of the ionic mechanisms underlying spontaneous electrical activity," *Journal of Experimental Biology*, vol. 203, no. 11, pp. 1633–1648, 2000.

[47] R. Courjaret and B. Lapied, "Complex intracellular messenger pathways regulate one type of neuronal α-bungarotoxin-resistant nicotinic acetylcholine receptors expressed in insect neurosecretory cells (dorsal unpaired median neurons)," *Molecular Pharmacology*, vol. 60, no. 1, pp. 80–91, 2001.

[48] R. Courjaret, F. Grolleau, and B. Lapied, "Two distinct calcium-sensitive and -insensitive pkc up- and down-regulate an α-bungarotoxin-resistant nAChR1 in insect neurosecretory cells (DUM neurons)," *European Journal of Neuroscience*, vol. 17, no. 10, pp. 2023–2034, 2003.

[49] C. Lavialle-Defaix, B. Moignot, C. Legros, and B. Lapied, "How does calcium-dependent intracellular regulation of voltage-dependent sodium current increase the sensitivity to the oxadiazine insecticide indoxacarb metabolite decarbomethoxylated JW062 (DCJW) in insect pacemaker neurons?" *Journal of Pharmacology and Experimental Therapeutics*, vol. 333, no. 1, pp. 264–272, 2010.

[50] B. Lapied, F. Grolleau, and D. B. Sattelle, "Indoxacarb, an oxadiazine insecticide, blocks insect neuronal sodium channels," *British Journal of Pharmacology*, vol. 132, no. 2, pp. 587–595, 2001.

[51] F. Grolleau, L. Gamelin, M. Boisdron-Celle, B. Lapied, M. Pelhate, and E. Gamelin, "A possible explanation for a neurotoxic effect of the anticancer agent oxaliplatin on neuronal voltage-gated sodium channels," *Journal of Neurophysiology*, vol. 85, no. 5, pp. 2293–2297, 2001.

[52] F. Grolleau, M. Stankiewicz, L. Birinyi-Strachan et al., "Electrophysiological analysis of the neurotoxic action of a funnel-web spider toxin, δ-atracotoxin-hv1a, on insect voltage-gated Na^+ channels," *Journal of Experimental Biology*, vol. 204, no. 4, pp. 711–721, 2001.

[53] B. Lapied, M. Stankiewicz, F. Grolleau, H. Rochat, E. Zlotkin, and M. Pelhate, "Biophysical properties of scorpion alpha-toxin-sensitive background sodium channel contributing to the pacemaker activity in insect neurosecretory cells (DUM neurons)," *European Journal of Neuroscience*, vol. 1, pp. 1449–1460, 1999.

[54] M. Stankiewicz, F. Grolleau, H. Rochat, E. Zlotkin, M. Pelhate, and B. Lapied, "Insect background sodium channel as a new target for scorpion alpha toxin," *Pesticide Science*, vol. 55, pp. 1021–1026, 1999.

[55] F. Grolleau, M. Stankiewicz, E. Kielbasiewicz et al., "Indirect activation of neuronal noncapacitative Ca^{2+} entry is the final step involved in the neurotoxic effect of *Tityus serrulatus* scorpion β-toxin," *European Journal of Neuroscience*, vol. 23, no. 6, pp. 1465–1478, 2006.

[56] Y. Pichon and J. J. Callec, "Further studies on synaptic transmission in insects. i. external recording of synaptic potentials in a single giant axon of the cockroach, *Periplaneta americana* l," *Journal of Experimental Biology*, vol. 52, no. 2, pp. 257–265, 1970.

[57] J. J. Callec, J. C. Guillet, Y. Pichon, and J. Boistel, "Further studies on synaptic transmission in insects. ii. relations between sensory information and its synaptic integration at the level of a single giant axon in the cockroach," *Journal of Experimental Biology*, vol. 55, no. 1, pp. 123–149, 1971.

[58] B. Hue, M. Pelhate, J. J. Callec, and J. Chanelet, "Postsynaptic effects of 4-aminopyridine in the sixth abdominal ganglion of the cockroach," *European Journal of Pharmacology*, vol. 49, no. 3, pp. 327–329, 1978.

[59] B. Hue, *Electrophysiologie et pharmacologie de la transmission synaptique dans le système nerveux central de la blatte* Periplaneta americana *L.*, Ph.D. thesis, Universite d'Angers, France, 1983.

[60] B. Hue and J. J. Callec, "Electrophysiology and phramacology of synaptic transmission in the central nervous system of the cockroach," in *Cockroaches as Models for Neurobiology: Applications in Biomedical Research*, I. Huber, E. P. Masler, and B. R. Rao, Eds., pp. 149–168, CRC Press , Boca Raton, Fla, USA, 1990.

[61] B. Hue, "Functional assay for gaba receptor subtypes of a cockroach giant interneuron," *Archives of Insect Biochemistry and Physiology*, vol. 18, no. 3, pp. 147–157, 1991.

[62] H. Le Corronc, B. Lapied, and B. Hue, "M2-like presynaptic receptors modulate acetylcholine release in the cockroach (*Periplaneta americana*) central nervous system," *Journal of Insect Physiology*, vol. 37, no. 9, pp. 647–652, 1991.

[63] T. Piek, B. Hue, H. Le Corronc, P. Mantel, M. Gobbo, and R. Rocchi, "Presynaptic block of transmission in the insect cns by mono- and di-galactosyl analogues of vespulakinin 1, a wasp (*Paravespula maculifrons*) venom neurotoxin," *Comparative Biochemistry and Physiology. C*, vol. 105, no. 2, pp. 189–196, 1993.

[64] I. D. Harrow, B. Hue, M. Pelhate, and D. B. Sattelle, "α-bungarotoxin blocks excitatory post-synaptic potentials in an identified insect interneurone," *Journal of Physiology*, vol. 295, pp. 63–64, 1979.

[65] V. A. Chiappinelli, B. Hue, L. Mony, and D. B. Sattelle, "α-bungarotoxin blocks nicotinic transmission at an identified invertebrate central synapse," *Journal of Experimental Biology*, vol. 141, pp. 61–71, 1989.

[66] M. Stankiewicz, A. Hamon, R. Benkhalifa et al., "Effects of a centipede venom fraction on insect nervous system, a native xenopus oocyte receptor and on an expressed drosophila muscarinic receptor," *Toxicon*, vol. 37, no. 10, pp. 1431–1445, 1999.

[67] V. Corbel, M. Stankiewicz, J. Bonnet, F. Grolleau, J. M. Hougard, and B. Lapied, "Synergism between insecticides permethrin and propoxur occurs through activation of presynaptic muscarinic negative feedback of acetylcholine release in the insect central nervous system," *Neurotoxicology*, vol. 27, no. 4, pp. 508–519, 2006.

[68] M. E. de Lima, F. Couraud, B. Lapied, M. Pelhate, C. R. Diniz, and H. Rochat, "Photoaffinity labeling of scorpion toxin receptors associated with insect synaptosomal Na^+ channels," *Biochemical and Biophysical Research Communications*, vol. 151, no. 1, pp. 187–192, 1988.

Kinetic and Reaction Pathway Analysis in the Application of Botulinum Toxin A for Wound Healing

Frank J. Lebeda,[1,2] Zygmunt F. Dembek,[3] and Michael Adler[4]

[1] *Integrated Toxicology Division, US Army Medical Research Institute of Infectious Diseases (USAMRIID), 1425 Porter Street, Fort Detrick, MD 21702, USA*
[2] *USAMRMC, Combat Casualty Care Research Program, ATTN: MCMR-RTC, 504 Scott Street, Fort Detrick, MD 21702-5011, USA*
[3] *Division of Medicine, USAMRIID, 1425 Porter Street, Fort Detrick, MD 21702-5011, USA*
[4] *Neurobehavioral Toxicology Branch, Analytical Toxicology Division, US Army Medical Research Institute of Chemical Defense, Aberdeen Proving Ground, Edgewood Area, MD 21010, USA*

Correspondence should be addressed to Frank J. Lebeda, frank.lebeda@amedd.army.mil

Academic Editor: Martha L. Hale

A relatively new approach in the treatment of specific wounds in animal models and in patients with type A botulinum toxin is the focus of this paper. The indications or conditions include traumatic wounds (experimental and clinical), surgical (incision) wounds, and wounds such as fissures and ulcers that are signs/symptoms of disease or other processes. An objective was to conduct systematic literature searches and take note of the reactions involved in the healing process and identify corresponding pharmacokinetic data. From several case reports, we developed a qualitative model of how botulinum toxin disrupts the vicious cycle of muscle spasm, pain, inflammation, decreased blood flow, and ischemia. We transformed this model into a minimal kinetic scheme for healing chronic wounds. The model helped us to estimate the rate of decline of this toxin's therapeutic effect by calculating the rate of recurrence of clinical symptoms after a wound-healing treatment with this neurotoxin.

1. Introduction

As characterized by Hanchanale and coworkers [1], the perception of botulinum toxin A has been transformed "from poison to a healing agent." Much of our present knowledge about this toxin comes from the toxicological literature. Information concerning botulinum neurotoxin serotypes, molecular structures, substrate specificities, mechanisms of zinc-dependent peptide hydrolysis, ion channel formation, and other detailed topics has been extensively reviewed [2–4]. Of the seven immunologically distinct serotypes (A–F) from *Clostridium botulinum* and several other species, type A is the best characterized and is among the most potent of all toxins. The neurotoxin is initially expressed as a single polypeptide of nearly 1300 amino acid residues (MW ~150 kDa). Crude toxin extracts (MW ranges from ~300 to 900 kDa) contain several nontoxic ancillary proteins that form a complex with the neurotoxin. When ingested, these additional proteins are thought to protect the neurotoxin against austere environments such as those found in the certain regions of the gastrointestinal tract [5]. The neurotoxin is posttranslationally modified to form two chains that are covalently bridged with a disulfide bond. The light (L) chain (MW ~50 kDa) has zinc-dependent proteolytic activity, while the heavy (H) chain contains the translocation and binding domains. Subsequent to binding to specific receptors (SV2) [6] at peripheral cholinergic nerve terminals, the receptor-toxin complex is internalized into a membrane-bound compartment that undergoes a drop in pH. This acidification initiates a series of interrelated reactions. Conformational changes occur that allow the insertion of the H-chain into this compartment's membrane. As a result, the disulfide bond that links the L and H chains is reduced, an ion channel is formed, and the presumed proteolytic active moiety, the L-chain, is translocated into the neuroplasm. When the type A toxin substrate, SNAP-25, is selectively cleaved, synaptic vesicle-mediated neurotransmission is blocked that could eventually lead to fatal paralysis.

Since the 1980s, the therapeutic potential of this toxin has been exploited. Extraocular muscles have been injected with the partially purified neurotoxin as an adjunct or alternative to surgical correction in treating strabismus [7, 8]. The chemodenervation effects of this most poisonous of poisons [9] have been used to relax hyperkinetic striated muscle groups to diminish the effects of dystonia and related diseases [10]. Currently, BOTOX has been approved by the U.S. Food and Drug Administration (FDA) for the following indications: strabismus, blepharospasm, cervical dystonia, upper limb spasticity, maxillary hyperhidrosis, chronic migraine [11], and urinary incontinence [12]. These indications along with the temporary enhancement in the appearance (cosmesis) with BOTOX COSMETIC of moderate to severe wrinkles in adults [13, 14] introduces the theme of muscle immobilization in terms of a desired therapeutic outcome. Immobilization has been characterized as a fundamental principle of wound healing [15]. Advantage has also been taken of this toxin's chemoimmobilization property to improve the healing of wounds.

In contrast to the relatively vast amounts of information regarding this toxin's structure and mechanism of action, the newer, off-label uses for botulinum toxin have been less extensively reviewed. To gain further insight regarding the scope of these efforts, we have gathered and examined biomedical research articles by conducting systematic searches of the relevant literature in PubMed, in a manner similar to that of Steele and Madoff [16]. We have examined studies that range from descriptive observations to randomized controlled clinical trials to obtain more information about the components and processes involved in wound healing and the related time courses of action of botulinum toxin A.

The processes observed clinically on the wound healing effects of the type A toxin are at an early stage of our understanding. This proposal is substantiated by evidence-based reviews that critically evaluate this toxin's effects with different indications [17, 18]. We previously noted [19, 20] that only a few clinical studies have focused on kinetic analyses. Constructing even partial models for the clinically observed effects by this toxin remains a challenge. To advance our understanding, we have selected some of those clinical studies that have examined the timing of this toxin's effects.

2. Methods

2.1. Literature Searches. botXminer, the botulinum reference tool of clostridial neurotoxin citations in Entrez-PubMed/MEDLINE [20], was initially used to search in article titles, abstracts, and MeSH headings for the words "wound" and "heal" or "healing." A more extensive list of 29 wound-related keywords was then generated: anal, angiogenesis, collagen, cytokine, fibroblast, fibroblastic, fibrosis, fissure, flap, glycosaminoglycan, heal, healing, hemorrhoid, hemorrhoidectomy, hypertrophic, incision, inflammation, inflammatory, keloid, lesion, repair, scar, scarring, sphincterotomy, surgical, tendon, tensile, ulcer, and wound. This controlled vocabulary was used in the batch mode [21] to search botXminer for additional related citations. Another set of filter terms were used to find time-course-related information about this toxin. This set included 26 terms: clearance, day, decay, decline, delay, diffusion, duration, follow up, frequency, hour, hr, interval, kinetic, latency, minute, month, onset, period, persistence, recurrence, repeat, resistance, sec, time, week, and year.

Within the two lists in the batch matrix search, $(a_1, a_2, \ldots, a_m)$ and $(b_1, b_2, \ldots, b_n)$, the terms undergo the OR operation ($\bigcup$) which can be represented in a general form of (a_1 OR a_2 OR, etc.). In addition, the lists are combined with the AND operation ($\bigcap$) [21] which results in a batch query that can be represented by

$$\left(a_1 \bigcup a_2 \bigcup \cdots a_m\right) \bigcap \left(b_1 \bigcup b_2 \bigcup \cdots b_n\right). \quad (1)$$

Summaries from the two sets of terms were returned by botXminer in the form of tables, histograms, and lists. Lists of citations were subsequently manually examined. Additional keywords and phrases within the more than 70 downloaded text files were automatically searched with file search assistant (v. 3.1, 2009, AKS-Labs, Raleigh, NC, USA).

2.2. Analysis of Kinetic Data. Data from the clinical literature that were analyzed were fitted to an exponential function

$$y = y_0 + (a)\exp\left(-k_{\text{decay}}t\right), \quad (2)$$

where y is the cumulative number of patients who are free of symptoms at time $= t$, y_0 is the cumulative number of patients who are symptom-free at $t = \infty$, a is a preexponential constant, and k_{decay} is the rate constant for the decay of this response. SigmaPlot (v. 11.0, 2008, Systat Software, Inc. Chicago, Ill, USA) was used to conduct a least-squared fit for the values of y_0, a, and k_{decay}. The 95% confidence intervals for y values were also calculated. This equation is commonly used for simulating the decay rate of a reactant from a single model compartment.

2.3. Nomenclature. The FDA has approved generic, nonproprietary names for commercial formulations of botulinum toxin [22–24]. For botulinum toxin type A, BOTOX (Allergan, Calif, USA) is onabotulinumtoxinA, DYSPORT (Ipsen Biopharm Limited Co., UK) is abobotulinumtoxinA, and Xeomin (Merz Pharma GmbH & Co KGaA., Germany) is incobotulinumtoxinA [25]. For botulinum toxin type B, MYOBLOC/NeuroBloc (Solstice Neuroscience, Inc., Pa, USA; Eisai Ltd., UK) is now rimabotulinum toxin B [26]. The changes in nomenclature emphasize the different potencies and the noninterchangeable unit dosages of these distinct brand name products. As reviewed by Alberto [24], these distinctions in names emphasize the differences in manufacturing and formulation techniques that may contribute to differences in the pharmacokinetics, efficacy, safety, and antigenicity among these products.

In the present paper, partially purified toxin with non-toxic or accessory proteins is referred to as botulinum toxin type A to distinguish it from botulinum neurotoxin A (BoNT/A), the pure holotoxin.

2.4. Sources of Error and Uncertainty. The lists of selective keywords are not intended to be exhaustive but serve as a starting point for the present work. Additional terms, such as proctology and coloproctology [27], can be used in more comprehensive studies.

Software development involves verification and validation. Verification confirms that, for example, the equations being coded are producing the correct calculations. Software can be validated when it can model the results that best fit existing data, and is subsequently reinforced by further data obtained experimentally. For kinetically related clinical problems, the underlying processes that need to be included are still uncertain. Furthermore, mathematical models are not designed to replace validation by basic research experiments or clinical observations. Rather, models are meant to enhance validation procedures by providing stimuli for new ideas, hypotheses, and perspectives on the problems being examined.

3. Results and Discussion

3.1. Literature Search for Botulinum Toxin A and Wound Healing. A preliminary search of botXminer, using the query "wound AND (heal OR healing)" for years 1980–2010, returned over 150 citations about half of which were true positives due to the large number of references related to tetanus (false positives). From the list of true positive citations, additional keywords were identified.

A variety of indications were found, in which botulinum toxin A has been used for wound healing and related conditions. These examples included experimental cutaneous scars in animal models [15, 28] and in clinical studies: chronic anal fissures [29, 30], cleft lip surgical repair [31], traumatic head lacerations or elective excisions of forehead masses [32], focal fold granuloma [33], hypertrophic scarring [34], pressure ulcers [35, 36], Raynaud's phenomenon (vasospastic ischemia of the digits, digital ischemia, including chronic ulcers) [37], and self-mutilation injuries in Lesch-Nyhan syndrome [38]. Another healing application of botulinum toxin A, referred to as protective ptosis, is used against persistent corneal ulcers, burns, and other ophthalmic-related problems [39, 40].

Conducting a matrix batch search in which "tetanus" was filtered out, using 26 time-related terms along with the 29 wound healing related terms, yielded 671 unique citations. From this filtered output, we concentrated on references dealing with wound conditions and indications in which botulinum has been used for therapeutic purposes in which some mechanistic, dosage, and/or kinetic information was also available (Methods, Figure 1).

3.2. Botulinum Toxin A and the Components of the Healing Process. The normal wound-healing process has been described as being comprised of four overlapping phases: haemostasis, inflammation, tissue proliferation, and remodeling [41]. If any of these processes are disrupted, healing is impeded leading to a chronic wound state. The interference by botulinum toxin in reducing muscle movement has helped to define healing phases further. For example, a vicious cycle involving inflammation, pain, and muscle spasm was first noted to be the underlying cause for the development of chronic anal fissures [29, 42]. Subsequently, low blood flow and ischemia were added to this cycle [43–45]. Additional components of the healing process have been identified for other conditions as presented in this section.

Scar formation is a hallmark of wound healing, and it usually causes significant physical, psychological, and cosmetic problems. Hypertrophic scarring is a common, refractory dermal disease that is manifested by the abnormal appearance of wound healing which can be the result of different types of injuries [34, 46, 47]. In the study by Xiao et al. [46], 19 patients were treated once a month over 3 months with 1.8–35 U botulinum toxin A (Hengli/CBTX-A, Lanzou Biochemical Co., China [48]). Improvements in wound healing were based on subjective grading by patients and plastic surgeons. Scores were assigned before treatment for the associated erythema, pliability (lesion softening), and the severity of itching. After a 6-month followup of the 19 patients participating in that study, 15 gave an overall assessment of their lesion improvement as "good," and seven others rated their improvement as "excellent." Some critical comments provided by the authors included the lack of control subjects, the study was not double blinded, and a small patient population size. Finally, there was only a relatively short follow-up time of 6 months so that no determination of the total time course of toxin action could be established.

A number of quantitative parameters may be accessed to evaluate the effectiveness of wound healing by botulinum toxin A. Increased metabolic activity and inflammation during the healing process induce muscle contractions around the edges of the skin wound [32, 46]. The major role of botulinum toxin A in this healing process is to prevent the repeated, small contractions that produce "microtraumas" near the hypertrophic scar and thereby decrease the tensile force (muscle activity) during scar formation. Traditional surgical techniques that align incisions along Langer's lines do not prevent repeated contractions [15]. The development of fibrosis also involves the deposition of extracellular collagen and glycosaminoglycans that can cause the scar to hypertrophy, invert, and become hyperpigmented resulting in poor color matching of this tissue with the neighboring skin [15, 28]. Other parameters for wound healing include size of wound, amount of and infiltration of inflammatory cells, blood vessel proliferation, and wound thickness [28].

Additional cellular and molecular mechanisms of healing by the formation of scar tissue (traumatic cicatrisation) are beginning to be elucidated [46]. Transforming growth factor $\beta1$ (TGF- $\beta1$) is a fibrotic cytokine that stimulates cellular growth, differentiation, and adherence and leads to the collagen deposition. This cytokine initiates these processes by extracellularly binding to a coupled pair of

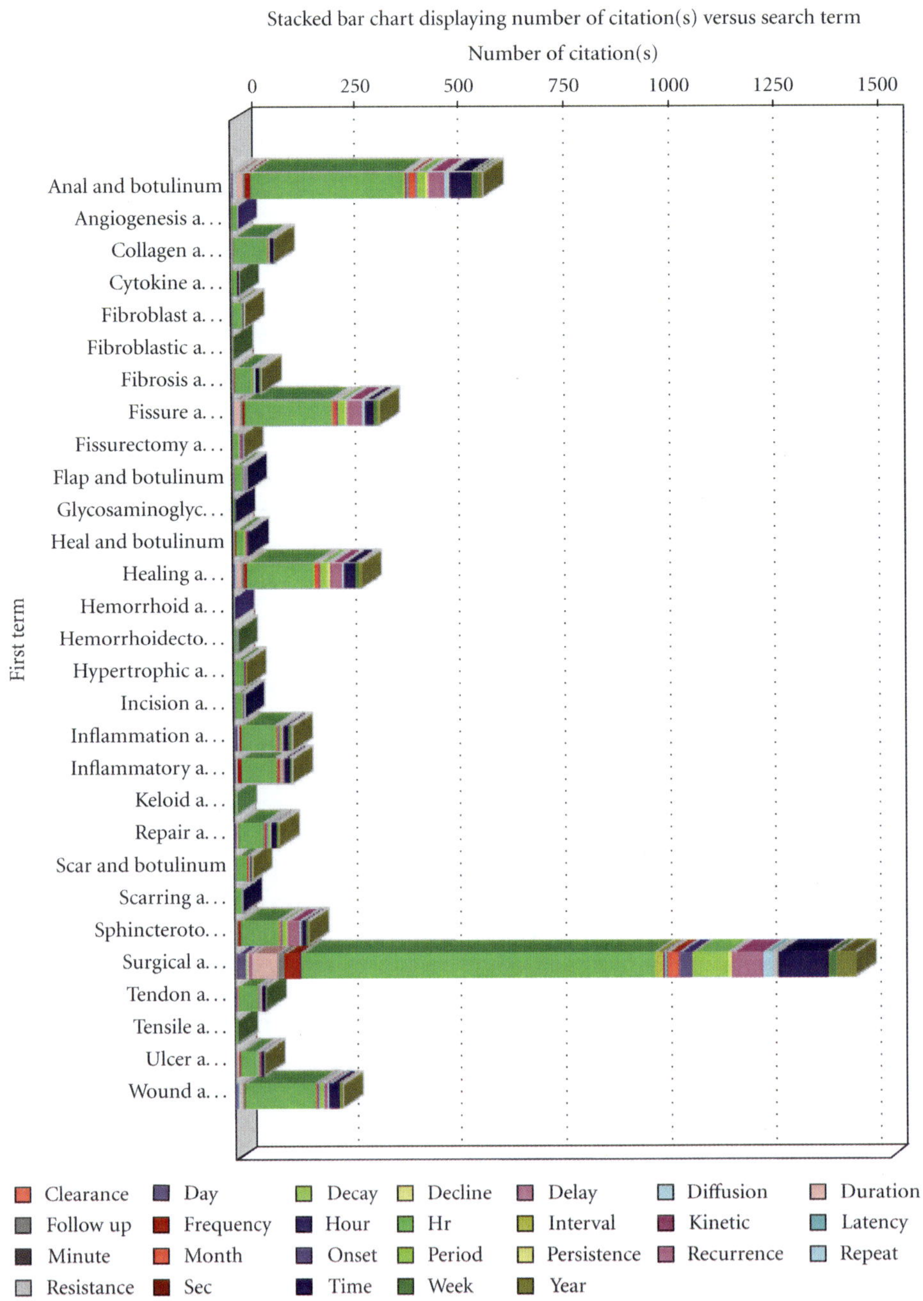

Figure 1: Example output from a botXminer database search. The numbers of botulinum toxin citations are shown for each of the combined 29 wound-healing (first term) and 26 time-related terms (legend) that were associated with 671 unique citations. The wound-related keywords associated with "botulinum" are associated with histograms that represent the different numbers of articles found in these multiple searches. The color-coded, time-related keywords used in these searches are simultaneously displayed in these histograms. Each "a..." in the left-hand labels signifies "and botulinum."

serine-threonine kinases. On binding, one receptor recruits and phosphorylates the other. This signaling pathway eventually stimulates transcription of the collagen gene and the formation of hypertrophic scars. Because human fibroblasts derived from hypertrophic scars overexpress and secrete TGF-β1, another wound-healing effect of botulinum toxin A has been speculated to be inhibiting the secretion of TGF-β1 [47]. Similarly, suramin, an antifibrotic polysulfonated naphthylurea compound, has been reported to promote wound healing by antagonizing TFG-β1 in muscle-derived fibroblasts [49].

The circulatory system is also affected by the apparent ability of botulinum toxin to enhance wound healing. Using a rat model for wounds, Yoo's group [50] observed that pretreatment with botulinum toxin A increased dorsal skin flap survival and concluded that this process was caused by increased perfusion. Because this toxin inhibits secretion of norepinephrine from sympathetic vasodilator

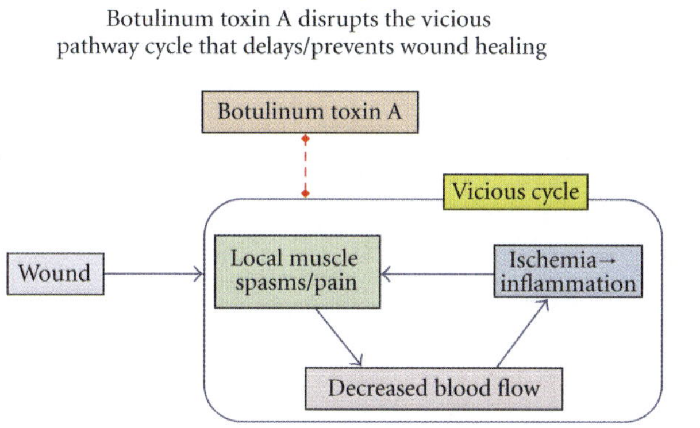

FIGURE 2: Botulinum toxin is depicted to disrupt the vicious pathway cycle that delays or prevents the healing of moderate wounds. This cycle involving spasm, pain, diminished blood flow, ischemia, and inflammation is blocked by the inhibition of chemical transmission at neuromuscular junctions by botulinum toxin A [29, 42, 43]. Dashed line is inhibitory action.

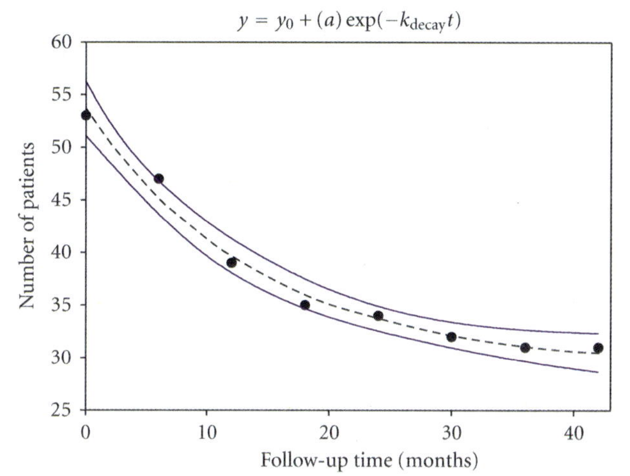

FIGURE 3: Time course of recurrence of CAF symptoms in some patients (22 of 53) in a 42-month follow-up study [55]. Initially ($t = 0$, i.e., 6 months after injection), all 53 patients were symptom-free for 6 months after injection of 10–20 U BOTOX. The fitted values from (2) (see text) are $y_0 = 29.2$, $a = 24.4$, and $k_{decay} = 0.85$ years^{-1}. The y-axis represents the number of symptom-free patients. Dashed line is fitted data; solid lines are 95% C.I.

and vasoconstrictor neurons [51, 52], the effect of botulinum toxin A may involve increased perfusion by decreasing sympathetic vasoconstriction in the skin flaps, thus promoting skin flap survival.

3.3. Kinetic Data for Onset and Duration of Healing Effects Produced by Botulinum Toxin A. The protective effects of botulinum toxin-induced ptosis have been used for the conditions of recalcitrant corneal ulcers and other surface disorders as an alternative to the surgical practice of partially sewing the eyelids together (tarsorrhaphy) [39]. This secondary healing effect is produced when botulinum toxin A is injected into eye muscles, typically the levator palpebrae superioris (LPS) muscles [53]. This therapeutic application has been the subject of studies that have also generated kinetic data [39]. From an open-label, multicentered study with 16 ophthalmic patients who received 5 U BOTOX in the LPS muscle, the time to "suitable" ptosis was 4.0 ± 0.5 days (mean ± SE, range: 2–8 days), and the duration of this ptosis was 46.0 ± 12 days (1–206 days) [39]. A similar number of patients who received a single, lower dose (2.5 U) had a comparable mean time to ptosis (3.6 days) and a shorter, mean duration (16 days). Diplopia was the only adverse effect experienced by five patients. Although statistical analyses with more patients are required to make more definitive conclusions, these trends are not unexpected but are, nevertheless, remarkable because a twofold change of a low dose apparently resulted in appreciable differences in duration.

3.4. Kinetic Analysis of Recurrence of Symptoms. Chronic anal fissure (CAF) is a painful condition caused by spasms of the internal sphincter smooth muscles. The traditional surgical approach has been sphincterotomy that can result in the adverse effect of incontinence [30]. Traditional nonsurgical approaches that have been used include sitz bath, topical anaesthesia, nitroglycerin, isosorbide dinitrate, nifedipine, Diltiazem, L-arginine gel, hyperbaric oxygen, and botulinum toxin A [43]. The first use of botulinum toxin as a medical alternative for CAF was conducted by Jost and Schimrigk [29]. For this indication, we chose what has been described as one of the longest follow-up studies using botulinum toxin (type A) in the treatment of CAF [54].

We analyzed data for the time course of recurrence of CAF symptoms in patients in a 42-month follow-up study [55, Table 1]. As illustrated in Figure 3, at the beginning of the followup (at $t = 0$), all 53 patients were symptom-free for 6 months after one to two injections of 10–20 U BOTOX. Subsequently, 22 of 53 patients showed a recurrence of symptoms. Most patients (31 of 53) did not undergo recurrence indicating that they remained healed during this follow-up period. From the nonlinear fit of these data to (2), the fitted values ± SEMs are $y_0 = 29.2 \pm 1.2$, $a = 24.4 \pm 1.3$. The k_{decay} (decay rate constant) is $7.08 \times 10^{-2} \pm 1.07 \times 10^{-2}$ month^{-1}, 1.64×10^{-6} min^{-1} (see below), or 0.85 years^{-1} (see Table 1). The value of $1/k_{decay}$ or τ is 14.1 months, and the corresponding value of $t_{1/2} (= \tau \ln 2)$ is 9.8 months or 294 days.

The long-term success rate was only 31/53 (58%) or a 42% rate of recurrence [30]. From Arroyo's group [54], recurrence rate of 12% occurred initially, and a rate of 53% at the 3-year follow-up point. Bilateral fissurectomies of the internal anal sphincter combined with toxin injections [56] have been reported to have a high success rate although the follow-up time in that study was limited to 1 year. Also, it was not determined whether surgery itself produced a similar rate of healing.

An interpretation of the single exponential decay curve during the 42-month followup (Figure 3) is that it reflects a zero-order elimination or inactivation step of the persistent, intraneuronally located toxin [57]. This step is described by the rate constant of decay, k_{decay}, in Figure 4 and k_e in a previous publication [58]. The table summarizes the processes displayed in Figure 4 and highlights the recurrence of symptoms that may be used to gauge the slow elimination

TABLE 1: Summary of processes involved in wound healing as described in text. Recurrence of symptoms results from long-term observations [55] was analyzed in the present paper and is highlighted in bold.

Parameter	Relative rates	Rate constant symbol	Units	Value
Onset of initial wounding	Very fast	k_1	$msec^{-1}$ or sec^{-1}	N.A.[a]
Development of chronic wound	Moderate	k_2	$days^{-1}$ or $weeks^{-1}$	N.A.
Healing of acute wound	Slow	k_3	$weeks^{-1}$ or $months^{-1}$	N.A.
Healing of chronic wound	Very slow	k_4	$years^{-1}$	N.A.
Recurrence of symptoms [55], [Figure 3]	**Very slow**	$\mathbf{k_{decay}}$	$\mathbf{years^{-1}}$	**0.85**
4-step reaction [19]				
Diffusion toxin to receptors	Moderate	k_5	min^{-1}	0.001
Binding of toxin	Fast	k_B	min^{-1}	0.058
Translocation of toxin	Fast	k_T	min^{-1}	0.141
Toxic reaction (lysis)	Fast	k_L	min^{-1}	0.013

[a] N.A., because data are not presently available, order of magnitude estimates are given.

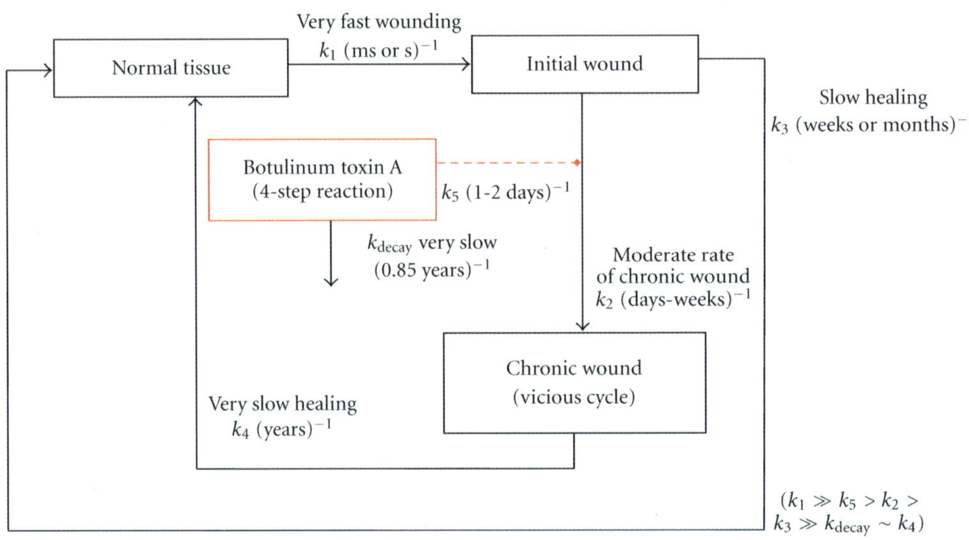

FIGURE 4: A minimal kinetic model for enhanced wound healing with botulinum toxin. Wounding of the normal tissue state is assumed to occur most rapidly leading to an initial wound state of the tissue. Healing from a significant wound is typically a slow process taking weeks or months. In the meantime, without treatment, this system enters, at a moderate rate, into a vicious cycle state (Figure 2) from which its escape represents a very slow healing process. With botulinum toxin treatment, this cycle is blocked thus allowing the tissue to return to the normal state by the slow healing route. The four-step reaction of toxin binding, translocation, internalization, and toxicity is described elsewhere [19]. A competing reaction is depicted as the slow decay or the inactivation rate of this toxin (k_{decay}) that leads to a recurrence of symptoms.

or inactivation of the type A botulinum toxin. Notably, this rate may be comparable to the slow rates of healing of some chronic wounds.

Alternatively, the long-lived toxic effect may be related to the rate of restoration of intact SNAP-25 intracellular levels or a combination of a slow degradation and a persistent inhibitory action of the SNAP-25 BoNT/A cleavage product [59]. The value of $t_{1/2}$ of 294 days is comparable to the recurrence times of 444 ± 132 days (mean ± S.D.; range 270–718 days [60]) for achalasia patients after receiving a single injection of 80 U BOTOX. On the other hand, our calculated decay rate constant of $1.64 \times 10^{-6}\,min^{-1}$ is about 1000 times slower than the estimated rate constant for decay of efficacy ($1.1 \times 10^{-3}\,min^{-1}$) in a single dystonic patient [58, 61, 62]. This difference may be due to several factors, among which are the different patient populations, the muscles being injected, the conditions being treated, and the assessment methods.

4. Future Directions

While the above studies show encouraging trends in support of using botulinum toxin A in wound-healing paradigms, additional studies are necessary. Overall, more prospective clinical studies of these treatments with botulinum toxin A are needed. Evidence from blinded, randomized, placebo-controlled, multicentered studies will help determine if these toxin treatments have significant benefit and if the minimal adverse reactions can be sustained.

Future trials should also use larger populations of more homogeneous (standardized) patients and control subjects, plan to examine long-term outcomes, and conduct cost-benefit analyses [63]. Although randomized controlled trials are considered the gold standard of clinical research [64], assessing them using criteria for standardizing phase III trials remains a substantial challenge [65]. Moreover, there is also a need for additional controlled studies to clearly establish an advantage of botulinum products over other methods.

Retrospective meta-analysis studies are also needed for all of these new treatments. An outcome of one of these analyses was the low probability that type A botulinum toxin or calcium channel blockers were found to be more effective in treating CAF than nitroglycerin ointment in 182 patients [30]. Another example is Shao et al.'s analysis [44] which determined that for 279 CAF patients the traditional surgical procedure of lateral internal sphincterotomy (LIS) was more effective than BOTOX in healing chronic anal fissure. While LIS produced a higher rate of minor anal incontinence, botulinum toxin was associated with a higher rate of recurrent disease. For those patients who had a high risk of incontinence, local injection of the toxin was considered appropriate.

Computational modeling and simulation studies at different levels of granularity (i.e., detail) should also be beneficial. Starting with existing minimal kinetic models [19, 66], dose-dependent kinetic models could be developed to predict the time course (onset, duration, and recurrence of symptoms) and the extent of botulinum toxin A's effectiveness. Kinetic models could help to identify what research gaps exist and which ones can be experimentally or clinically resolved. One gap that could be experimentally verified is to determine if the intracellular diffusion of botulinum toxin A [67] is influenced by other coinjected materials, for example, epinephrine and local anesthetics (lidocaine, Xylocaine), compounds that have been considered in controlling local diffusion and predicting the extent of this toxin's paralytic effect [15, 32].

As more realistic physiological-pharmacological models are developed, more free parameters and more sources of error, assumptions, and caveats will need to be evaluated. Potentially confounding factors associated with wounds include cell viability, alkali conditions [41], the generation of reactive oxygen species, and inflammation that is related to low blood flow and ischemia [45]. Changes in the ion flow through transmembrane channels and in metabolism could also have roles in wound healing. Another confounding factor is the well known, persistent muscle weakness (up to 5 years) that results from protracted patient immobilization due to critical illness polyneuropathy or myopathy [68, 69]. This persisting weakness and residual neurologic deficits are likely due to denervation, combined with catabolic muscle wasting and potential myopathic changes [68]. It remains for future studies to differentiate these physiological deficits from botulinum toxin-induced effects in either a botulism patient or with therapeutic treatments with this toxin.

The tissues involved in the healing process in cytoskeletal architectures and in membrane structures associated with various organs also need to be considered. Neurophysiological abnormalities, such as transient denervation-induced muscle fibrillations and presynaptic alterations producing muscle fasciculations, may also need to be considered. Other complicating factors in the healing process could also involve the biomechanical dynamic properties of soft tissue (e.g., stiffness) in response to stress and strain, and tissue anisotropy (directionality of nonhomogeneous material).

5. Summary/Conclusions

This succinct review examines the soft tissue wound-healing properties of botulinum toxin. When viewed from the perspective of treating neurologic and other disorders, it is noteworthy that the efficacy of this toxin is predicted to be transient as the toxin's effect wanes, while for wound healing, a permanent resolution is expected. Further, with respect to wound healing, the concept is described that for some lesions, botulinum toxin interferes with the vicious cycle of muscle spasm, pain, inflammation, decreased blood flow, and ischemia [43]. A reaction pathway scheme is outlined to illustrate botulinum toxin's involvement in stopping the vicious cycle. A minimal kinetic scheme for healing chronic wounds is also presented that includes different macroscopic states of soft tissue conditions (normal, initial wound, and chronic wound), and quantitative estimates for the relevant rate constants are provided. A definitive validation of the results, that is, the minimal kinetic model for predicting the beneficial effects of type A toxin, awaits additional clinical data. Perhaps the most useful outcome is that our kinetic model is capable of identifying a measurable gap (decay rate of toxin's effect) in our attempt to comprehend how complex, interacting biological systems respond to environmental stressors.

Disclaimers

Opinions, interpretations, conclusions, and recommendations are those of the authors and are not necessarily endorsed by the U.S. Army. The content of this publication does not necessarily reflect the views or policies of the U.S. Army, nor does mention of trade names, commercial products, or organizations imply endorsement by the U.S. Government. This paper has been approved for public release.

References

[1] V. S. Hanchanale, A. R. Rao, F. L. Martin, and S. S. Matanhelia, "The unusual history and the urological applications of botulinum neurotoxin," *Urologia Internationalis*, vol. 85, no. 2, pp. 125–130, 2010.

[2] F. J. Lebeda and B. R. Singh, "Membrane channel activity and translocation of tetanus and botulinum neurotoxins," *Journal of Toxicology—Toxin Reviews*, vol. 18, no. 1, pp. 45–76, 1999.

[3] L. L. Simpson, "Identification of the major steps in botulinum toxin action," *Annual Review of Pharmacology and Toxicology*, vol. 44, pp. 167–193, 2004.

[4] G. Schiavo, M. Matteoli, and C. Montecucco, "Neurotoxins affecting neuroexocytosis," *Physiological Reviews*, vol. 80, no. 2, pp. 717–766, 2000.

[5] B. R. Singh, B. Li, and D. Read, "Botulinum versus tetanus neurotoxins: why is botulinum neurotoxin but not tetanus neurotoxin a food poison?" *Toxicon*, vol. 33, no. 12, pp. 1541–1547, 1995.

[6] M. Dong, F. Yeh, W. H. Tepp et al., "SV2 is the protein receptor for botulinum neurotoxin A," *Science*, vol. 312, no. 5773, pp. 592–596, 2006.

[7] A. B. Scott, "Botulinum toxin injection into extraocular muscles as an alternative to strabismus surgery," *Journal of Pediatric Ophthalmology and Strabismus*, vol. 17, no. 1, pp. 21–25, 1980.

[8] A. B. Scott, "Botulinum toxin injection into extraocular muscles as an alternative to strabismus surgery," *Ophthalmology*, vol. 87, no. 10, pp. 1044–1049, 1980.

[9] R. Kukreja and B. Singh, "Biologically active novel conformational state of botulinum, the most poisonous poison," *Journal of Biological Chemistry*, vol. 280, no. 47, pp. 39346–39352, 2005.

[10] O. R. Adam and J. Jankovic, "Treatment of dystonia," *Parkinsonism and Related Disorders*, vol. 13, supplement 3, pp. S362–S368, 2007.

[11] Allergan, Highlights of prescribing information, 2010, http://www.allergan.com/assets/pdf/botox_pi.pdf.

[12] US Food and Drug Administration, FDA approves Botox to treat specific form of urinary incontinence, 2011, http://www.fda.gov/NewsEvents/Newsroom/PressAnnouncements/ucm269509.htm.

[13] US Food and Drug Administration, OnabotulinumtoxinA (marketed as Botox/Botox Cosmetic), AbobotulinumtoxinA (marketed as Dysport) and RimabotulinumtoxinB (marketed as Myobloc) Information, 2009, http://www.fda.gov/Drugs/DrugSafety/PostmarketDrugSafetyInformationforPatientsandProviders/ucm175011.htm.

[14] J. D. A. Carruthers and J. A. Carruthers, "Treatment of glabellar frown lines with C. botulinum-A exotoxin," *Journal of Dermatologic Surgery and Oncology*, vol. 18, no. 1, pp. 17–21, 1992.

[15] H. G. Gassner, D. A. Sherris, and C. C. Otley, "Treatment of facial wounds with botulinum toxin A improves cosmetic outcome in primates," *Plastic and Reconstructive Surgery*, vol. 105, no. 6, pp. 1948–1955, 2000.

[16] S. R. Steele and R. D. Madoff, "Systematic review: the treatment of anal fissure," *Alimentary Pharmacology and Therapeutics*, vol. 24, no. 2, pp. 247–257, 2006.

[17] M. Naumann, Y. So, C. E. Argoff et al., "Assessment: botulinum neurotoxin in the treatment of autonomic disorders and pain (an evidence-based review): report of the Therapeutics and Technology Assessment Subcommittee of the American Academy of Neurology," *Neurology*, vol. 70, no. 19, pp. 1707–1714, 2008.

[18] D. M. Simpson, J. M. Gracies, H. K. Graham et al., "Assessment: botulinum neurotoxin for the treatment of spasticity (an evidence-based review): report of the Therapeutics and Technology Assessment Subcommittee of the American Academy of Neurology," *Neurology*, vol. 70, no. 19, pp. 1691–1698, 2008.

[19] F. J. Lebeda, M. Adler, K. Erickson, and Y. Chushak, "Onset dynamics of type A botulinum neurotoxin-induced paralysis," *Journal of Pharmacokinetics and Pharmacodynamics*, vol. 35, no. 3, pp. 251–267, 2008.

[20] U. Mudunuri, R. Stephens, D. Bruining, D. Liu, and F. J. Lebeda, "botXminer: mining biomedical literature with a new web-based application," *Nucleic Acids Research*, vol. 34, pp. W748–W752, 2006.

[21] R. Z. Cer, U. Mudunuri, R. M. Stephens, and F. J. Lebeda, "Mining the botulinum research literature," *Botulinum Journal*, vol. 1, no. 3, pp. 270–280, 2010.

[22] F. J. Lebeda, R. Z. Cer, R. M. Stephens, and U. Mudunuri, "Temporal characteristics of botulinum neurotoxin therapy," *Expert Review of Neurotherapeutics*, vol. 10, no. 1, pp. 93–103, 2010.

[23] B. Martin, "Botulinum toxin: the name game," 2009, http://bmartinmd.com/2009/08/botulinum-toxin-the-name-game.html.

[24] A. Alberto, "Terminology for preparations of botulinum neurotoxins: what a difference a name makes," *JAMA*, vol. 305, no. 1, pp. 89–90, 2011.

[25] Merz Pharmaceuticals, Medication Guide Xeomin (R) (Zeomin) (incobotulinumtoxinA) for injection, intramuscular, 2010, http://www.merzusa.com/pdf/Xeomin_Medication_Guide.pdf.

[26] US Food and Drug Administration, FDA gives update on botulinum toxin safety warnings; established names of drugs changed, 2009, http://www.fda.gov/NewsEvents/Newsroom/PressAnnouncements/ucm175013.htm.

[27] W. H. Jost and H. Muller-Lobeck, "Preoperative use of botulinum toxin in coloproctology: hypothesis and first results," *Colorectal Disease*, vol. 2, p. 55, 2010.

[28] B. J. Lee, J. H. Jeong, S. G. Wang, J. C. Lee, E. K. Goh, and H. W. Kim, "Effect of botulinum toxin type a on a rat surgical wound model," *Clinical and Experimental Otorhinolaryngology*, vol. 2, no. 1, pp. 20–27, 2009.

[29] W. H. Jost and K. Schimrigk, "Use of botulinum toxin in anal fissure," *Diseases of the Colon and Rectum*, vol. 36, no. 10, p. 974, 1993.

[30] R. Nelson, "Non surgical therapy for anal fissure," *Cochrane Database of Systematic Reviews*, no. 4, p. CD003431, 2006.

[31] T. T. Tollefson, C. M. Senders, J. M. Sykes, and P. J. Byorth, "Botulinum toxin to improve results in cleft lip repair," *Archives of Facial Plastic Surgery*, vol. 8, no. 3, pp. 221–222, 2006.

[32] H. G. Gassner, A. E. Brissett, C. C. Otley et al., "Botulinum toxin to improve facial wound healing: a prospective, blinded, placebo-controlled study," *Mayo Clinic Proceedings*, vol. 81, no. 8, pp. 1023–1028, 2006.

[33] L. A. Orloff and S. N. Goldman, "Vocal fold granuloma: successful treatment with botulinum toxin," *Otolaryngology—Head and Neck Surgery*, vol. 121, no. 4, pp. 410–413, 1999.

[34] X. Zhibo and Z. Miaobo, "Botulinum toxin type A affects cell cycle distribution of fibroblasts derived from hypertrophic scar," *Journal of Plastic, Reconstructive and Aesthetic Surgery*, vol. 61, no. 9, pp. 1128–1129, 2008.

[35] D. Intiso and M. Basciani, "Botulinum toxin type A in the healing of a chronic buttock ulcer in a patient with spastic paraplegia after spinal cord injury," *Journal of Rehabilitation Medicine*, vol. 41, no. 13, pp. 1100–1102, 2009.

[36] A. S. Naicker, S. A. Roohi, and J. L. Chan, "Botulinum toxin type A for rehabilitation after a spinal cord injury: a case report," *Journal of Orthopaedic Surgery*, vol. 17, no. 1, pp. 96–99, 2009.

[37] A. Fregene, D. Ditmars, and A. Siddiqui, "Botulinum toxin type A: a treatment option for digital ischemia in patients with Raynaud's phenomenon," *Journal of Hand Surgery*, vol. 34, no. 3, pp. 446–452, 2009.

[38] E. Dabrowski, S. A. Smathers, C. S. Ralstrom, M. A. Nigro, and J. P. Leleszi, "Botulinum toxin as a novel treatment for self-mutilation in Lesch-Nyhan syndrome," *Developmental Medicine and Child Neurology*, vol. 47, no. 9, pp. 636–639, 2005.

[39] M. F. Ellis and M. Daniell, "An evaluation of the safety and efficacy of botulinum toxin type A (BOTOX) when used to produce a protective ptosis," *Clinical and Experimental Ophthalmology*, vol. 29, no. 6, pp. 394–399, 2001.

[40] G. C. Gusek-Schneider and F. Erbguth, "Protective ptosis by botulinum A toxin injection in corneal affectations," *Klinische Monatsblätter für Augenheilkunde*, vol. 213, no. 1, pp. 15–22, 1998.

[41] G. Gethin, "The significance of surface pH in chronic wounds," *Wound Healing Science*, vol. 3, no. 3, pp. 52–56, 2007.

[42] W. H. Jost and K. Schimrigk, "Therapy of anal fissure using botulin toxin," *Diseases of the Colon and Rectum*, vol. 37, no. 12, pp. 1321–1324, 1994.

[43] R. Rajasundaram, R. Ayyathurai, S. Narayanan, and A. Maw, "Botulinum toxin A and chronic anal fissures—a literature review," *European Surgery*, vol. 38, no. 5, pp. 353–358, 2006.

[44] W. J. Shao, G. C. Li, and Z. K. Zhang, "Systematic review and meta-analysis of randomized controlled trials comparing botulinum toxin injection with lateral internal sphincterotomy for chronic anal fissure," *International Journal of Colorectal Disease*, vol. 24, no. 9, pp. 995–1000, 2009.

[45] Z. Zheng and M. A. Yenari, "Post-ischemic inflammation: molecular mechanisms and therapeutic implications," *Neurological Research*, vol. 26, no. 8, pp. 884–892, 2004.

[46] Z. Xiao, F. Zhang, and Z. Cui, "Treatment of hypertrophic scars with intralesional botulinum toxin type a injections: a preliminary report," *Aesthetic Plastic Surgery*, vol. 33, no. 3, pp. 409–412, 2009.

[47] Z. Xiao, F. Zhang, W. Lin, M. Zhang, and Y. Liu, "Effect of botulinum toxin type a on transforming growth factor $\beta 1$ in fibroblasts derived from hypertrophic scar: a preliminary report," *Aesthetic Plastic Surgery*, vol. 34, no. 4, pp. 424–427, 2010.

[48] F. J. Lebeda, R. Z. Cer, R. Stephens et al., "Time course of the effects of botulinum neurotoxin," in *Dystonia: Causes, Symptoms and Treatment*, J. Kurstot and M. Forsström, Eds., pp. 179–198, Nova Science, Hauppauge, NY, USA, 2010.

[49] Y. S. Chan, Y. Li, W. Foster, F. H. Fu, and J. Huard, "The use of suramin, an antifibrotic agent, to improve muscle recovery after strain injury," *American Journal of Sports Medicine*, vol. 33, no. 1, pp. 43–51, 2005.

[50] Y. S. Kim, T. S. Roh, W. J. Lee, W. M. Yoo, and K. C. Tark, "The effect of botulinum toxin A on skin flap survival in rats," *Wound Repair and Regeneration*, vol. 17, no. 3, pp. 411–417, 2009.

[51] J. L. Morris, P. Jobling, and I. L. Gibbins, "Differential inhibition by botulinum neurotoxin A of cotransmitters released from autonomic vasodilator neurons," *American Journal of Physiology—Heart and Circulatory Physiology*, vol. 281, no. 5, pp. H2124–H2132, 2001.

[52] J. L. Morris, P. Jobling, and I. L. Gibbins, "Botulinum neurotoxin A attenuates release of norepinephrine but not NPY from vasoconstrictor neurons," *American Journal of Physiology—Heart and Circulatory Physiology*, vol. 283, no. 6, pp. H2627–H2635, 2002.

[53] G. E. Wuebbolt and G. Drummond, "Temporary tarsorrhaphy induced with type A botulinum toxin," *Canadian Journal of Ophthalmology*, vol. 26, no. 7, pp. 383–385, 1991.

[54] A. Arroyo, F. Perez, P. Serrano, F. Candela, and R. Calpena, "Long-term results of botulinum toxin for the treatment of chronic anal fissure: prospective clinical and manometric study," *International Journal of Colorectal Disease*, vol. 20, no. 3, pp. 267–271, 2005.

[55] M. Minguez, B. Herreros, A. Espi et al., "Long-term follow-up (42 months) of chronic anal fissure after healing with botulinum toxin," *Gastroenterology*, vol. 123, no. 1, pp. 112–117, 2002.

[56] T. Scholz, F. H. Hetzer, D. Dindo, N. Demartines, P. A. Clavien, and D. Hahnloser, "Long-term follow-up after combined fissurectomy and Botox injection for chronic anal fissures," *International Journal of Colorectal Disease*, vol. 22, no. 9, pp. 1077–1081, 2007.

[57] J. E. Keller, E. A. Neale, G. Oyler, and M. Adler, "Persistence of botulinum neurotoxin action in cultured spinal cord cells," *FEBS Letters*, vol. 456, no. 1, pp. 137–142, 1999.

[58] F. J. Lebeda, M. Adler, Y. Chushak et al., "Botulinum neurotoxin: a kinetic analysis," in *Proceedings of the Scientific Conference on Chemical and Biological Defense Research*, pp. 1–18, CBRNIAC, Hunt Valley, Md, USA, 2006.

[59] R. Eleopra, V. Tugnoli, O. Rossetto, D. de Grandis, and C. Montecucco, "Different time courses of recovery after poisoning with botulinum neurotoxin serotypes A and E in humans," *Neuroscience Letters*, vol. 256, no. 3, pp. 135–138, 1998.

[60] S. Leelakusolvong, T. Sinpeng, S. Pongprasobchai, T. Tanwandee, U. Kachintorn, and S. Manatsathit, "Effect of botulinum toxin injection for achalasia in Thai patients," *Journal of the Medical Association of Thailand*, vol. 89, supplement 5, pp. S67–S72, 2006.

[61] D. Dressler and F. A. Saberi, "Botulinum toxin: mechanisms of action," *European Neurology*, vol. 53, no. 1, pp. 3–9, 2005.

[62] D. Dressler, F. A. Saheri, and E. R. Barbosa, "Botulinum toxin: mechanisms of action," *Arquivos de Neuro-Psiquiatria*, vol. 63, no. 1, pp. 180–185, 2005.

[63] Z. Waseem, C. Boulias, A. Gordon, F. Ismail, G. Sheean, and A. D. Furlan, "Botulinum toxin injections for low-back pain and sciatica," *Cochrane Database of Systematic Reviews*, vol. 1, p. CD008257, 2011.

[64] E. N. Kiehna, R. M. Starke, N. Pouratian, and A. S. Dumont, "Standards for reporting randomized controlled trials in neurosurgery: a review," *Journal of Neurosurgery*, vol. 114, no. 2, pp. 280–285, 2011.

[65] D. Moher, S. Hopewell, K. F. Schulz et al., "CONSORT 2010 explanation and elaboration: updated guidelines for reporting parallel group randomised trials," *Journal of Clinical Epidemiology*, vol. 63, no. 8, pp. e1–e37, 2010.

[66] L. L. Simpson, "Kinetic studies on the interaction between botulinum toxin type A and the cholinergic neuromuscular junction," *Journal of Pharmacology and Experimental Therapeutics*, vol. 212, no. 1, pp. 16–21, 1980.

[67] F. J. Lebeda and M. Adler, "Hydrodynamic models for the diffusivity of type A botulinum neurotoxin," *Botulinum Journal*, vol. 1, no. 4, pp. 393–406, 2010.

[68] S. N. Fletcher, D. D. Kennedy, I. R. Ghosh et al., "Persistent neuromuscular and neurophysiologic abnormalities in long-term survivors of prolonged critical illness," *Critical Care Medicine*, vol. 31, no. 4, pp. 1012–1016, 2003.

[69] G. Hermans, B. de Jonghe, F. Bruyninckx, and G. van den Berghe, "Clinical review: critical illness polyneuropathy and myopathy," *Critical Care*, vol. 12, no. 6, p. 238, 2008.

6

Neurodegeneration in Alzheimer Disease: Role of Amyloid Precursor Protein and Presenilin1 Intracellular Signaling

Mario Nizzari,[1] Stefano Thellung,[1] Alessandro Corsaro,[1] Valentina Villa,[1] Aldo Pagano,[2] Carola Porcile,[3] Claudio Russo,[3] and Tullio Florio[1]

[1] *Section of Pharmacology, Department of Internal Medicine and Center of Excellence for Biomedical Research, University of Genova, 16132 Genova, Italy*
[2] *IRCCS Azienda Ospedaliera Universitaria San Martino-Istituto Nazionale per la Ricerca sul Cancro (IST), Università di Genova, 16132 Genova, Italy*
[3] *Department of Health Sciences, University of Molise, 86100 Campobasso, Italy*

Correspondence should be addressed to Claudio Russo, claudo.russo@unimol.it and Tullio Florio, tullio.florio@unige.it

Academic Editor: Wei Zheng

Alzheimer disease (AD) is a heterogeneous neurodegenerative disorder characterized by (1) progressive loss of synapses and neurons, (2) intracellular neurofibrillary tangles, composed of hyperphosphorylated Tau protein, and (3) amyloid plaques. Genetically, AD is linked to mutations in few proteins amyloid precursor protein (APP) and presenilin 1 and 2 (PS1 and PS2). The molecular mechanisms underlying neurodegeneration in AD as well as the physiological function of APP are not yet known. A recent theory has proposed that APP and PS1 modulate intracellular signals to induce cell-cycle abnormalities responsible for neuronal death and possibly amyloid deposition. This hypothesis is supported by the presence of a complex network of proteins, clearly involved in the regulation of signal transduction mechanisms that interact with both APP and PS1. In this review we discuss the significance of novel finding related to cell-signaling events modulated by APP and PS1 in the development of neurodegeneration.

1. Introduction

Alzheimer disease (AD) is a neurodegenerative disease clinically characterized by progressive dementia, and, neuropathologically, by loss of synapses and neurons, gliosis, and the presence of both amyloid plaques and neurofibrillary tangles. The main amyloid components of plaques are a family of short peptides (Aβ) of 40 or 42 amino acids, in the most common forms, derived from the proteolysis of the type I protein, amyloid β precursor protein (*AβPP*), upon sequential cleavage by β- and γ-secretases [1]. γ-secretase has been characterized as a multiprotein complex in which presenilins 1 and 2 have a regulatory role [1]. Familial AD forms (FADs) are caused by the overexpression or by mutations in the *AβPP* gene, or by mutations on the presenilins (*presenilins 1 and 2*).

The molecular mechanisms underlying the development of AD are not yet known, and also the physiological role of AβPP is still unclear [2].

In particular, it is still debated whether presenilins (PSs) familial mutations cause gain or loss of function in the γ-secretase complex. PS mutations have been presumed to cause FAD by enhancing production of the more toxic Aβ42 over the Aβ40 isoform, thereby conferring a toxic gain of function [3]. However, a number of recent studies have shown that clinically relevant PS mutations impair Aβ40 production without affecting Aβ42 production, leading to the revised view that pathogenic PS mutations consistently shift the cleavage specificity of the mutant protein to favor production of Aβ42 at the cost of Aβ40 [4, 5]. On the other hand, it has been recently suggested that, at least, some FAD-associated PS mutations can cause a nearly complete loss of

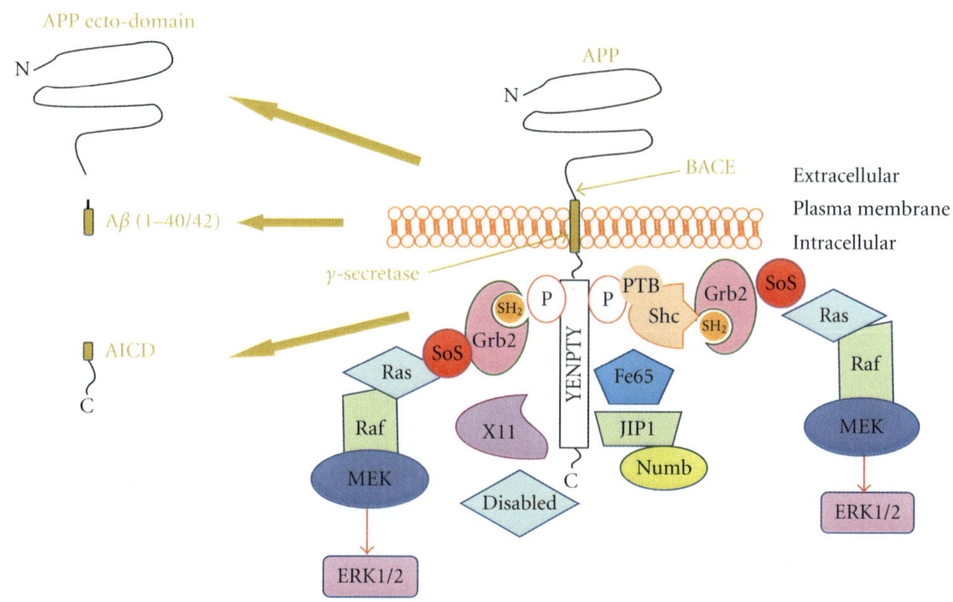

Figure 1: Schematic representation of AβPP processing, the adaptor proteins interacting with its intracellular domain and the pathway leading to ERK1/2 activation. In the left panels is reported the transmembrane protein APP, before and after ITS sequential beta secretase (BACE) and gamma secretase cleavage, with its final products, AICD, APP ectodomain, and beta amyloid peptide (1–40/1–42). In the right part of the figure are indicated the protein interacting with APP intracellular domain, upon or independently from tyrosine phosphorylation. The adaptor proteins Shc and Grb2 through their phosphotyrosine-binding domain (PTB) and src homology domain (SH2) are able to directly bind tyrosine-phosphorylated APP, resulting in the recruitment of the components of the MAP kinase cascade (SoS, ras, Raf, MEK) leading to ERK1/2 activation. Grb2 may participate in this pathway either by direct binding to APP or being recruited by Shc. Alteration in ERK1/2 activity induced in this way may contribute to neurodegeneration in AD. Transduction pathway adaptors (X11, disabled, Fe65, JIP1, and Numb) that bind APP in the absence of tyrosine phosphorylation depicted are also shown.

the mutant protein's ability to support γ-secretase activity rather than an absolute or relative overproduction of Aβ42 [6]. Hence, a loss of function can be associated to a shift of the cleavage specificity (Aβ42 at the cost of Aβ40), or to another unknown target substrate of the γ-secretase activity. In this case, the loss of PS function may be a primary event, in the adult mammalian brain, triggering a putative pathogenic cascade which leads to neurodegeneration in AD [7].

Several studies suggest a relevant role for AβPP in maintaining active synapses, and recent evidence has indicated the presence of AβPP in the postsynaptic density, where it may interact with NMDA receptors, thus supporting the observation that NMDA receptors regulated trafficking and processing of AβPP, although *via* a controversial mechanism of action [8].

Moreover, recent findings have also suggested that AβPP, through an NPTY motif located in its cytodomain, and PSs form functional complexes with different signaling protein, supporting the hypothesis that AβPP and PS1 are at the centre of a complex network of interactions, likely involved in multiple cell-signaling events which are still unknown (Figures 1 and 2) [9, 10]. Even apolipoprotein E (ApoE), which is the most relevant risk factor for developing late-onset AD, rather than being a mere Aβ chaperone, might be involved in complex-signaling pathways through its multiple receptors (LRPs), such as those bearing to the low-density lipoprotein receptor family (LDLR) (for review see [11]). LRPs participate in neuronal functions modulating neurotransmission and thus synaptic stability [12], and several data indicate that LRPs could modulate AβPP processing through the regulation of its endocytic trafficking, implying a possible association between LRPs activity and AD onset (Figure 3) [13]. Taken together, these data suggest a model that links the functions of AβPP, PSs, and LRPs in physiological and pathophysiological conditions as relevant actors in neuronal intracellular signaling.

This review will focus on the involvement of AβPP in cell signaling, exploring the possibility that posttranslational modifications on its C-terminal domain may modulate, together with PSs and LRPs, intracellular pathways involved in cell-cycle progression that in postmitotic neurons may induce neurodegeneration.

2. APP Processing, Interacting Proteins, and Intracellular Signalling

The main amyloid components of senile plaques result from the proteolytic processing of AβPP by β-secretase (BACE1), leading to the formation of C-terminal fragments (CTFs) that are subsequently cleaved by the "γ-secretase-complex" which is responsible for the formation of Aβ (40 or 42 amino acids in length) and the AβPP intracellular domain peptide (AICD) of 58 or 56 amino acids (Figure 1) [1].

These amyloid peptides are considered mainly responsible for the neurodegeneration that occurs in AD. Thus,

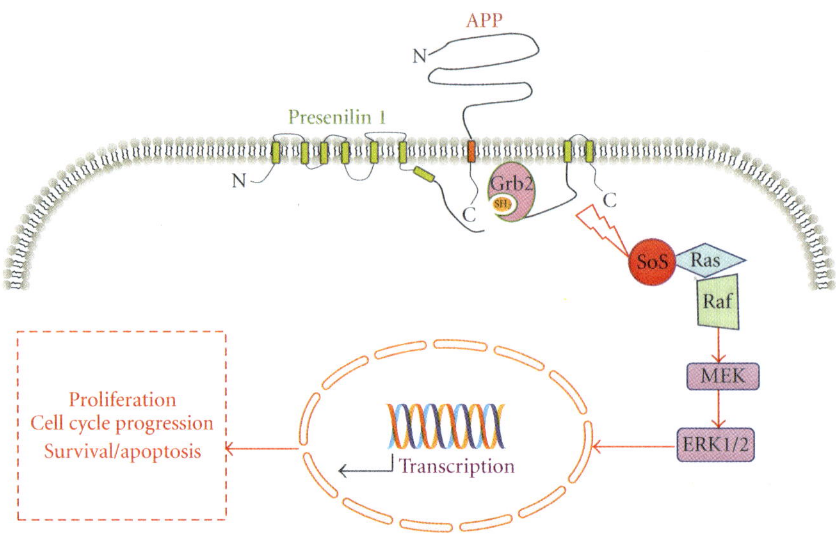

FIGURE 2: Schematic representation of the intracellular pathway by which AβPP and PS1 control the activation of the MAPK/ERK1/2 cascade and their final biological effects. In the figure is specified the interaction between APP intracellular domain and PS1 C-terminus, with the adaptor protein Grb2. Grb2 can bind simultaneously to APP and PS1 (as measured in FRET experiments) leading to the MAPK ERK1/2 cascade activation. In AD an aberrant activation of ERK1/2 induced by APP and/or PS1 can determine the tentative activation of the cell cycle that, in postmitotic neurons, may induce cells to undergo apoptosis.

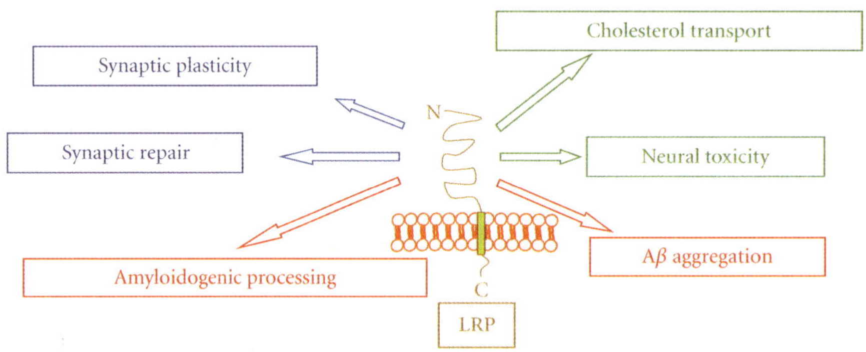

FIGURE 3: Role of LPR8 activation in normal brain functioning and in neurodegeneration during AD. In the figure are indicated the different roles in which LRP8 transmembrane protein is involved, in the healthy brain and AD pathogenesis.

the "amyloid hypothesis" sustains that the first step during AD development is the accumulation and the subsequent deposition of Aβ peptides [1, 2, 10, 14–23].

The generation of Aβ40/42 peptides, by the sequential proteolytic activity of β- and γ-secretases, is enhanced by mutations in AβPP and PSs, and it may be prevented by the action of a third protease, the α-secretase, that cleaves AβPP within the Aβ region, thus resulting in the formation of a different subset of CTFs (α-CTFs) that upon γ-cleavage generate shorter and nonamyloidogenic fragments [24].

However, from the point of view of the signaling activity of CTFs, it is still unclear whether α- and β-stubs or the AICD fragments generated by γ-secretase might represent protective or pathologically related molecule [25].

As far as AICD fragments are concern, it was reported that, after binding Fe65 (Figure 1), an adaptor protein mediating assembly of multimolecular complexes through a variety of protein-interaction domains, and the histone acetyltransferase Tip60, AICD translocate into the nucleus where it acts as gene transcription regulators [24, 26–29]. However, this latter event is still debated, because AICD displays a very short half-life and a poorly characterized *in vivo* transcriptional activity [30].

Recent data have demonstrated that AβPP may signal to the nucleus also using a β-secretase-independent mechanism that involves membrane sequestration and phosphorylation of Tip60 [31].

More recently, Stante et al. have suggested that the presence of Fe65 into the nucleus may have a protective role, and that its translocation depends on AβPP. They propose that DNA repair defects could significantly contribute to the neurodysfunction and neurodegeneration observed in AD, and that an involvement of the Fe65-APP complex in the response of the cells to DNA damage and in the DNA repair machinery could represent a possible mechanism contributing to neuronal degeneration observed in AD pathology [32].

Indeed, new data suggest that, during embryonic development, AICD release, triggered by extracellular signals activating the β-secretase-dependent cleavage, may be involved in the control of neurogenesis [33]. Conversely, Vogt and Coll showed that the overexpression of AICD in mice caused abnormal neuronal networks and increased seizure susceptibility [34]. Other studies demonstrated that AICD may induce the expression of neprilysin, an enzyme known for its specific Aβ-degrading activity, through a direct modulation of its promoter [35].

At the same time, it is noteworthy that the C-terminal portion of AβPP and in particular the last 20 amino acids in the cytoplasmic tail which contains the well-known YENPTY (Figure 1) motif present in several receptor tyrosine kinase (TK) is a docking site for different intracellular proteins involved in signal transduction. Traditionally, this sequence was described as internalization motif, while now it has been recognized to play a central role also in the regulation of multiple interactions with intracellular proteins [9, 36]. In particular, in receptor TK, tyrosine residue can be phosphorylated to generate the NPXpY motif, which represents a docking site for several intracellular adaptor proteins through the phosphortyrosine-binding domain (PTB). Similarly, the adaptor proteins Shc and Grb2 can bind AβPP (or its CTFs) in the presence of phosphorylated tyrosine in this motif (Figure 1). However, AβPP (or its CTFs) and the AβPP-related proteins, APLP1 and APLP2, can also interact with several other signalling proteins, including X11 [37], Fe65 [37, 38], mDab [39], c-Abl [40], JIP-1 [41], and Numb [36, 41], (Figure 1) independently of the phosphorylation of the tyrosine residue within the YENPTY motif. From a functional point of view, the interaction between the neuron-specific adaptor protein Fe65 and AβPP via the second PTB domain of Fe65 [37, 38] was shown to modulate AβPP processing, favoring the generation of Aβ and AβPP trafficking, in several cell lines [26, 42]. Another adaptor that binds to AβPP is mDAB. It is a protein related to the reelin pathway and interacting with YENPTY motif through a PTB domain. mDAB is active during embryogenesis, where it regulates the position of neurons in the brain laminar structure [43], and mDAB binding increases the amounts of mature AβPP and Aβ formation [44]. On the contrary, X11 stabilizes AβPP conformation in membrane, inhibiting Aβ secretion in cultured cells [45], likely impairing AβPP trafficking to sites containing active γ-secretase complexes [46]. JIP's are member of JNK-scaffolding family proteins kinases, implicated in different signal pathway, including neuronal apoptosis. JNK-interacting proteins JIP1b and JIP2 bind to the cytoplasmic tail of AβPP. The expression of JIP1b stabilizes immature AβPP and decreases the AβPP ectodomain, Aβ40/β42 and CTFs abundance [47].

All these observations suggest that some of these protein-protein interactions may play a role in the modulation of the amyloidogenic pathway and thus might have a role in neurodegeneration.

The role of Aβ peptides as unique cause of neuronal toxicity and AD is highly debated, and recent data have challenged the "amyloid only" hypothesis, questioning the role of APP and PSs as mere amyloid productors. The central role of APP and PSs in the genesis of AD is unquestionable; however, phenotypical heterogeneity among patients, and even among familial patients with the same genetic mutation, is commonly observed, implying that other genes might have a role in regulating the onset and severity of the neurodegeneration in FAD and, likely, in sporadic AD. For these reasons, considering that APP and PSs are key players in a complex network of interactions with many different intracellular adaptors, it is tempting to hypothesize that, in parallel to amyloid formation, APP and PSs may induce neurodegeneration through specific alterations in neuronal signaling pathways [48].

In this context, it was reported that other two adaptor proteins, which have been involved in the regulation of the amyloidogenic pathway, ShcA and growth factor receptor-bound protein 2 (Grb2) are able to interact with the cytodomain of AβPP in the presence of specific tyrosine 682 phosphorylation in the YENPTY motif of AβPP cytodomain [36, 49]. ShcA (or ShcC) adaptors connect growth factor receptors to specific signaling pathways (typically Ras/ERK1/2 pathway but also PI3K/Akt signalling) and are involved in cell proliferation differentiation and apoptosis and neuronal development [50, 51]. Also the role of Grb2 in Ras-signaling pathway is well known as well as its involvement in the activation of the mitogen-activated protein kinase (MAPK) pathways cascade (Figures 1 and 2) [50, 52–54]. It is worth noting that ERK1/2 activity is increased in AD brains [55–57] and that activated MAPKs have been involved in the abnormal hyperphosphorylation of Tau in AD [58].

The pathogenic correlation between Shc/Grb2 binding to AβPP during AD development is supported by the observation that the complexes AβPP (or CTFs)/ShcA or Grb2 are significantly increased in AD brain as compared to controls [55]. The increased phosphorylation/activation of ERK1/2, often described in AD brain, is also observed in thrombin-activated astrocytes [55], suggesting that, in this model, ERK1/2 may be activated by AβPP through ShcA. These data give prominence to the biological importance of AβPP phosphorylation for its functions and the regulation of intracellular adaptor binding as events responsible for the induction of glial-associated mitogenic pathway. Furthermore, ERK1/2, activated by Aβ *in vitro*, plays a role in AβPP processing and phosphorylates Tau in a PHF-Tau similar manner [59]. However, it is conceivable that a different signaling Aβ-independent might as well activate tau phosphorylation by ERK1/2 via the intracellular signaling regulated by the AβPP/CTFs-Shc-Grb2 pathway (Figure 1).

AβPP cytodomain also interacts with other proteins directly linked to signal transduction mechanisms. In particular, AβPP binds to the heterotrimeric GTP-binding protein Go [60–63] that comprises up to 1% of all membrane-associated proteins in the developing nervous system [55]. There is evidence that AβPP cytodomain binds proteins involved in cell-cycle regulation such as AβPP-binding protein 1 (APP-BP1) [64] and p-21-activated kinase 3 (PAK3) [65] which is a serine/threonine kinase involved in DNA synthesis and neuronal apoptosis. These data are consistent with a model in which AβPP is a component of a Go multiprotein complex, including PAK3, to transduce extracellular signals to the cytoplasm. In this model, the FAD APP-mediated pathway, leading to tentative neuronal cell-cycle activation (see below), consists of the APP-Go-PAK3 formation, followed by the activation of the AβPP-BP1 through JNK [25].

Considering all these aspects, it is possible to hypothesize that posttranslational modifications of AβPP, or in its CTFs, such as a selective phosphorylation, might couple them, to different cellular pathways. These observation supports the hypothesis that AβPP may act as a receptor/transducer molecule in multiple cell-signaling events, the comprehension of which may have implications either for the normal biological function of AβPP, for its processing and for its pathological role in the genesis of AD [66–68].

3. Presenilins Modulation of Intracellular Signaling

Presenilins 1 and 2 are multitransmembrane proteins that, associated to nicastrin, APH-1 and PEN-2, form high-molecular γ-secretase complex, involved in Aβ production *via* intramembrane cleavage of AβPP (Figures 1 and 2) [69–71]. These proteins are highly expressed in brain but have been detected also in several different tissues. Amount of PSs are localized in the nuclear membrane, kinetochores, and centrosomes [72, 73]. At present more than 182 different mutations (and some deletions) in PS1 have been associated with inherited early onset AD (Alzheimer disease and Frontotemporal Dementia Mutation Database 2006) [56, 74, 75] while only 13 mutations have been found in PS2 that are definitively linked to FAD [15, 16, 76].

Besides their involvement in Aβ formation, PSs regulate the cleavage of other signaling receptors and transducers such as Notch-1, ErbB4, DC44, and LDL-receptor-related proteins and cadherins [1, 69, 77–79]. PSs also affect different other signaling molecules, such as wingless-type MMTV integration site family (Wnt) signal transduction pathway, which is evolutionary conserved and controls many events during the embryogenesis [80]. At cellular level, this pathway regulates morphology, proliferation, and motility of the cell. Wnt pathway plays a central role during tumorigenesis, and the inappropriate activation of this pathway has been observed in several human cancers [81]. It has been shown that Wnt-ligand-mediated signaling leads to the accumulation of cytosolic β-catenin. Cytosolic β-catenin will then translocate into the nucleus to bind to members of the T-cell factor (Tcf)/lymphoid-enhancing factor (Lef) family of DNA-binding proteins leading to the transcription of Wnt target genes. In the absence of Wnt ligand, axin recruits CK1 causing the initiation of the β-catenin phosphorylation cascade by glycogen synthase kinase-3 β (GSK-3β). Phosphorylated β-catenin is recognized by β-transducin repeat-containing protein (β-TrCP) and degraded by the proteosome, reducing the level of cytosolic β-catenin. It was reported that β-catenin interacts with PSs, and that PS1 promotes β-catenin degradation regulating phosphorylation by cyclin-dependent kinase 5 (CDK5) and GSK-3β [82–84]. Importantly, GSK-3β was implicated in various neurological disorders, including AD [85]. Gosal and Coll showed that AICD-overexpressing transgenic mice may have an abnormal activation of GSK-3β. These mice exhibit AD-like characteristics, including hyperphosphorylation and aggregation of tau, neurodegeneration, and working memory deficits that are prevented by treatment with lithium [86].

In cultured cells expressing PSs FAD mutants, the intracellular trafficking of β-catenin is altered, while in cells from PS-null animals cytosolic β-catenin levels and β-catenin-mediated Lef/Tcf signaling are increased [83], thus resulting in the activation of the downstream target cyclin D1 and accelerated entry into the S phase of the cell cycle [87].

Another relevant role for PSs is Notch processing. Notch signaling is involved in cell fate regulation, cell differentiation, proliferation, and apoptosis as well as neurodegeneration [88, 89]. Notch is a membrane receptor whose C-terminal domain (NICD), upon interaction with appropriate ligands, translocates into the nucleus where it activates the CSL family of transcription factors. NICD formation depends on γ-secretase complex as the AICD fragment of AβPP [78].

PSs play a role in apoptosis, since FAD mutants cause cell death or induce secondary events that may lead to apoptosis [90]. Animals, in which PS1 and PS2 genes are deleted, show deficit in learning, memory, synaptic function and neuronal death [91]. The processes beneath these effects are unknown, but the findings that PS1 interacts with anti-apoptotic member of Bcl-2 family might indicate a possible mechanism [92, 93].

PS1 is also essential for efficient N-cadherin trafficking from ER to plasma membrane. Cadherins, including E-cadherin and neuronal cadherin (N-cadherin), are a family of type I transmembrane proteins that mediate Ca^{2+}-dependent cell-cell adhesion, and recognition [94, 95]. PS1-mediated delivery of N-cadherin to the plasma membrane is important to exert its physiological function, including the control of the state of cell-cell contact [96].

PS1 is involved in the intramembrane cleavage of CD44, a cell surface adhesion molecule for the extracellular matrix components which is implicated in a wide variety of physiological and pathological processes including the regulation of tumor cell growth and metastasis [70].

Recently, also the low-density receptor-related protein (LRP) has been shown to be cleaved by a γ-secretase-like activity [97]. It is important to note that LRPs receptors are activated by apolipoprotein E, a well-known risk factor for the developing of late onset AD in carriers of the ε_4 alleles [98, 99]. It is, however, still unknown if the processing by γ-secretase and the apolipoprotein E-mediated signaling on neuronal LRPs might modulate a single pathway, and which is the physiological significance for these processes.

PS1 also modulates basal level of ERK1/2 activity through a ras-Raf-MEK-dependent pathway activated by a direct binding with the SH2 domain of Grb2 (Figure 2) [100–102]. ERK family is one of the most ubiquitous cellular signaling mechanisms, whose activation links extracellular stimuli to cell proliferation, survival, and differentiation, but also cell death and apoptosis [103–105]. In this respect, it is worth of note to observe, as mentioned above, that ERK1/2 pathway is also modulated by AβPP (Figures 1 and 2).

Taken together, these data suggest that PS1 and/or AβPP are able to modulate different intracellular signalling pathway through a plethora of intracellular mediators; when the signaling activated by PS1 and AβPP become dysfunctional in neurons, in particular the activation of the cell cycle-machinery induced by ERK1/2, the neurodegenerative process may be activated (Figure 2).

4. AβPP, Presenilins, and Cell Cycle

The hypothesis that cell-cycle abnormalities and aberrant neuron cell-cycle reentering may cause neuronal death in AD is supported by different experimental findings including AD patients brain analysis and data obtained by *in vitro* experiments.

Chromosome missegregation and trisomy 21 mosaicism have been associated with mutations in AβPP and PSs [72]. Aberrant expression of cell-cycle proteins and tetraploidy in neurons from AD patients have been described [106]. In AD brains, the activation of several cell-cycle components has been detected, including cdc2, cdk4, p16, Ki-67, cyclin B1 and cyclin D, p25 (the regulatory subunit of cdk5) [107, 108], as well as the increased expression activity of genes encoding for cell-cycle proteins [109]. It was observed that hippocampal pyramidal and basal forebrain neurons, in AD brain show markers of DNA replication [110], and it was speculated that the state of tetraploidy is lethal to neurons [110].

Increasing observations suggest that aberrant activation of cell cycle may affect the formation of neurofibrillary tangles with hyperphosphorylation of Tau protein in AD brain. It is well known that p25/cdk5 complex hyperphosphorylates Tau and reduces its ability to associate with microtubules [107]. On the other hand, cell-cycle activation can lead to apoptosis [108], and several studies showed the activation of caspases in AD brain [111–113]. Finally, cell-cycle defects represent a major neuropathological feature also in transgenic animal models of AD [108, 110, 114, 115].

As previously discussed [73], AβPP regulates ERK1/2 levels, its phosphorylation/translocation to the centrosome, and cell proliferation rate.

Additionally, in the same study, we showed that also PS1 interacts with Grb2 in the centrosomes and modulates ERK1/2 signaling. Thus, the proposed hypothesis is that both AβPP and PS1 participate in the same signaling pathway through Grb2 binding. Since many regulatory molecules are found at centrosomes, it was postulated that centrosomes might serve as signaling machinery modulating different cell functions [98]. In particular, since Grb2, AβPP, PS1, and pERK1/2 are all detectable in mitotic centrosomes, it is conceivable that these structures might anchor signal transduction pathways, integrate signals, and facilitate its conversion, into cellular functions (Figure 2).

In this scenario, it was proposed that PS1 and AβPP may determine the activation of ERK1/2 that, in turn, was responsible for the initiation of the cell cycle [73]; when these events occur in postmitotic neurons, the impossibility to complete cell division leads inevitably to neuronal apoptosis.

5. AβPP, Presenilins, and LRPs

Low-density lipoprotein receptors (LDLRs) are type I integral membrane proteins currently composed of 10 members. LDLR possesses a wide array of ligands with different functions from cellular cholesterol uptake in the liver to cell specification and neuronal positioning during embryogenesis. ApoE, complexed in HDL and VLDL, is the major ligand for these receptors, and, being the ε_4 allele of APOE gene, the most relevant risk for the development of late-onset AD, several studies support a role for these receptors in the pathogenesis of AD [116]. Although the molecular mechanisms underlying the association between ApoE alleles and AD development have not yet been completely elucidated, ApoE, along with its receptor-LDLR and LDL-receptors related protein (LRP), was reported to modulate Aβ production and clearance. Lack of LDLRs increased amyloid deposition and impaired cognitive behavior in AD transgenic mice [117]. ApoE colocalizes in amyloid deposits in brain parenchyma [118], and its lipidation state affects the ability to bind Aβ [119].

Beside its role as Aβ chaperone, ApoE might modulate specific internalization and signaling events via binding to its receptors. Some of them possess shared adaptors with AβPP; in particular Fe65 and JIP1 bind to LRP8, LRP1, and megalin. Indeed γ-secretase cleavage regulates the intramembrane proteolysis of LRP8, LRP1, and of SOR-1/LRP11. It is tempting to speculate that LRPs could affect AβPP processing and signaling (and vice versa) through γ-secretase and ApoE-mediated stimuli.

LRPs possess at least one NPxY motif in their cytoplasmic tail (except SOR-1/LRP11), and this motif, present in AβPP as well, is critically required for receptor interaction with adaptors proteins and for internalization. It has been recently demonstrated that several LRPs family members modulate AβPP processing by affecting different aspects of AβPP trafficking [120]. For example, LRP8 is a member of the LDLR family that is highly expressed in the brain [121]. It has been recently proposed that the physiological role of LRP8 might include the regulation of signal transduction pathways rather than endocytosis of lipoproteins and other ligands [116]. It is known that LRP8 interacts with AβPP, enhancing the level of AβPP at the cell surface, and reducing its internalization [122, 123]. Overexpression of LRP8 induces an increase in AβPP association with lipid rafts and decreases AβPP-CTFs levels [116].

ApoE was reported to induce Dab1 phosphorylation and ERK1/2 activation and JNK inhibition *via* LRPs. This pathway depends on the presence of Ca^{++} influx through the NMDA receptor, but it is independent of Dab1 [124].

Overall these data indicate a likely involvement of LRP8 as modulator of AβPP processing, by affecting its endocytic trafficking and the proportion of AβPP present in lipid rafts. These events may have consequence on the γ-secretase-mediated cleavage of AβPP and on its neurodegeneration-related signaling activity.

Upon binding, LRP8 transduces reelin signaling during neuronal development [125], and recent evidence has indicated that it interacts with the NR2A and NR2B subunits of NMDA receptor [126], being involved in neuronal functions such as maturation of NMDA receptor composition in the hippocampus, and the regulation of long-term potentiation [127]. Importantly, it has been determined that LRP8 ligand reelin is found in neuritic plaques of transgenic mice overexpressing AβPP [128], suggesting a possible association with AD. Subsequently, a novel interaction between reelin and AβPP was discovered, leading to increase in the cell surface levels of AβPP and affecting AβPP processing and Aβ production [8]. It was shown that reelin signaling in excitatory synapses can restore normal synaptic plasticity, which is impaired by oligomeric Aβ peptides at concentrations within the range detectable in the brains of AD patients. At high concentrations of Aβ peptides, reelin can no longer overcome the Aβ-induced functional suppression, and this condition coincides with a complete blockade of the reelin-dependent phosphorylation of NR2 subunits in NMDA receptors. This reversal requires the LRP receptor-dependent activation of tyrosine kinases of the Src family. It was proposed a model in which Aβ, reelin, and LRP receptors modulate neurotransmission and thus synaptic stability as opposing regulators of synaptic gain [12]. A schematic representation of potential roles of LRPs in normal brain function and in neurodegenerative processes is depicted in Figure 3.

6. Small Nuclear RNA in AD

Recent discoveries in molecular genetics of mammalian genome have shed light on a widespread transcription of noncoding regions, devoted to the regulation of the protein-coding genome expression. The mechanisms of action of these transcripts are various and different in nature, although all of them are devoted to the regulation of fundamental genetic pathways involved in the determination of the cell phenotype [129–132].

Alternative splicing is a central component of human brain complexity whose regulatory mechanisms are still largely unclear. The recent discovery of factors that control alternative splicing might contribute to clarify the molecular basis of physiological and pathological processes [133]. In two recent works, we described the discovery of two novel RNA polymerase III-dependent, noncoding RNAs (ncRNA) transcripts, named 17A and 38A. In particular, it was shown that the expression of 17A induces an alternative splicing of GABA-B2 receptor leading to the formation of a non-functional protein. The ncRNA 17A is normally expressed in the human brain but is highly upregulated in the brain of AD patients. The stable expression of 17A in SH-SY5Y neuroblastoma cells enhances the secretion of Aβ and the Aβ x-42/Aβ x-40 peptide ratio. Indeed the synthesis of 17A is upregulated in response to inflammatory stimuli, suggesting that it may be induced by AD-related inflammation and that it could contribute to neurodegeneration in AD [134].

In the other study, we found that IL1-α-dependent up-regulation of another ncRNA, named 38A, drives the synthesis of an alternatively spliced form of the potassium channel-interacting protein (KCNIP4). The alternative KCNIP4 isoform cannot interact with the γ-secretase complex, resulting in modification of γ-secretase activity, AβPP processing, and increased secretion of β-amyloid enriched in the more toxic Aβ x-42 species.

This alternative splicing shift is observed at high frequency in tissue from AD patients, suggesting that RNA polymerase III transcribed ncRNA may be upstream determinants of alternative splicing of significantly proteins involved in the brain homeostasis and that their inflammation-dependent overexpression may induce alterations in the Aβ production contributing to the neurodegeneration during AD development [135].

In this context, a more detailed investigation of ncRNA functional mechanisms might allow to identify new molecular connections with neurodegenerative diseases like those identified in AD.

7. Environmental Factors and AD Pathoetiology

In recent years, several data have showed evidence that environmental and/or nutritional factors may play a causal, disruptive, and/or protective role in the development of AD although the initiating molecular events are not entirely known. While a direct causal role for aluminum or other transition metals (copper, zinc, and iron) in AD has not yet been definitively demonstrated, epidemiological evidence suggests that elevated levels of these metals in the brain may be linked to the development or progression of the neurodegenerative processes during AD [136].

Aluminum role in AD has been investigated for decades. Recent studies have identified aluminum in early neurofibrillary tangle (NFT) of hippocampal CA1 neurons from brains of aged patients [137]. However, aluminum contribution to AD remains controversial, lacking physiological mechanistic role.

Iron deposition in the brain is another important proposed mechanisms in the pathophysiology AD. Excessive iron can contribute to the formation of free radicals, leading to lipid peroxidation and neurotoxicity, which can result in cell membrane damage and cell death [138]. Recently, it has been shown that iron concentration in AD patients brain was significantly higher than those of nondemented controls. In particular iron deposition in parietal cortex and hippocampus at the early stage of AD were positively correlated with the severity of patients cognitive impairment [139].

Also zinc was reported to accelerate the aggregation of the Aβ peptides and to play a role in the control of inflammatory responses. Inflammation clearly occurs in pathologically vulnerable regions of the AD brain with increased expression of acute phase proteins and proinflammatory cytokines which are hardly evident in normal brain and that could participate in the induction of neuronal death. In particular, cytokine expression may be regulated by zinc availability, so influencing inflammatory network phenotypic expression [140].

New lines of study show that lead exposures in early life has been implicated in subsequent progression of amyloidogenesis in rodents during old age. This exposure resulted in an increase in proteins associated with AD pathology: AβPP and Aβ peptide [141].

Recent work has shown that *in vitro* metal ligands such as clioquinol (CQ) increase the intracellular level of copper. The increase in intracellular copper was correlated with a dramatic and rapid decrease in levels of extracellular Aβ including Aβ1–40 and 1–42 [142]. It has been previously reported that CQ/copper complexes trigger the activation of PI3K and its downstream modulator Akt and the inhibition of glycogen synthase kinase 3 that in turn potentiated ERK1/2 phosphorylation [143, 144].

It is not clear if and how environmental factors take part to pathway discussed in this review, in which both AβPP and PS1 participate in the same signaling pathway leading, through Grb2 binding, to ERK1/2 activation and neurodegeneration. However, we may speculate that ERK1/2 activation by copper may contribute to the signal transduction system activated by AβPP, and PSs.

8. Concluding Remarks

The toxicity of Aβ peptides, eventually triggered or modulated by environmental or genetic factors, is a central dogma in AD genesis, which has been recently challenged by new achievements [48]. In particular, AβPP and PS1 participate in a plethora of protein-protein interactions and signaling pathways, suggesting that beside their implication for amyloid formation might also modulate specific cell signaling events involved in neuronal homeostasis that in a pathological context may lead to neurodegeneration.

In this scenario, it is under investigation the possible contribution of other receptors, such as LRPs, which interact with AβPP, could modulate its processing, are often target of γ-secretase cleavage, and share with AβPP relevant adaptors such as Fe65 and JIP1. It is tempting to hypothesize that the role of ApoE isoform 4 in AD, rather than being linked only to Aβ formation and clearing, might be also due to a specific receptor-mediated function which hampers AβPP physiological signaling and homeostatic control. In this vision, a unique pathway in which ApoE isoform 4, LRPs, AβPP, and PSs share common signal transduction events may represent the keystone that may explain Aβ formation and neurodegeneration.

We would like to underline that, among these events, AβPP and PSs may affect ERK1/2 signaling through ShcA/Grb2 transduction system, with a net relevance for cell-cycle regulation that in postmitotic neurons may lead to cell death. Also some LRPs, as possible modulators of AβPP processing by affecting its endocytic trafficking and the proportion of AβPP present in lipid rafts, as well as the activity of the γ-secretase complex, could modulate ERK1/2 signaling via ShcA/Grb2 or through parallel pathways.

A parallel and complementary issue is given by the brain complexity and by the largely unexplored world of noncoding genome. The tip of the iceberg hides potentially relevant genomic control systems that may explain the widespread phenotypic variability, even among familial patients, observed in AD.

A more deep understanding of these complexes mechanism is necessary, in order to open new prospects for therapeutic applications in neurodegenerative disorders.

References

[1] T. E. Golde and C. B. Eckman, "Physiologic and pathologic events mediated by intramembranous and juxtamembranous proteolysis," *Science's STKE*, vol. 2003, no. 172, p. RE4, 2003.

[2] D. J. Selkoe and M. B. Podlisny, "Deciphering the genetic basis of Alzheimer's disease," *Annual Review of Genomics and Human Genetics*, vol. 3, pp. 67–99, 2002.

[3] J. Hardy and D. J. Selkoe, "The amyloid hypothesis of Alzheimer's disease: progress and problems on the road to therapeutics," *Science*, vol. 297, no. 5580, pp. 353–356, 2002.

[4] D. J. Selkoe and M. S. Wolfe, "Presenilin: running with scissors in the membrane," *Cell*, vol. 131, no. 2, pp. 215–221, 2007.

[5] M. S. Wolfe, "When loss is gain: reduced presenilin proteolytic function leads to increased Aβ42/Aβ40. Talking point on the role of presenilin mutations in Alzheimer disease," *EMBO Reports*, vol. 8, no. 2, pp. 136–140, 2007.

[6] E. A. Heilig, W. Xia, J. Shen, and R. J. Kelleher, "A presenilin-1 mutation identified in familial Alzheimer disease with cotton wool plaques causes a nearly complete loss of γ-secretase activity," *Journal of Biological Chemistry*, vol. 285, no. 29, pp. 22350–22359, 2010.

[7] J. Shen and R. J. Kelleher III, "The presenilin hypothesis of Alzheimer's disease: evidence for a loss-of-function pathogenic mechanism," *Proceedings of the National Academy of Sciences of the United States of America*, vol. 104, no. 2, pp. 403–409, 2007.

[8] H. S. Hoe, Z. Fu, A. Makarova et al., "The effects of amyloid precursor protein on postsynaptic composition and activity," *Journal of Biological Chemistry*, vol. 284, no. 13, pp. 8495–8506, 2009.

[9] E. F. da Cruz e Silva and O. A. da Cruz e Silva, "Protein phosphorylation and APP metabolism," *Neurochemical Research*, vol. 28, no. 10, pp. 1553–1561, 2003.

[10] B. De Strooper and W. Annaert, "Proteolytic processing and cell biological functions of the amyloid precursor protein," *Journal of Cell Science*, vol. 113, no. 11, pp. 1857–1870, 2000.

[11] G. Bu, "Apolipoprotein e and its receptors in Alzheimer's disease: pathways, pathogenesis and therapy," *Nature Reviews Neuroscience*, vol. 10, no. 5, pp. 333–344, 2009.

[12] M. S. Durakoglugil, Y. Chen, C. L. White, E. T. Kavalali, and J. Herz, "Reelin signaling antagonizes β-amyloid at the synapse," *Proceedings of the National Academy of Sciences of the United States of America*, vol. 106, no. 37, pp. 15938–15943, 2009.

[13] T. Wagner and C. U. Pietrzik, "The role of lipoprotein receptors on the physiological function of APP," *Experimental Brain Research*. In press.

[14] T. E. Golde, "Alzheimer disease therapy: can the amyloid cascade be halted?" *Journal of Clinical Investigation*, vol. 111, no. 1, pp. 11–18, 2003.

[15] E. Levy-Lahad, W. Wasco, P. Poorkaj et al., "Candidate gene for the chromosome 1 familial Alzheimer's disease locus," *Science*, vol. 269, no. 5226, pp. 973–977, 1995.

[16] E. I. Rogaev, R. Sherrington, E. A. Rogaeva et al., "Familial Alzheimer's disease in kindreds with missense mutations in a gene on chromosome 1 related to the Alzheimer's disease type 3 gene," *Nature*, vol. 376, no. 6543, pp. 775–778, 1995.

[17] L. Bertram, M. Hiltunen, M. Parkinson et al., "Family-based association between alzheimer's disease and variants in UBQLN1," *The New England Journal of Medicine*, vol. 352, no. 9, pp. 884–894, 2005.

[18] L. Bertram, M. Hsiao, M. B. McQueen et al., "The LDLR locus in alzheimer's disease: a family-based study and meta-analysis of case-control data," *Neurobiology of Aging*, vol. 28, no. 1, pp. e4–e1, 2007.

[19] L. Bertram, M. Hsiao, K. Mullin et al., "ACAT1 is not associated with Alzheimer's disease in two independent family-based samples," *Molecular Psychiatry*, vol. 10, no. 6, pp. 522–524, 2005.

[20] L. Bertram, M. Parkinson, M. B. McQueen et al., "Further evidence for LBP-1c/CP2/LSF association in Alzheimer's disease families," *Journal of Medical Genetics*, vol. 42, no. 11, pp. 857–862, 2005.

[21] L. Bertram and R. E. Tanzi, "The genetic epidemiology of neurodegenerative disease," *Journal of Clinical Investigation*, vol. 115, no. 6, pp. 1449–1457, 2005.

[22] B. C. Dickerson, D. H. Salat, D. N. Greve et al., "Increased hippocampal activation in mild cognitive impairment compared to normal aging and AD," *Neurology*, vol. 65, no. 3, pp. 404–411, 2005.

[23] R. E. Tanzi and L. Bertram, "Twenty years of the Alzheimer's disease amyloid hypothesis: a genetic perspective," *Cell*, vol. 120, no. 4, pp. 545–555, 2005.

[24] N. Zambrano, J. D. Buxbaum, G. Minopoli et al., "Interaction of the phosphotyrosine interaction/phosphotyrosine binding-related domains of Fe65 with wild-type and mutant Alzheimer's β-amyloid precursor proteins," *Journal of Biological Chemistry*, vol. 272, no. 10, pp. 6399–6405, 1997.

[25] R. L. Neve and D. L. McPhie, "The cell cycle as a therapeutic target for Alzheimer's disease," *Pharmacology and Therapeutics*, vol. 111, no. 1, pp. 99–113, 2006.

[26] K. Ando, K. I. Iijima, J. I. Elliott, Y. Kirino, and T. Suzuki, "Phosphorylation-dependent regulation of the interaction of amyloid precursor protein with Fe65 affects the production of β-amyloid," *Journal of Biological Chemistry*, vol. 276, no. 43, pp. 40353–40361, 2001.

[27] X. Cao and T. C. Sudhof, "A transcriptively active complex of APP with Fe65 and histone acetyltransferase Tip60," *Science*, vol. 293, no. 5534, Article ID 1436, 2001.

[28] X. Cao and T. C. Sudhof, "Dissection of amyloid-β precursor protein-dependent transcriptional transactivation," *Journal of Biological Chemistry*, vol. 279, no. 23, pp. 24601–24611, 2004.

[29] A. Kinoshita, C. M. Whelan, C. J. Smith, O. Berezovska, and B. T. Hyman, "Direct visualization of the gamma secretase-generated carboxyl-terminal domain of the amyloid precursor protein: association with Fe65 and translocation to the nucleus," *Journal of Neurochemistry*, vol. 82, no. 4, pp. 839–847, 2002.

[30] S. S. Hebert, L. Serneels, A. Tolia et al., "Regulated intramembrane proteolysis of amyloid precursor protein and regulation of expression of putative target genes," *EMBO Reports*, vol. 7, no. 7, pp. 739–745, 2006.

[31] M. R. Hass and B. A. Yankner, "A γ-secretase-independent mechanism of signal transduction by the amyloid precursor protein," *Journal of Biological Chemistry*, vol. 280, no. 44, pp. 36895–36904, 2005.

[32] M. Stante, G. Minopoli, F. Passaro, M. Raia, L. D. Vecchio, and T. Russo, "Fe65 is required for Tip60-directed histone H4 acetylation at DNA strand breaks," *Proceedings of the National Academy of Sciences of the United States of America*, vol. 106, no. 13, pp. 5093–5098, 2009.

[33] Q. H. Ma, T. Futagawa, W. L. Yang et al., "A TAG1-APP signalling pathway through Fe65 negatively modulates neurogenesis," *Nature Cell Biology*, vol. 10, no. 3, pp. 283–294, 2008.

[34] D. L. Vogt, D. Thomas, V. Galvan, D. E. Bredesen, B. T. Lamb, and S. W. Pimplikar, "Abnormal neuronal networks and seizure susceptibility in mice overexpressing the APP intracellular domain," *Neurobiology of Aging*, vol. 32, no. 9, pp. 1725–1729, 2009.

[35] N. D. Belyaev, N. N. Nalivaeva, N. Z. Makova, and A. J. Turner, "Neprilysin gene expression requires binding of the amyloid precursor protein intracellular domain to its promoter: implications for Alzheimer disease," *EMBO Reports*, vol. 10, no. 1, pp. 94–100, 2009.

[36] P. E. Tarr, R. Roncarati, G. Pelicci, P. G. Pelicci, and L. D'Adamio, "Tyrosine phosphorylation of the β-amyloid precursor protein cytoplasmic tail promotes interaction with Shc," *Journal of Biological Chemistry*, vol. 277, no. 19, pp. 16798–16804, 2002.

[37] J. P. Borg, J. Ooi, E. Levy, and B. Margolis, "The phosphotyrosine interaction domains of X11 and FE65 bind to distinct sites on the YENPTY motif of amyloid precursor protein," *Molecular and Cellular Biology*, vol. 16, no. 11, pp. 6229–6241, 1996.

[38] F. Fiore, N. Zambrano, G. Minopoli, V. Donini, A. Duilio, and T. Russo, "The regions of the Fe65 protein homologous to the phosphotyrosine interaction/phosphotyrosine binding domain of Shc bind the intracellular domain of the Alzheimer's amyloid precursor protein," *Journal of Biological Chemistry*, vol. 270, no. 52, pp. 30853–30856, 1995.

[39] B. W. Howell, L. M. Lanier, R. Frank, F. B. Gertler, and J. A. Cooper, "The disabled 1 phosphotyrosine-binding domain binds to the internalization signals of transmembrane glycoproteins and to phospholipids," *Molecular and Cellular Biology*, vol. 19, no. 7, pp. 5179–5188, 1999.

[40] N. Zambrano, P. Bruni, G. Minopoli et al., "The β-amyloid precursor protein APP is tyrosine-phosphorylated in cells expressing a constitutively active form of the Abl protoncogene," *Journal of Biological Chemistry*, vol. 276, no. 23, pp. 19787–19792, 2001.

[41] M. H. Scheinfeld, R. Roncarati, P. Vito, P. A. Lopez, M. Abdallah, and L. D'Adamio, "Jun NH2-terminal kinase (JNK) interacting protein 1 (JIP1) binds the cytoplasmic domain of the Alzheimer's β-amyloid precursor protein (APP)," *Journal of Biological Chemistry*, vol. 277, no. 5, pp. 3767–3775, 2002.

[42] S. L. Sabo, A. F. Ikin, J. D. Buxbaum, and P. Greengard, "The Alzheimer amyloid precursor protein (APP) and FE65, an APP-binding protein, regulate cell movement," *Journal of Cell Biology*, vol. 153, no. 7, pp. 1403–1414, 2001.

[43] B. W. Howell, R. Hawkes, P. Soriano, and J. A. Cooper, "Neuronal position in the developing brain is regulated by mouse disabled-1," *Nature*, vol. 389, no. 6652, pp. 733–737, 1997.

[44] L. Parisiadou and S. Efthimiopoulos, "Expression of mDab1 promotes the stability and processing of amyloid precursor protein and this effect is counteracted by X11α," *Neurobiology of Aging*, vol. 28, no. 3, pp. 377–388, 2007.

[45] J. P. Borg, Y. Yang, M. De Taddeo-Borg, B. Margolis, and R. S. Turner, "The X11α protein slows cellular amyloid precursor protein processing and reduces aβ40 and aβ42 secretion," *Journal of Biological Chemistry*, vol. 273, no. 24, pp. 14761–14766, 1998.

[46] B. Rogelj, J. C. Mitchell, C. C. Miller, and D. M. McLoughlin, "The X11/Mint family of adaptor proteins," *Brain Research Reviews*, vol. 52, no. 2, pp. 305–315, 2006.

[47] H. Taru, Y. Kirino, and T. Suzuki, "Differential roles of JIP scaffold proteins in the modulation of amyloid precursor protein metabolism," *Journal of Biological Chemistry*, vol. 277, no. 30, pp. 27567–27574, 2002.

[48] J. Hardy, "The amyloid hypothesis for Alzheimer's disease: a critical reappraisal," *Journal of Neurochemistry*, vol. 110, no. 4, pp. 1129–1134, 2009.

[49] D. Zhou, C. Noviello, C. D'Ambrosio, A. Scaloni, and L. D'Adamio, "Growth factor receptor-bound protein 2 interaction with the tyrosine-phosphorylated tail of amyloid β precursor protein is mediated by its Src homology 2 domain," *Journal of Biological Chemistry*, vol. 279, no. 24, pp. 25374–25380, 2004.

[50] E. Cattaneo and P. G. Pelicci, "Emerging roles for SH2/PTB-containing Shc adaptor proteins in the developing mammalian brain," *Trends in Neurosciences*, vol. 21, no. 11, pp. 476–481, 1998.

[51] L. Luzi, S. Confalonieri, P. P. Di Fiore, and P. G. Pelicci, "Evolution of Shc functions from nematode to human," *Current Opinion in Genetics and Development*, vol. 10, no. 6, pp. 668–674, 2000.

[52] D. Dankort, B. Maslikowski, N. Warner et al., "Grb2 and Shc adapter proteins play distinct roles in Neu (ErbB-2)-induced mammary tumorigenesis: implications for human breast cancer," *Molecular and Cellular Biology*, vol. 21, no. 5, pp. 1540–1551, 2001.

[53] L. A. Puto, K. Pestonjamasp, C. C. King, and G. M. Bokoch, "p21-activated kinase 1 (PAK1) interacts with the Grb2 adapter protein to couple to growth factor signaling," *Journal of Biological Chemistry*, vol. 278, no. 11, pp. 9388–9393, 2003.

[54] V. Venezia, M. Nizzari, E. Repetto et al., "Amyloid precursor protein modulates ERK-1 and -2 signaling," *Annals of the New York Academy of Sciences*, vol. 1090, pp. 455–465, 2006.

[55] C. Russo, V. Dolcini, S. Salis et al., "Signal transduction through tyrosine-phosphorylated C-terminal fragments of amyloid precursor protein via an enhanced interaction with Shc/Grb2 adaptor proteins in reactive astrocytes of Alzheimer's disease brain," *Journal of Biological Chemistry*, vol. 277, no. 38, pp. 35282–35288, 2002.

[56] C. Russo, V. Venezia, S. Salis, V. Dolcini, and G. Schettini, "Molecular aspects of neurodegeneration in Alzheimer's disease," *Functional Neurology*, vol. 17, no. 2, pp. 65–70, 2002.

[57] C. Russo, E. Violani, S. Salis et al., "Pyroglutamate-modified amyloid β-peptides—aβN3(pE)—strongly affect cultured neuron and astrocyte survival," *Journal of Neurochemistry*, vol. 82, no. 6, pp. 1480–1489, 2002.

[58] H. M. Roder, P. A. Eden, and V. M. Ingram, "Brain protein kinase PK40(erk) converts TAU into a PHF-like form as found in Alzheimer's disease," *Biochemical and Biophysical Research Communications*, vol. 193, no. 2, pp. 639–647, 1993.

[59] S. Guise, D. Braguer, G. Carles, A. Delacourte, and C. Briand, "Hyperphosphorylation of tau is mediated by erk activation during anticancer drug-induced apoptosis in neuroblastoma cells," *Journal of Neuroscience Research*, vol. 63, no. 3, pp. 257–267, 2001.

[60] E. Brouillet, A. Trembleau, D. Galanaud et al., "The amyloid precursor protein interacts with G(o) heterotrimeric protein within a cell compartment specialized in signal transduction," *Journal of Neuroscience*, vol. 19, no. 5, pp. 1717–1727, 1999.

[61] B. T. Edmonds, C. R. Moomaw, J. T. Hsu, C. Slaughter, and L. Ellis, "The p38 and p34 polypeptides of growth cone particle membranes are the α- and β-subunits of G proteins," *Developmental Brain Research*, vol. 56, no. 1, pp. 131–136, 1990.

[62] U. Giambarella, T. Yamatsuji, T. Okamoto et al., "G protein βγ complex-mediated apoptosis by familial Alzheimer's disease mutant of APP," *The EMBO Journal*, vol. 16, no. 16, pp. 4897–4907, 1997.

[63] I. Nishimoto, T. Okamoto, Y. Matsuura et al., "Alzheimer amyloid protein precursor complexes with brain GTP-binding protein G(o)," *Nature*, vol. 362, no. 6415, pp. 75–79, 1993.

[64] N. Chow, J. R. Korenberg, X. N. Chen, and R. L. Neve, "APP-BP1, a novel protein that binds to the carboxyl-terminal region of the amyloid precursor protein," *Journal of Biological Chemistry*, vol. 271, no. 19, pp. 11339–11346, 1996.

[65] D. L. McPhie, R. Coopersmith, A. Hines-Peralta et al., "DNA synthesis and neuronal apoptosis caused by familial Alzheimer disease mutants of the amyloid precursor protein are mediated by the p21 activated kinase PAK3," *Journal of Neuroscience*, vol. 23, no. 17, pp. 6914–6927, 2003.

[66] M. Nizzari, V. Venezia, P. Bianchini et al., "Amyloid precursor protein and presenilin 1 interaction studied by FRET in human H4 cells," *Annals of the New York Academy of Sciences*, vol. 1096, pp. 249–257, 2007.

[67] V. Venezia, M. Nizzari, P. Carlo, A. Corsaro, T. Florio, and C. Russo, "Amyloid precursor protein and presenilin involvement in cell signaling," *Neurodegenerative Diseases*, vol. 4, no. 2-3, pp. 101–111, 2007.

[68] V. Venezia, C. Russo, E. Repetto et al., "Apoptotic cell death and amyloid precursor protein signaling in neuroblastoma SH-SY5Y cells," *Annals of the New York Academy of Sciences*, vol. 1030, pp. 339–347, 2004.

[69] B. De Strooper, "Aph-1, Pen-2, and nicastrin with presenilin generate an active γ-secretase complex," *Neuron*, vol. 38, no. 1, pp. 9–12, 2003.

[70] D. Murakami, I. Okamoto, O. Nagano et al., "Presenilin-dependent γ-secretase activity mediates the intramembranous cleavage of CD44," *Oncogene*, vol. 22, no. 10, pp. 1511–1516, 2003.

[71] D. J. Selkoe, "Presenilin, notch, and the genesis and treatment of Alzheimer's disease," *Proceedings of the National Academy of Sciences of the United States of America*, vol. 98, no. 20, pp. 11039–11041, 2001.

[72] J. Li, M. Xu, H. Zhou, J. Ma, and H. Potter, "Alzheimer presenilins in the nuclear membrane, interphase kinetochores, and centrosomes suggest a role in chromosome segregation," *Cell*, vol. 90, no. 5, pp. 917–927, 1997.

[73] M. Nizzari, V. Venezia, E. Repetto et al., "Amyloid precursor protein and presenilin1 interact with the adaptor GRB2 and

modulate ERK1,2 signaling," *Journal of Biological Chemistry*, vol. 282, no. 18, pp. 13833–13844, 2007.

[74] S. Gandy, J. Naslund, and C. Nordstedt, "Alzheimer's disease: molecular consequences of presenilin-1 mutation," *Nature*, vol. 411, no. 6838, pp. 654–656, 2001.

[75] C. Russo, G. Schettini, T. C. Saido et al., "Presenilin-1 mutations in Alzheimer's disease," *Nature*, vol. 405, no. 6786, pp. 531–532, 2000.

[76] M. Ezquerra, A. Lleo, M. Castellvi et al., "A novel mutation in the PSEN2 gene (T430M) associated with variable expression in a family with early-onset Alzheimer disease," *Archives of Neurology*, vol. 60, no. 8, pp. 1149–1151, 2003.

[77] S. Baulac, M. J. LaVoie, W. T. Kimberly et al., "Functional γ-secretase complex assembly in Golgi/trans-Golgi network: interactions among presenilin, nicastrin, Aph1, Pen-2, and γ-secretase substrates," *Neurobiology of Disease*, vol. 14, no. 2, pp. 194–204, 2003.

[78] R. Kopan and A. Goate, "A common enzyme connects Notch signaling and Alzheimer's disease," *Genes and Development*, vol. 14, no. 22, pp. 2799–2806, 2000.

[79] E. H. Schroeter, J. A. Kisslinger, and R. Kopan, "Notch-1 signalling requires ligand-induced proteolytic release of intracellular domain," *Nature*, vol. 393, no. 6683, pp. 382–386, 1998.

[80] T. C. Dale, "Signal transduction by the Wnt family of ligands," *Biochemical Journal*, vol. 329, no. 2, pp. 209–223, 1998.

[81] K. E. Spink, P. Polakis, and W. I. Weis, "Structural basis of the Axin-adenomatous polyposis coli interaction," *The EMBO Journal*, vol. 19, no. 10, pp. 2270–2279, 2000.

[82] P. Marambaud, J. Shioi, G. Serban et al., "A presenilin-1/γ-secretase cleavage releases the E-cadherin intracellular domain and regulates disassembly of adherens junctions," *The EMBO Journal*, vol. 21, no. 8, pp. 1948–1956, 2002.

[83] P. Marambaud, P. H. Wen, A. Dutt et al., "A CBP binding transcriptional repressor produced by the PS1/ ε-cleavage of N-Cadherin is inhibited by PS1 FAD mutations," *Cell*, vol. 114, no. 5, pp. 635–645, 2003.

[84] Z. Zhang, H. Hartmann, V. M. Do et al., "Destabilization of β-catenin by mutations in presenilin-1 potentiates neuronal apoptosis," *Nature*, vol. 395, no. 6703, pp. 698–702, 1998.

[85] C. J. Phiel, C. A. Wilson, V. M. Lee, and P. S. Klein, "GSK-3α regulates production of Alzheimer's disease amyloid-β peptides," *Nature*, vol. 423, no. 6938, pp. 435–439, 2003.

[86] K. Ghosal, D. L. Vogt, M. Liang, Y. Shen, B. T. Lamb, and S. W. Pimplikar, "Alzheimer's disease-like pathological features in transgenic mice expressing the APP intracellular domain," *Proceedings of the National Academy of Sciences of the United States of America*, vol. 106, no. 43, pp. 18367–18372, 2009.

[87] X. Xia, S. Qian, S. Soriano et al., "Loss of presenilin 1 is associated with enhanced β-catenin signaling and skin tumorigenesis," *Proceedings of the National Academy of Sciences of the United States of America*, vol. 98, no. 19, pp. 10863–10868, 2001.

[88] S. Artavanis-Tsakonas, M. D. Rand, and R. J. Lake, "Notch signaling: cell fate control and signal integration in development," *Science*, vol. 284, no. 5415, pp. 770–776, 1999.

[89] B. Osborne and L. Miele, "Notch and the immune system," *Immunity*, vol. 11, no. 6, pp. 653–663, 1999.

[90] G. Thinakaran and A. T. Parent, "Identification of the role of presenilins beyond Alzheimer's disease," *Pharmacological Research*, vol. 50, no. 4, pp. 411–418, 2004.

[91] C. A. Saura, S. Y. Choi, V. Beglopoulos et al., "Loss of presenilin function causes impairments of memory and synaptic plasticity followed by age-dependent neurodegeneration," *Neuron*, vol. 42, no. 1, pp. 23–36, 2004.

[92] A. Albericit, D. Moratto, L. Benussi et al., "Presenilin 1 protein directly interacts with Bcl-2," *Journal of Biological Chemistry*, vol. 274, no. 43, pp. 30764–30769, 1999.

[93] B. J. Passer, L. Pellegrini, P. Vito, J. K. Ganjei, and L. D'Adamio, "Interaction of Alzheimer's presenilin-1 and presenilin-2 with Bcl-X(L). A potential role in modulating the threshold of cell death," *Journal of Biological Chemistry*, vol. 274, no. 34, pp. 24007–24013, 1999.

[94] B. M. Gumbiner, "Regulation of cadherin adhesive activity," *Journal of Cell Biology*, vol. 148, no. 3, pp. 399–403, 2000.

[95] T. Yagi and M. Takeichi, "Cadherin superfamily genes: functions, genomic organization, and neurologic diversity," *Genes and Development*, vol. 14, no. 10, pp. 1169–1180, 2000.

[96] K. Uemura, N. Kitagawa, R. Kohno et al., "Presenilin 1 is involved in maturation and trafficking of N-cadherin to the plasma membrane," *Journal of Neuroscience Research*, vol. 74, no. 2, pp. 184–191, 2003.

[97] P. May, Y. K. Reddy, and J. Herz, "Proteolytic processing of low density lipoprotein receptor-related protein mediates regulated release of its intracellular domain," *Journal of Biological Chemistry*, vol. 277, no. 21, pp. 18736–18743, 2002.

[98] E. H. Corder, A. M. Saunders, W. J. Strittmatter et al., "Gene dose of apolipoprotein E type 4 allele and the risk of Alzheimer's disease in late onset families," *Science*, vol. 261, no. 5123, pp. 921–923, 1993.

[99] W. J. Strittmatter, A. M. Saunders, D. Schmechel et al., "Apolipoprotein E: high-avidity binding to β-amyloid and increased frequency of type 4 allele in late-onset familial Alzheimer disease," *Proceedings of the National Academy of Sciences of the United States of America*, vol. 90, no. 5, pp. 1977–1981, 1993.

[100] D. E. Kang, I. S. Yoon, E. Repetto et al., "Presenilins mediate phosphatidylinositol 3-kinase/AKT and ERK activation via select signaling receptors: selectivity of PS2 in platelet-derived growth factor signaling," *Journal of Biological Chemistry*, vol. 280, no. 36, pp. 31537–31547, 2005.

[101] H. K. Kim, M. J. Jeong, M. Y. Kong et al., "Inhibition of Shc/Grb2 protein-protein interaction suppresses growth of B104-1-1 tumors xenografted in nude mice," *Life Sciences*, vol. 78, no. 3, pp. 321–328, 2005.

[102] M. Y. Kim, J. H. Park, E. J. Choi, and H. S. Park, "Presenilin acts as a positive regulator of basal level activity of ERK through the Raf-MEK1 signaling pathway," *Biochemical and Biophysical Research Communications*, vol. 332, no. 2, pp. 609–613, 2005.

[103] G. L. Johnson and R. Lapadat, "Mitogen-activated protein kinase pathways mediated by ERK, JNK, and p38 protein kinases," *Science*, vol. 298, no. 5600, pp. 1911–1912, 2002.

[104] J. M. Kyriakis, "Making the connection: coupling of stress-activated ERK/MAPK (extracellular-signal-regulated kinase/mitogen-activated protein kinase) core signalling modules to extracellular stimuli and biological responses," *Biochemical Society Symposium*, vol. 64, pp. 29–48, 1999.

[105] N. Sawe, G. Steinberg, and H. Zhao, "Dual roles of the MAPK/ERK1/2 cell signaling pathway after stroke," *Journal of Neuroscience Research*, vol. 86, no. 8, pp. 1659–1669, 2008.

[106] E. Y. Lee, C. Y. Chang, N. Hu et al., "Mice deficient for Rb are nonviable and show defects in neurogenesis and

haematopoiesis," *Nature*, vol. 359, no. 6393, pp. 288–294, 1992.

[107] G. N. Patrick, L. Zukerberg, M. Nikolic, S. de La Monte, P. Dikkes, and L. H. Tsai, "Conversion of p35 to p25 deregulates Cdk5 activity and promotes neurodegeneration," *Nature*, vol. 402, no. 6762, pp. 615–622, 1999.

[108] I. Vincent, M. Rosado, and P. Davies, "Mitotic mechanisms in Alzheimer's disease?" *Journal of Cell Biology*, vol. 132, no. 3, pp. 413–425, 1996.

[109] N. Chow, C. Cox, L. M. Callahan, J. M. Weimer, L. Guo, and P. D. Coleman, "Expression profiles of multiple genes in single neurons of Alzheimer's disease," *Proceedings of the National Academy of Sciences of the United States of America*, vol. 95, no. 16, pp. 9620–9625, 1998.

[110] Y. Yang, D. S. Geldmacher, and K. Herrup, "DNA replication precedes neuronal cell death in Alzheimer's disease," *Journal of Neuroscience*, vol. 21, no. 8, pp. 2661–2668, 2001.

[111] A. K. Raina, A. Hochman, X. Zhu et al., "Abortive apoptosis in Alzheimer's disease," *Acta Neuropathologica*, vol. 101, no. 4, pp. 305–310, 2001.

[112] L. A. Selznick, D. M. Holtzman, B. H. Han et al., "In situ immunodetection of neuronal caspase-3 activation in Alzheimer disease," *Journal of Neuropathology and Experimental Neurology*, vol. 58, no. 9, pp. 1020–1026, 1999.

[113] C. Stadelmann, T. L. Deckwerth, A. Srinivasan et al., "Activation of caspase-3 in single neurons and autophagic granules of granulovacuolar degeneration in Alzheimer's disease: evidence for apoptotic cell death," *American Journal of Pathology*, vol. 155, no. 5, pp. 1459–1466, 1999.

[114] A. Dranovsky, I. Vincent, L. Gregori et al., "Cdc2 phosphorylation of nucleolin demarcates mitotic stages and Alzheimer's disease pathology," *Neurobiology of Aging*, vol. 22, no. 4, pp. 517–528, 2001.

[115] Y. Yang, N. H. Varvel, B. T. Lamb, and K. Herrup, "Ectopic cell cycle events link human Alzheimer's disease and amyloid precursor protein transgenic mouse models," *Journal of Neuroscience*, vol. 26, no. 3, pp. 775–784, 2006.

[116] M. P. Marzolo and G. Bu, "Lipoprotein receptors and cholesterol in APP trafficking and proteolytic processing, implications for Alzheimer's disease," *Seminars in Cell and Developmental Biology*, vol. 20, no. 2, pp. 191–200, 2009.

[117] D. Cao, K. Fukuchi, H. Wan, H. Kim, and L. Li, "Lack of LDL receptor aggravates learning deficits and amyloid deposits in Alzheimer transgenic mice," *Neurobiology of Aging*, vol. 27, no. 11, pp. 1632–1643, 2006.

[118] M. P. Burns, W. J. Noble, V. Olm et al., "Co-localization of cholesterol, apolipoprotein E and fibrillar Aβ in amyloid plaques," *Molecular Brain Research*, vol. 110, no. 1, pp. 119–125, 2003.

[119] T. Tokuda, M. Calero, E. Matsubara et al., "Lipidation of apolipoprotein E influences its isoform-specific interaction with Alzheimer's amyloid β peptides," *Biochemical Journal*, vol. 348, no. 2, pp. 359–365, 2000.

[120] P. G. Ulery, J. Beers, I. Mikhailenko et al., "Modulation of β-amyloid precursor protein processing by the low density lipoprotein receptor-related protein (LRP). Evidence that LRP contributes to the pathogenesis of Alzheimer's disease," *Journal of Biological Chemistry*, vol. 275, no. 10, pp. 7410–7415, 2000.

[121] D. H. Kim, H. Iijima, K. Goto et al., "Human apolipoprotein E receptor 2: a novel lipoprotein receptor of the low density lipoprotein receptor family predominantly expressed in brain," *Journal of Biological Chemistry*, vol. 271, no. 14, pp. 8373–8380, 1996.

[122] R. A. Fuentealba, M. I. Barria, J. Lee et al., "ApoER2 expression increases abeta production while decreasing amyloid precursor protein (APP) endocytosis: possible role in the partitioning of APP into lipid rafts and in the regulation of gamma-secretase activity," *Molecular Neurodegeneration*, vol. 2, 14 pages, 2007.

[123] H. S. Hoe, D. C. Harris, and G. W. Rebeck, "Multiple pathways of apolipoprotein E signaling in primary neurons," *Journal of Neurochemistry*, vol. 93, no. 1, pp. 145–155, 2005.

[124] H. S. Hoe, D. Wessner, U. Beffert, A. G. Becker, Y. Matsuoka, and G. W. Rebeck, "F-spondin interaction with the apolipoprotein E receptor ApoEr2 affects processing of amyloid precursor protein," *Molecular and Cellular Biology*, vol. 25, no. 21, pp. 9259–9268, 2005.

[125] H. S. Hoe, J. L. Kea, R. S. Carney et al., "Interaction of reelin with amyloid precursor protein promotes neurite outgrowth," *Journal of Neuroscience*, vol. 29, no. 23, pp. 7459–7473, 2009.

[126] H. S. Hoe, A. Pocivavsek, G. Chakraborty et al., "Apolipoprotein E receptor 2 interactions with the N-Methyl-D-aspartate receptor," *Journal of Biological Chemistry*, vol. 281, no. 6, pp. 3425–3431, 2006.

[127] M. Sinagra, D. Verrier, D. Frankova et al., "Reelin, very-low-density lipoprotein receptor, and apolipoprotein E receptor 2 control somatic NMDA receptor composition during hippocampal maturation in vitro," *Journal of Neuroscience*, vol. 25, no. 26, pp. 6127–6136, 2005.

[128] A. Botella-Lopez, F. Burgaya, R. Gavin et al., "Reelin expression and glycosylation patterns are altered in Alzheimer's disease," *Proceedings of the National Academy of Sciences of the United States of America*, vol. 103, no. 14, pp. 5573–5578, 2006.

[129] D. Dahary, O. Elroy-Stein, and R. Sorek, "Naturally occurring antisense: transcriptional leakage or real overlap?" *Genome Research*, vol. 15, no. 3, pp. 364–368, 2005.

[130] J. S. Mattick, "RNA regulation: a new genetics?" *Nature Reviews Genetics*, vol. 5, no. 4, pp. 316–323, 2004.

[131] E. M. Reis, H. I. Nakaya, R. Louro et al., "Antisense intronic non-coding RNA levels correlate to the degree of tumor differentiation in prostate cancer," *Oncogene*, vol. 23, no. 39, pp. 6684–6692, 2004.

[132] R. Yelin, D. Dahary, R. Sorek et al., "Widespread occurrence of antisense transcription in the human genome," *Nature Biotechnology*, vol. 21, no. 4, pp. 379–386, 2003.

[133] A. Pagano, M. Castelnuovo, F. Tortelli, R. Ferrari, G. Dieci, and R. Cancedda, "New small nuclear RNA gene-like transcriptional units as sources of regulatory transcripts," *Plos Genetics*, vol. 3, no. 2, pp. 174–184, 2007.

[134] S. Massone, I. Vassallo, G. Fiorino et al., "17A, a novel non-coding RNA, regulates GABA B alternative splicing and signaling in response to inflammatory stimuli and in Alzheimer disease," *Neurobiology of Disease*, vol. 41, no. 2, pp. 308–317, 2011.

[135] S. Massone, I. Vassallo, M. Castelnuovo et al., "RNA polymerase III drives alternative splicing of the potassium channel-interacting protein contributing to brain complexity and neurodegeneration," *Journal of Cell Biology*, vol. 193, no. 5, pp. 851–866, 2011.

[136] I. Shcherbatykh and D. O. Carpenter, "The role of metals in the etiology of Alzheimer's disease," *Journal of Alzheimer's Disease*, vol. 11, no. 2, pp. 191–205, 2007.

[137] J. R. Walton, "Evidence for participation of aluminum in neurofibrillary tangle formation and growth in Alzheimer's

disease," *Journal of Alzheimer's Disease*, vol. 22, no. 1, pp. 65–72, 2010.

[138] G. Casadesus, M. A. Smith, X. Zhu et al., "Alzheimer disease: evidence for a central pathogenic role of iron-mediated reactive oxygen species," *Journal of Alzheimer's Disease*, vol. 6, no. 2, pp. 165–169, 2004.

[139] Y. Qin, W. Zhu, C. Zhan et al., "Investigation on positive correlation of increased brain iron deposition with cognitive impairment in Alzheimer disease by using quantitative MR **R2**′ mapping," *Journal of Huazhong University of Science and Technology*, vol. 31, no. 4, pp. 578–585, 2011.

[140] S. Vasto, G. Candore, F. Listi et al., "Inflammation, genes and zinc in Alzheimer's disease," *Brain Research Reviews*, vol. 58, no. 1, pp. 96–105, 2008.

[141] S. Joshi, R. S. Guleria, J. Pan, D. DiPette, and U. S. Singh, "Heterogeneity in retinoic acid signaling in neuroblastomas: role of matrix metalloproteinases in retinoic acid-induced differentiation," *Biochimica et Biophysica Acta*, vol. 1772, no. 9, pp. 1093–1102, 2007.

[142] G. Filiz, K. A. Price, A. Caragounis, T. Du, P. J. Crouch, and A. R. White, "The role of metals in modulating metalloprotease activity in the AD brain," *European Biophysics Journal*, vol. 37, no. 3, pp. 315–321, 2008.

[143] A. Caragounis, T. Du, G. Filiz et al., "Differential modulation of Alzheimer's disease amyloid β-peptide accumulation by diverse classes of metal ligands," *Biochemical Journal*, vol. 407, no. 3, pp. 435–450, 2007.

[144] A. R. White, T. Du, K. M. Laughton et al., "Degradation of the Alzheimer disease amyloid β-peptide by metal-dependent up-regulation of metalloprotease activity," *Journal of Biological Chemistry*, vol. 281, no. 26, pp. 17670–17680, 2006.

The Association between Chronic Arsenic Exposure and Hypertension: A Meta-Analysis

Tanvir Abir,[1] Bayzidur Rahman,[2] Catherine D'Este,[3] Farooq A,[4] and Abul Hasnat Milton[1]

[1] *Centre for Clinical Epidemiology and Biostatistics (CCEB), The School of Medicine and Public Health, Faculty of Health, The University of Newcastle, Newcastle, NSW 2008, Australia*
[2] *The School of Public Health and Community Medicine, Faculty of Medicine, The University of New South Wales, Sydney, NSW 2052, Australia*
[3] *Biostatistics, School of Medicine and Public Health, The University of Newcastle, Newcastle, NSW 2008, Australia*
[4] *Research and Education Department, ASPETAR-Qatar Orthopaedic and Sports Medicine Hospital, P.O. Box 29992, Doha, Qatar*

Correspondence should be addressed to Abul Hasnat Milton, milton.hasnat@newcastle.edu.au

Academic Editor: Habibul Ahsan

Background. There is inconclusive evidence from cross-sectional and cohort studies that arsenic exposure is a risk factor involved in the development of hypertension. *Methods.* A database search, using several keywords, was conducted to identify relevant studies. Separate odds ratio estimates for arsenic exposure with concentration only and arsenic exposure with duration, including biomarker, were extracted from studies that met all inclusion criteria. The extracted odds ratios (OR) comparing the highest exposure categories with the lowest in each study were pooled using the random effects methods of meta-analysis. Heterogeneity of odds ratios in the included studies were analyzed using I^2 statistics. *Results.* Eight studies were analyzed. Using the exposure as arsenic concentration in the drinking water, the OR estimate was 1.9 (95% CI: 1.2–3.0), with the $I^2 = 92\%$, while using the exposure as concentration and duration, the OR estimate was 1.4 (95% CI: 0.95–2.0) with the $I^2 = 80\%$. Meta-regression was done and the quality of exposure measurement was found to be significantly associated with the effect measure. For a one unit increase in the score from exposure assessment, the odds ratio decreased by 6%. No publication bias was evident. The only major weaknesses of this study were heterogeneity across studies and small sample size. *Conclusions.* The study findings provide limited evidence for a relationship between arsenic and hypertension. In summary, the relationship between arsenic exposure and hypertension is still inconclusive and needs further validation through prospective cohort studies.

1. Introduction

Arsenic is a known carcinogen [1], and increasing evidence also suggests a possible role of chronic arsenic exposure in the development of chronic diseases, including cardiovascular diseases [2]. Cardiovascular diseases associated with high levels of arsenic in the drinking water include atherosclerosis, hypertension, cerebrovascular diseases, ischemic heart diseases, and peripheral vascular disease [3, 4].

The possible role of chronic arsenic exposure in the development of hypertension has been previously reported from Taiwan, Bangladesh, and the United States [5–7]. These studies reported that individuals drinking arsenic-contaminated water for a long period of time might be at higher risk of developing hypertension compared to those unexposed to arsenic, and the effects were dose dependent.

Hypertension is one of the major risk factors for cardiovascular diseases [8] and is considered a major public health problem worldwide [9]. A total of 972 million adults were reported to have hypertension in 2000 and that number is estimated to increase by 60%, to a total of 1.56 billion, by the year 2025 [9]. The economic costs associated with hypertension are also very high.

To date, only a few cross-sectional and cohort studies have investigated the association between hypertension and chronic arsenic exposure [10]. Therefore, it is important from the public health perspective to explore the role of chronic arsenic exposure in development and prevention of hypertension. In this study, we conducted a meta-analysis that included all relevant cross-sectional and cohort studies of chronic arsenic exposure and hypertension. The meta-analysis provides greater precision in estimating risk especially when data are scarce and inconclusive. Our analysis includes a careful assessment of the possible effects of study quality as well as other biases on the meta-analysis results.

2. Materials and Methods

2.1. Literature Search. We used a comprehensive search strategy to identify all relevant studies. The research question was defined as "Is there any association between chronic arsenic exposure and hypertension?" This question was then broken down to cover specific search terms such as "hypertension," "chronic arsenic exposure," "arsenite," "arsenosis," "arsenicosis," "diastolic," and "systolic." Each term was included in one or more searches. The search was first carried out in Ovid MEDLINE and Google Scholar in September 2009, without limitation on the time of publication. We also replicated the search in EMBASE and PubMed, but no additional references were identified through these databases. The search was last updated in February 2012 to locate new studies published after the initial search. No new studies on this topic had been published. The references cited in the collected list of articles were also hand-searched for additional relevant studies.

2.2. Selection of Studies. The included studies (1) were observational studies, that is, cross-sectional, case control or cohort studies, of chronic arsenic exposure through drinking water and hypertension, (2) reported a relative risk (RR) or odds ratio (OR), or such parameters could be estimated from the published data, and (3) measured arsenic, using a laboratory technique.

Two investigators (T. A. and R. E. Y.) screened the initial list of articles to identify articles that were irrelevant and, therefore, discarded from the list. To facilitate faster screening, articles were first judged on the basis of their titles, where obviously irrelevant articles were discarded. The abstracts of the remaining articles were then read by three investigators (T. A., B. R., and A. H. M.) to ensure that the main subject of the study was related to arsenic exposure and hypertension. Articles whose abstracts showed that the study was not relevant to the objective of the meta-analysis were discarded. Final screening of the articles was based on the full content. After the screening, information for the articles was extracted and a quality evaluation was done.

2.3. Data Extraction. A data extraction format was prepared to extract relevant information from the individual studies. The data items extracted from each study were

(i) general information: first author's name and affiliation, year of publication, country, and region in which the study was conducted;

(ii) study design: population, number and sources of study participants, and type of study;

(iii) exposure and outcome measurement: analytical methods for measuring arsenic, speciation of arsenic, duration of arsenic exposure, relevant information on individual level of exposure assessment, and measurement of hypertension;

(iv) analysis: covariates for adjustment in multivariate models, adjusted and unadjusted or stratified effect estimates (i.e., RR and OR) and 95% confidence intervals (CIs). If a study did not report CIs, the standard error and the resulting CI from the *P* value were estimated [11], where possible.

For cross-sectional studies, ORs were extracted as the estimate of the effect of arsenic exposure. For cohort studies, the RRs were used.

2.4. Quality of the Studies. Each article was evaluated in a standardised manner to assess its individual qualities. Quality assessment was facilitated through the use of a standardised questionnaire which was developed specifically for this study. The questionnaire was a comprehensive scoring instrument based on critical appraisal principles and understanding of the methodological issues of population selection, measurement of arsenic exposure and outcome, adjustment for potential confounders, and appropriateness of analysis. Each criterion was given weighted scores to evaluate the quality of the studies in comparison to each other, with key factors being given specific scores. Although the scoring in itself can be subjective, it enables comparisons among the studies. Three independent readers (T. A., R. E. Y., and A. F.) scored each of the studies and were blinded to the others' assessments. Any significant disagreement between the readers was resolved through discussion. For minor differences, the average score was used as the agreed score. This resulted in a single agreed score for each characteristic of each paper.

The maximum score value that could be assigned to each study was 100, and this score summarised the overall quality of the study. The score was the weighted sum of four major domains of quality: selection issues (score weight 20%), measurement issues (of exposure and outcome, score weight 50%), adjustment of confounding factors (score weight 20%) and analysis (score weight 10%). The analysis section was given the least weight because if the other three sections were of good quality but the analysis was not carried out properly, the data could often be reanalyzed. Two scoring systems were developed, one for cross-sectional studies and one for prospective studies. Each of the studies was subjectively assessed and scored using these instruments.

3. Statistical Analysis

To assess the interrater reliability of the study quality scores, reliability and reproducibility were analyzed by computing intraclass correlation coefficients (ICCs) for absolute agreement between raters on each quality domain along with the overall score.

To conduct the meta-analysis, ORs were extracted from cohort studies and used to estimate the effects, with the exception of one cohort study where the RR was used instead. For studies where several measures of association were reported, associations which related hypertension to amount of arsenic intake, or to arsenic intake combined with duration of exposure, were considered. Pooled ORs were estimated by comparing the highest exposure category to the lowest one combined for males and females.

The meta-analysis included checking for heterogeneity of the ORs, checking for influential studies, checking for asymmetry and publication biases, and checking for relationships between the log of effect measures and the article's quality scores.

Effect estimates (ORs) were pooled using DerSimonian and Laird's inverse-variance-weighted random effects method [12]. Heterogeneity was measured using the I^2-statistic [13], which describes the proportion of total variation in study estimates that is due to heterogeneity [13]. The influence of each study on the pooled effect measure was examined by repeating the meta-analysis while omitting each study one by one.

A Funnel plot was used to check for potential publication bias [14]. This was also objectively measured using Begg's statistic [15]. A random effect metaregression was conducted using the logs of the effect measures (OR) as the outcome variable and the study quality score as the explanatory variable to assess the possible impact of study quality on the effect measures. These random effect models were fitted with two additive variance components: within study variance and between study residuals [16, 17]. All meta-analysis was conducted using STATA version 11.0 SE.

4. Results

4.1. Literature Survey. The database search yielded 85 articles, 10 of which investigated the association between chronic arsenic exposure and hypertension. Two of these articles were excluded from the meta-analysis because the full texts were not available. Thus, the final meta-analysis comprised eight studies: seven analytical cross-sectional studies and one prospective cohort study. Of these eight studies, two reported arsenic concentration only as exposure, two reported arsenic concentration and duration of drinking arsenic-contaminated water as a combined exposure value, and three reported arsenic concentration and arsenic concentration and duration of exposure separately. Table 1 provides a summary of the relevant studies.

4.2. Quality Scoring. The average total scores and average per criterion scores for quality assessment are summarized in Table 2. The scores are percentages out of the highest possible score per criterion. The one cohort study scored better in the domains of *Selection* and *Outcome* compared to the other seven cross-sectional studies. The cohort study had a *Selection* score of 18.7 (of 20 possible), while the cross-sectional studies averaged 15.8. The cohort had an *Outcome* score of 16 (of 20 possible), while the 7 cross-sectional studies averaged 14.7. In particular, the study by Zierold et al. [18] scored low in this domain (1.3) due to missing details in the report. The 7 cross-sectional studies scored higher in the *Exposure* (cross-sectional = 24.3, cohort = 20, of 30 possible) and *Confounders* (cross-sectional = 18.6, cohort = 10, of 20 possible) domains. The *Analysis* (cohort = 9.3, cross-sectional = 10, of 10 possible) domain scores were similar; but, overall, the cross-sectional studies (total score = 84.1) scored higher than the cohort study (total score = 74). Good interobserver agreement on the total quality scores was verified by the intraclass correlation coefficient (ICC). The total score ICC was 0.88 (95% CI: 0.62–0.98). The highest agreement was seen among scores for the *Exposure* (ICC = 0.87 95% CI: .56–.98) and *Outcome* (ICC = 0.96 95% CI: 0.64–1.00) domains, and the lowest for the *Analysis* (ICC = 0.001 95% CI: −0.24–0.78) domain. The low ICC, however, was due to one rater's disagreement on one study, but there was perfect agreement among the raters on the rest of the studies. Other domains showed moderate agreement: the ICC for *Confounders* was 0.59 (95% CI: −0.19–0.90) while that for *Selection* was 0.66 (95% CI: −0.01–0.93).

The eight selected studies were scored based on criteria that were specifically developed to assess their quality. The cohort study by Wang et al. [5] scored a total of 74 points, having scored well on *Selection* and *Exposure* but not on *Confounder* criteria. The seven cross-sectional studies had an average score of 84.1 (range = 61 to 93.3). Overall, the cross-sectional studies scored higher than the prospective cohort study for the *Confounders* and *Exposure* criteria but scored lower for the *Selection* and *Outcome* criteria. The summary of scores is presented in Table 2.

4.3. Adjustment of Potential Confounders. The studies differed in the adjustment of potential confounders, such as age, sex, and body mass index, as well. Such differences may add to the heterogeneity of the conclusions presented in the articles.

5. Risk Estimate and Meta-Analysis

The pooled OR of studies using arsenic concentration as the exposure measure was 1.9 (95% CI: 1.2–3.0), while the pooled estimate for OR of studies using arsenic concentration and duration including biomarker as the exposure was 1.4 (95% CI: 0.95–2.0). For the arsenic concentration studies, the I^2 was 92% ($P < 0.001$), while, for the concentration and duration studies, I^2 was 80% ($P < 0.001$). A P value <0.001 suggests a strong heterogeneity across studies. The meta-analysis results are presented with forest plots in Figure 1. In the forest plots, the point estimate for one study is represented by the centre of each rectangle. The size of the rectangle is relative to the weight of the point estimate when the results are pooled. The length of the horizontal line through the rectangle represents the 95% confidence interval of the point estimate. The pooled estimate is represented by the diamond on the lower portion of the plot. The vertical axis through the diamond represents the point estimate, and the horizontal end corners are the upper and lower 95% confidence boundaries.

5.1. Influence Analysis. The results of the influence analysis showed that no single study exerted a disproportionate influence on the pooled estimate for either arsenic concentration or arsenic concentration and duration (Figure 2).

Table 1: Findings from hypertension and chronic exposure to arsenic studies.

Reference	Study design and sample size	Location and population	Exposure assessment	Outcome assessment	Variables adjusted for	Findings: Exposure categories	Findings: Prevalence	Findings: Odds ratios (95% CI)
Chen et al. [19]	Cross-sectional: 382 men and 516 women of age over 30 and residing in arseniasis hyperendemic villages of Taiwan Exposed: 779 (drunk artesian well for some time) Unexposed: 119 (never used artesian well)	Taiwan	Long-term arsenic exposure calculated, structured questionnaire, and measured arsenic concentration in well water Cumulative arsenic exposure index was used	WHO protocol: Systolic blood pressure ≥160 mm Hg, Diastolic blood pressure ≥95 mm Hg AND/OR history of hypertension regularly treated with antihypertensive drugs	Age, sex, body mass index, fasting serum triglyceride levels, diabetes mellitus, proteinuria	0 years 1–10 years 11–20 years 21–30 years >30 years 0 μg/L 10–700 μg/L 710–900 μg/L >900 μg/L Unknown 0 μg/L-years 100–6300 μg/L years 6400–10800 μg/L-years 10900–14700 μg/L-years 14800–18500 μg/L-years >18500 μg/L-years Unknown	Case: 5.0% Case: 3.8% Case: 15.4% Case: 24.7% Case: 27.7% Case: 5.0% Case: 20.0% Case: 28.8% Case: 19.2% Case: 17.0% Case: 5.0% Case: 4.9% Case: 12.8% Case: 22.1% Case: 26.5% Case: 29.2% Case: 17.0%	1.0 1.1 (0.2–4.6) 3.2 (1.2–8.2) 3.0 (1.2–7.3) 1.9 (0.7–6.0) 1.0 2.5 (1.0–6.2) 3.6 (1.4–9.1) **2.6 (1.0–6.9)*** 1.7 (0.7–4.6) 1.0 0.9 (0.2–3.3) 2.4 (0.8–6.9) 3.6 (1.4–9.6) 3.6 (1.4–9.3) **2.8 (1.1–7.1)*** 1.7 (0.7–4.6)
Rahman et al. [21]	Cross-sectional: 1595 residents 30 years or older Exposed: 1481 (had a history of arsenic-contaminated drinking water) Unexposed: 114 (had no history of arsenic-contaminated drinking water)	Bangladesh	Arsenic concentration measured in artesian well water and consumption was assessed by structured questionnaire to estimate time-weighted mean arsenic levels (mg/L) for each subject	Systolic blood pressure ≥140 mm Hg, AND diastolic blood pressure ≥90 mm Hg	Age, sex, body mass index	Unexposed <500 μg/L 500–1000 μg/L >1000 μg/L Unexposed <1000 μg/L 1000–5000 μg/L 5000–10000 μg/L >10000 μg/L	Case: 7.9% Case: 8.0% Case: 16.1% Case: 19.5% Case: 7.9% Case: 5.5% Case: 12.0% Case: 14.3% Case: 22.9%	1.0 1.2 (0.6–2.3) 2.2 (1.1–4.3) **2.5 (1.2–4.9)*** 1.0 0.8 (0.3–1.7) 1.5 (0.7–2.9) 2.2 (1.1–4.4) **3.0 (1.5–5.8)*** Dose response among exposed *P* value <0.001

Table 1: Continued.

Reference	Study design and sample size	Location and population	Exposure assessment	Outcome assessment	Variables adjusted for	Findings: Exposure categories	Findings: Prevalence	Findings: Odds ratios (95% CI)
Zieroldet al. [18]	Cross-sectional: 1185 residents from Wisconsin, USA, who are 35 years or older and were drinking from private well water supply for 20 or more years Exposed: 40 (>2 μg/L) Unexposed: 34 (<2 μg/L)	Wisconsin, USA	Questionnaire survey for life-time history, usual drinking water consumption, use of water-treatment systems and family health history. Length of exposure estimated between July 2000 and January 2002	Self-reported	Gender, age, smoking status, body mass index	<2 μg/L 2 μg/L–10 μg/L >10 μg/L		1.0 1.2 (0.8–1.6) **1.7 (1.1–2.5)***
Wang et al. [5]	Prospective cohort: 18940 residents 40 years or older followed up for an average of 12 years Exposed: 2264 (residents from arsenic-exposed areas and drinking from tube wells) Unexposed: 16676 (residents from unexposed areas and drinking from tap water)	Taiwan	In one area, median arsenic concentration of the shared artesian well was used as exposure, whereas, in other area, the exposure was the arsenic level in the participants' own tube wells. People using tap water or drinking water with <10 μg/L of arsenic were considered unexposed.	Systolic blood pressure ≥160 mm Hg, diastolic blood pressure ≥95 mm Hg, OR history of hypertension regularly treated with antihypertensive agents	Age, gender	<10 μg/L 10–49 μg/L 50–499 μg/L >500 μg/L —	Case: 8.1% Case: 22.0%	1.0 **2.4 (2.1–2.7)***

Table 1: Continued.

Reference	Study design and sample size	Location and population	Exposure assessment	Outcome assessment	Variables adjusted for	Findings: Exposure categories	Findings: Prevalence	Findings: Odds ratios (95% CI)
Chen [25]	Cross-sectional: 11,458 men and women from Bangladesh who are 18 years or older	Bangladesh		Systolic blood pressure ≥140 mm Hg Diastolic blood pressure ≥90 mm Hg Systolic blood pressure ≥140 mm Hg AND/OR Diastolic blood pressure ≥90 mm Hg Pulse pressure ≥55 mm Hg	Age, gender, body mass index, cigarette smoking status, education length	0.1–7.0	Case: 6.7%	1.0
						7.3–39.0	Case: 9.3%	1.50 (1.20–1.88)
						40.0–91.0	Case: 7.7%	1.24 (0.99–1.57)
						92.0–179.0	Case: 8.1%	1.32 (1.05–1.66)
						180.0–864.0	Case: 7.7%	1.25 (0.99–1.57)
						0.1–7.0	Case: 9.1%	1.0
						7.3–39.0	Case: 9.9%	1.15 (0.94–1.41)
						40.0–91.0	Case: 8.9%	1.05 (0.85–1.29)
						92.0–179.0	Case: 8.7%	1.02 (0.83–1.26)
						180.0–864.0	Case: 8.8%	1.07 (0.87–1.31)
						0.1–7.0	Case: 11.9%	1.0
						7.3–39.0	Case: 13.8%	1.24 (1.04–1.49)
						40.0–91.0	Case: 12.0%	1.07 (0.89–1.29)
						92.0–179.0	Case: 12.1%	1.08 (0.90–1.30)
						180.0–864.0	Case: 12.2%	**1.11 (0.92–1.33)***
						0.1–7.0	Case: 9.0%	1.00
						7.3–39.0	Case: 11.4%	1.33 (1.10–1.62)
						40.0–91.0	Case: 11.0%	1.27 (1.04–1.55)
						92.0–179.0	Case: 10.4%	1.19 (0.98–1.45)
						180.0–864.0	Case: 10.6%	1.20 (0.99–1.47)
						<48.1	Case: 7.2%	1.00
						48.1–227.8	Case: 8.2%	1.19 (0.95–1.50)
						227.9–585.8	Case: 8.1%	1.28 (1.01–1.61)
						585.9–1494.0	Case: 8.3%	1.26 (1.00–1.58)
						>1494.1	Case: 8.0%	1.15 (0.92–1.45)
						<48.1	Case: 10.2%	1.00
						48.1–227.8	Case: 8.5%	0.84 (0.68–1.04)
						227.9–585.8	Case: 9.1%	0.96 (0.78–1.18)
						585.9–1494.0	Case: 9.0%	0.93 (0.75–1.14)
						>1494.1	Case: 8.9%	0.91 (0.74–1.14)
						<48.1	Case: 13.2%	1.00
						48.1–227.8	Case: 11.9%	0.91 (0.75–1.09)
						227.9–585.8	Case: 12.3%	0.99 (0.82–1.19)
						585.9–1494.0	Case: 12.8%	1.01 (0.84–1.21)
						>1494.1	Case: 12.3%	**0.95 (0.79–1.14)***
						<48.1	Case: 9.1%	1.00
						48.1–227.8	Case: 11.6%	1.32 (1.10–1.62)
						227.9–585.8	Case: 10.8%	1.27 (1.04–1.55)

TABLE 1: Continued.

Reference	Study design and sample size	Location and population	Exposure assessment	Outcome assessment	Variables adjusted for	Findings: Exposure categories	Findings: Prevalence	Findings: Odds ratios (95% CI)
Chen [25]	Cross-sectional: 11,458 men and women from Bangladesh who are 18 years or older	Bangladesh			Age, gender, body mass index, cigarette smoking status, education length	585.9–1494.0	Case: 11.2%	1.19 (0.98–1.45)
						>1494.1	Case: 10.1%	1.20 (0.99–1.47)
				Systolic blood pressure ≥140 mm Hg		≤90.0	Case: 8.3%	1.00
						90.1–159.2	Case: 8.6%	1.14 (0.91–1.42)
						159.3–245.9	Case: 8.0%	1.12 (0.90–1.41)
						246.0–405.4	Case: 7.5%	1.11 (0.89–1.40)
						>405.4	Case: 6.6%	1.09 (0.86–1.39)
				Diastolic blood pressure ≥90 mm Hg		≤90.0	Case: 10.7%	1.00
						90.1–159.2	Case: 9.9%	1.00 (0.82–1.23)
						159.3–245.9	Case: 9.4%	1.06 (0.86–1.30)
						246.0–405.4	Case: 7.7%	0.87 (0.70–1.08)
						>405.4	Case: 7.7%	0.99 (0.80–1.24)
				Systolic blood pressure ≥140 mm Hg and/OR Diastolic blood pressure ≥90 mm Hg		≤90.0	Case: 14.0%	1.00
						90.1–159.2	Case: 13.6%	1.04 (0.87–1.24)
						159.3–245.9	Case: 12.4%	1.02 (0.85–1.22)
						246.0–405.4	Case: 11.1%	0.93 (0.77–1.12)
						>405.4	Case: 10.6%	0.99 (0.82–1.20)
				Pulse pressure ≥55 mm Hg		≤90.0	Case: 10.1%	1.00
						90.1–159.2	Case: 10.7%	1.07 (0.88–1.31)
						159.3–245.9	Case: 10.9%	1.10 (0.91–1.34)
						246.0–405.4	Case: 10.1%	1.05 (0.86–1.58)
						>405.4	Case: 10.1%	1.09 (0.89–1.34)
Huang et al. [20]	Cross-sectional: 488 women and 383 men southwestern coast of Taiwan whose age is 30 years or older	Taiwan	Percentage of inorganic arsenic in urine was used to determine exposure	WHO protocol: Systolic blood pressure ≥140 mm Hg, Diastolic blood pressure ≥90 mm Hg, and/or history of hypertension regularly treated with antihypertensive drugs	Age, gender, body mass index, cigarette smoke, alcohol consumption, triglyceride level, cumulative arsenic exposure	*InAs%		
						<4.53%		1.0
						4.53%–8.00%		0.72 (0.46–1.11)
						≥8.00%	Case: 37.3%	1.21 (0.79–1.85)
						CAE = 0 μg/L-year	Case: 30.6%	P for trend P-value:
						InAs%**	Case: 41.2%	0.35
						<61000	Case: 21.3%	1.0
						≥61000	Case: 22.0%	1.04 (0.43–2.48)
						CAE > 0 μg/L InAs%	Case: 38.6%	2.31 (1.19–4.48)*
						<61000%	Case: 56.5%	**2.84 (1.47–5.46)***
						≥61000		*$P < 0.05$ **$P < 0.01$

Table 1: Continued.

Reference	Study design and sample size	Location and population	Exposure assessment	Outcome assessment	Variables adjusted for	Findings: Exposure categories	Findings: Prevalence	Findings: Odds ratios (95% CI)
Chen et al. [6]	Cross-sectional: 10,910 participants from Bangladesh who are married, 18 years or older, and have had resided in the area for at least 5 years	Bangladesh	Arsenic concentration was measured in the wells to estimate time-weighted well arsenic concentration (TWA) combining the water use behaviour for, an average, last 10 years for men and 8.3 years for women	Overall population: Systolic hypertension ≥140 mm Hg Diastolic blood pressure ≥90 mm Hg Systolic hypertension ≥140 mm Hg and/or Diastolic blood pressure ≥90 mm Hg Pulse blood pressure ≥55 mm Hg	Age, gender, body mass index, cigarette smoking status, education length, daily water consumption	(Mean years exposed) 0.1 μg/L–8.0 μg/L (2.8 years)	Case: 7.3%	1.00
						8.1 μg/L–40.8 μg/L (23.2 years)	Case: 8.9%	1.39 (1.10–1.75)
						40.9 μg/L–91.0 μg/L (63.9 years)	Case: 8.0%	1.21 (0.96–1.54)
						91.1 μg/L–176.0 μg/L (128.1 years)	Case: 8.2%	1.28 (1.01–1.62)
						176.1 μg/L–864.0 μg/L (283.1 years)	Case: 7.6%	1.13 (0.90–1.44)
						0.1 μg/L–8.0 μg/L (2.8 years)	Case: 10.0%	1.00
						8.1 μg/L–40.8 μg/L (23.2 years)	Case: 8.9%	0.96 (0.77–1.2)
						40.9 μg/L–91.0 μg/L (63.9 years)	Case: 9.4%	1.01 (0.81–1.25)
						91.1 μg/L–176.0 μg/L (128.1 years)	Case: 8.5%	0.93 (0.75–1.16)
						176.1 μg/L–864.0 μg/L (283.1 years)	Case: 8.8%	0.97 (0.78–1.2)
						0.1 μg/L–8.0 μg/L (2.8 years)	Case: 12.9%	1.00
						8.1 μg/L–40.8 μg/L (23.2 years)	Case: 12.9%	1.1 (0.90–1.33)
						40.9 μg/L–91.0 μg/L (63.9 years)	Case: 12.5%	1.03 (0.85–1.25)
						91.1 μg/L–176.0 μg/L (128.1 years)	Case: 11.9%	1.01 (0.83–1.22)
						176.1 μg/L–864.0 μg/L (283.1 years)	Case: 12.1%	**1.02 (0.84–1.23)***
						0.1 μg/L–8.0 μg/L (2.8 years)	Case: 9.1%	1.00
						8.1 μg/L–40.8 μg/L (23.2 years)	Case: 11.9%	1.39 (1.14–1.71)
						40.9 μg/L–91.0 μg/L (63.9 years)	Case: 10.6%	1.21 (0.99–1.49)
						91.1 μg/L–176.0 μg/L (128.1 years)	Case: 10.4%	1.19 (0.97–1.45)
						176.1 μg/L–864.0 μg/L (283.1 years)	Case: 10.7%	1.19 (0.97–1.46)

Table 1: Continued.

Reference	Study design and sample size	Location and population	Exposure assessment	Outcome assessment	Variables adjusted for	Findings: Exposure categories	Findings: Prevalence	Findings: Odds ratios (95% CI)
Chen et al. [6]	Cross-sectional: 10,910 participants from Bangladesh who are married, 18 years or older, and have had resided in the area for at least 5 years	Bangladesh		Subpopulation (≥5 years exposure): Systolic hypertension ≥140 mm Hg; Diastolic blood pressure ≥90 mm Hg; Systolic hypertension ≥140 mm Hg AND/OR Diastolic blood pressure ≥90 mm Hg; Pulse blood pressure ≥55 mm Hg	Age, gender, body mass index, cigarette smoking status, education length, daily water consumption	(Mean years exposed)		
						0.1 μg/L–8.0 μg/L (2.7 years)	Case: 7.6%	1.35 (1.02–1.77)
						8.1 μg/L–40.8 μg/L (23.2 years)	Case: 9.0%	1.28 (0.97–1.69)
						40.9 μg/L–91.0 μg/L (64.3 years)	Case: 8.9%	1.3 (0.99–1.72)
						91.1 μg/L–176.0 μg/L (127.2 years)	Case: 8.4%	1.12 (0.85–1.47)
						176.1 μg/L–864.0 μg/L (284.7 years)	Case: 7.7%	1.00
						0.1 μg/L–8.0 μg/L (2.7 years)	Case: 10.2%	0.94 (0.72–1.22)
						8.1 μg/L–40.8 μg/L (23.2 years)	Case: 8.8%	1.07 (0.83–1.38)
						40.9 μg/L–91.0 μg/L (64.3 years)	Case: 10.2%	0.93 (0.72–1.20)
						91.1 μg/L–176.0 μg/L (127.2 years)	Case: 8.4%	1.00 (0.78–1.28)
						176.1 μg/L–864.0 μg/L (284.7 years)	Case: 9.1%	1.00
						0.1 μg/L–8.0 μg/L (2.7 years)	Case: 12.9%	1.06 (0.84–1.34)
						8.1 μg/L–40.8 μg/L (23.2 years)	Case: 12.6%	1.12 (0.89–1.41)
						40.9 μg/L–91.0 μg/L (64.3 years)	Case: 13.7%	1.03 (0.82–1.30)
						91.1 μg/L–176.0 μg/L (127.2 years)	Case: 12.0%	1.05 (0.84–1.31)
						176.1 μg/L–864.0 μg/L (284.7 years)	Case: 12.5%	1.00
						0.1 μg/L–8.0 μg/L (2.7 years)	Case: 8.7%	1.5 (1.16–1.91)
						8.1 μg/L–40.8 μg/L (23.2 years)	Case: 11.9%	1.34 (1.04–1.73)
						40.9 μg/L–91.0 μg/L (64.3 years)	Case: 11.1%	1.35 (1.05–.71)
						91.1 μg/L–176.0 μg/L (127.2 years)	Case: 10.9%	1.24 (0.97–1.59)
						176.1 μg/L–864.0 μg/L (284.7 years)	Case: 10.5%	

TABLE 1: Continued.

Reference	Study design and sample size	Location and population	Exposure assessment	Outcome assessment	Variables adjusted for	Exposure categories	Findings Prevalence	Odds ratios (95% CI)
Jones et al. [22]	Prospective cohort: 4167 adults (men) of age 20 years or older who participated in the survey from 2003 to 2008	USA	Total arsenic concentration (μg/L) in urine was used as exposure level	Overall population: Systolic hypertension ≥140 mm Hg Diastolic blood pressure ≥90 mm Hg	Sex, age, race/ethnicity, education, BMI, smoking status, continine, serum folate, vitamin12, diabetes, and alcohol consumption	Total arsenic (μg/L) <4.2	4.2–8.3 >8.3–17.1	>17.1
						Model 2 1.03 (0.96–1.10)	1.00 1.09 (0.84–1.41)	1.33 (0.99–1.80) **1.22 (0.91–1.64)***
						Total arsenic minus arsenobetaine ((μg/L)	<3.1 3.1–5.8	>5.8–10.8 >10.8
						Model 2 1.05 (0.96–1.14)	1.00 1.07 (0.81–1.42)	1.34 (0.95–1.89) 1.30 (092–1.83)
						Dimethylarsinate ((μg/L)	<2.0 2.0–3.6	>3.6–6.0 >6.0
						Model 2 1.12 (1.01–1.23)	1.00 1.06 (0.80–1.41)	1.21 (0.89–1.64) 1.29 (0.93–1.79)

* OR included in the meta-analysis.

**PMI: primary methylation index, InAs.

TABLE 2: Average quality scores on quality scores for studies included in the meta-analysis.

Categories of quality scoring (maximum points value)	Average (%) of the maximum category quality score (range)		ICC[a] for interobserver agreement (95% CI)
	Cross-sectional ($n = 7$)	Cohort studies ($n = 1$)	
Selection (20 points)	15.8 (14.7–16.0)	18.7	0.659 (−0.015–0.922)
Exposure (30 points)	24.3 (18.3–30.0)	20.0	0.870 (0.563–0.972)
Outcome (20 points)	14.7 (1.3–17.3)	16.0	0.958 (0.644–0.992)
Confounders (20 points)	18.6 (13.3–20.0)	10.0	0.578 (−0.188–0.902)
Analysis (10 points)	10 (10.0-10.0)	9.3	0.001 (−0.238–0.782)
Total quality score (100 points)	84.1 (61.0–93.3)	74.0	0.884 (0.620–0.975)

[a]ICC: intraclass correlation coefficient.

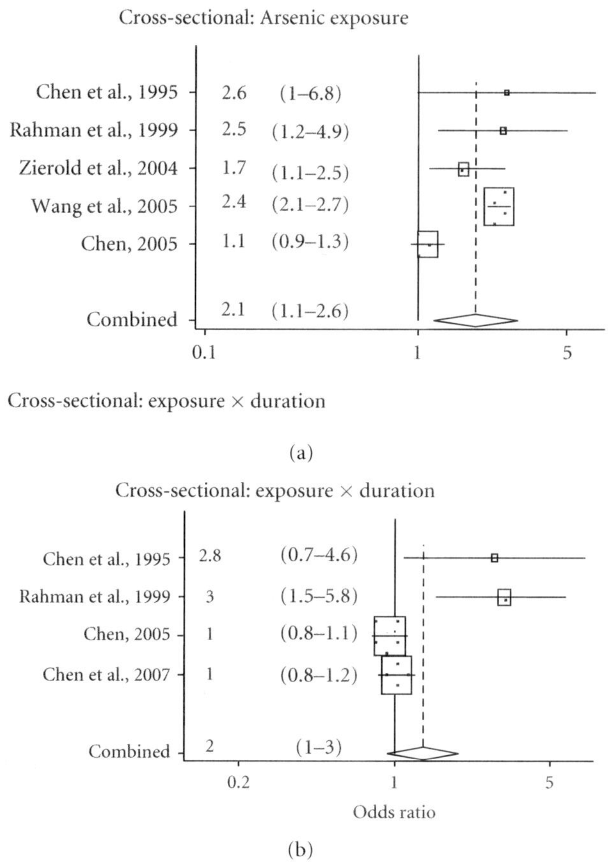

FIGURE 1: Forest plot of meta-analysis of arsenic and hypertension in cohort and cross-sectional studies.

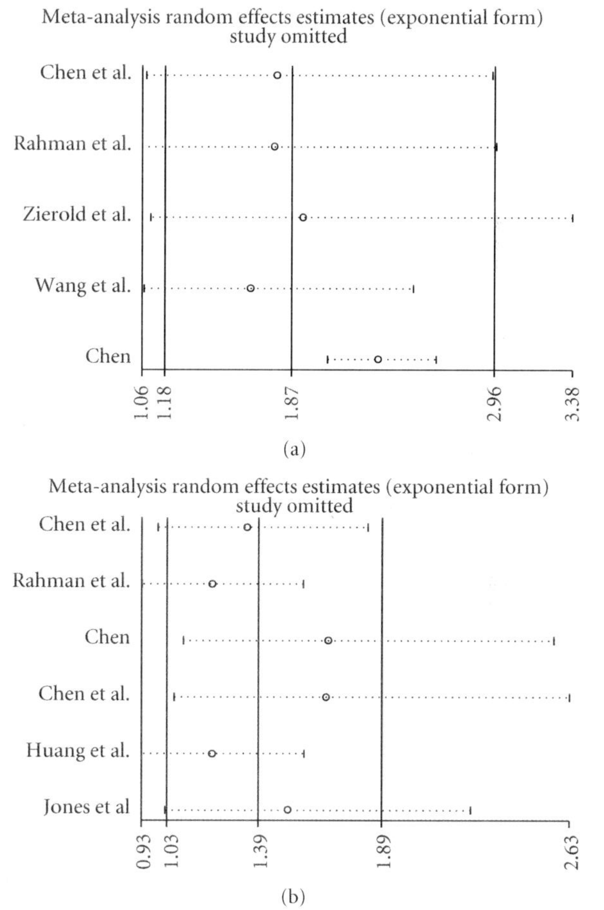

FIGURE 2: (a) Influence analysis for arsenic concentration as exposure assessment, (b) influence analysis for arsenic concentration and duration as exposure assessment.

5.2. Publication Bias. Investigation of the publication bias showed some evidence of positive results for the concentration and duration studies. The Egger's test P value for arsenic concentration studies was 1.00, while the Egger's test P value for the concentration and duration studies was 0.004. The funnel plot shows possible bias only for concentration and duration studies (Figure 3).

5.3. Metaregression. Using the scores from the *Quality* assessment, a metaregression was performed to verify the dependency of the *Outcome* measure on the quality scores. Of all the scoring criteria, the *Quality* of exposure measurement and total quality was significantly associated with the *Outcome* measure. For one unit increase in the score from the *Exposure* domain, the OR decreased by 6% ($P = 0.004$, 95% CI: 2.1%–10.7%).

6. Discussion

In the studies included in the meta-analysis, arsenic exposure was measured by different studies in different ways. Even when two studies used the same units of measurement,

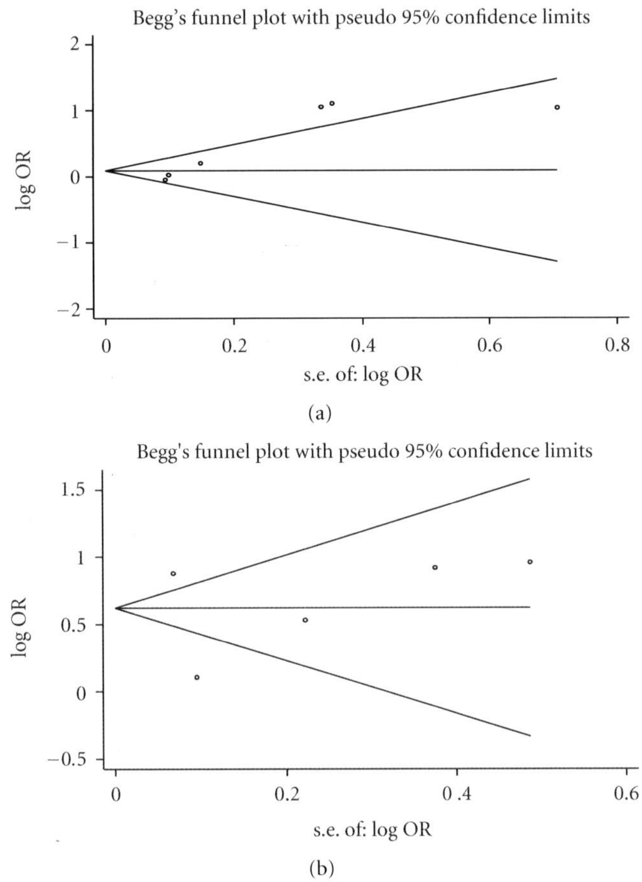

FIGURE 3: (a) Plot for arsenic concentration as exposure assessment, (b) funnel plot for arsenic concentration and duration as exposure assessment.

they may still have differed in categorization and definition of subjects being exposed to arsenic. The common units used were mg/L-year and μg/L. However, the definition of "*exposure*" differs from one study to another, since there is no agreement on how to express the duration of exposure or what quantities of arsenic constitute an exposure. This problem results from the fact that external validation of the methods used to determine exposure in studies is still problematic. In addition, while methods for detection of exposure to high levels of arsenic have been well characterized, measurement of arsenic exposure at low concentrations is still not very reliable. Furthermore, Wang et al. [5] and Chen et al. [19] have followed the WHO protocol for the measurement of blood pressure and have used the criteria of diastolic blood pressure >95 mm Hg or systolic blood pressure >160 mm Hg to define hypertension, while Huang et al. [20], Rahman et al. [21], and Chen et al. [6] specified hypertension as diastolic > 90 mm Hg or systolic >140 mm Hg. In the study by Jones et al. [22], they followed diastolic blood pressure >90 mm Hg or systolic blood pressure >140 mm Hg to define hypertension.

Overall, this meta-analysis suggests that chronic arsenic exposure is likely to be associated with hypertension. The pooled OR of arsenic concentration studies is 1.9 (95% CI: 1.2–3.0) and that for arsenic concentration and duration studies is 1.4 (95% CI: .95–2.0). The *P* values for homogeneity for arsenic exposure were significant at $P < 0.05$. The I^2 was 90% for arsenic concentration studies and 82.81% for arsenic concentration and duration studies. Investigation of publication bias showed some evidence of positive results for concentration and duration studies. The Egger's test *P* value for arsenic concentration studies was 0.828, while the *P* value for concentration and duration studies was 0.04.

Chen et al. [10] obtained similar results in their 2007 review of arsenic, diabetes, and hypertension. This paper included only four studies regarding arsenic exposure and hypertension and did not include a meta-analysis. In our meta-analysis, seven good quality studies were included that related arsenic exposure to hypertension using proper statistical analysis, with control groups (Table 1). As opposed to the report of Chen et al. [6], which only presented the results of their reviewed papers, the meta-analysis conducted here attempted to pool the reported ORs, tested for heterogeneity, and conducted a meta-regression. These are the major strengths of the current study. To the best of our knowledge, this is the first meta-analysis that has explored the association between hypertension and chronic arsenic exposure. One of the major limitations of this meta-analysis is the limited number of studies examining the association between hypertension and chronic arsenic exposure. These studies were also heterogeneous as reflected by the high values of the I^2 statistics. Thus, a random effects model was used in conducting the meta-analysis.

The adverse effects of arsenic on blood vessels have been demonstrated in previous studies which reported that constant exposure of rats and rabbits to arsenite caused a considerable increase in peripheral vascular resistance.

The eight studies evaluated in this paper have shown how varied the impact of arsenic on hypertension, depending on factors such as sex, age, body-mass index, diabetes, and triglyceride levels of the subject population. However, an increased risk for hypertension among arsenic exposed participants has not been consistently observed. For instance, Dastgiri et al. [23] reported a significant difference both for systolic and diastolic blood pressures between exposed and unexposed subjects, while Khan et al. [24] reported no significant effect. Inconsistent findings may be due to differences in measurement criteria both for exposure and outcome variables, or due to bias caused by limited consideration of potential confounders. Due to these inconsistencies, the increased prevalence of hypertension for a population that is exposed to high arsenic levels cannot yet be established.

7. Conclusions and Recommendations

This meta-analysis suggests a possible association between chronic arsenic exposure and hypertension. However, the small number of studies and limitations in study quality pose challenges to establishing causation between arsenic exposure and hypertension. Nevertheless, since a larger proportion of the rural Bangladeshi population drink arsenic contaminated water and the risk of hypertension is increasing among the general population, even a small association may lead to a large number of cases and a large population attributable risk. Therefore, the association deserves further investigation, preferably with cohort studies.

Conflict of Interests

The authors declare that there is no conflict of interests.

References

[1] NRDC, "Arsenic in drinking water," Natural Resources Defence Council, 2009 http://www.nrdc.org/water/drinking/qarsenic.asp#health.

[2] H. Y. Chiou, W. I. Huang, C. L. Su, S. F. Chang, Y. H. Hsu, and C. J. Chen, "Dose-response relationship between prevalence of cerebrovascular disease and ingested inorganic arsenic," *Stroke*, vol. 28, no. 9, pp. 1717–1723, 1997.

[3] C. O. Abernathy, D. J. Thomas, and R. L. Calderon, "Health effects and risk assessment of arsenic, a supplement at the 11th international symposium on trace elements in man and animals," *The American Society for Nutritional Sciences Journal of Nutrition*, vol. 133, pp. 1536S–1538S, 2003.

[4] D. R. Lewis, J. W. Southwick, R. Ouellet-Hellstrom, J. Rench, and R. L. Calderon, "Drinking water arsenic in Utah: a cohort mortality study," *Environmental Health Perspectives*, vol. 107, no. 5, pp. 359–365, 1999.

[5] C. H. Wang, C. L. Chen, L. I. Hsu et al., "Chronic arsenic exposure increases mortality from ischemic heart disease and stroke: a follow-up study on 26,851 residents in Taiwan," 2005.

[6] Y. Chen, P. Factor-Litvak, G. R. Howe et al., "Arsenic exposure from drinking water, dietary intakes of B vitamins and folate, and risk of high blood pressure in Bangladesh: a population-based, cross-sectional study," *The American Journal of Epidemiology*, vol. 165, no. 5, pp. 541–552, 2007.

[7] C.-J. Chen, L.-I. Hsu, C.-H. Wang et al., "Biomarkers of exposure, effect, and susceptibility of arsenic-induced health hazards in Taiwan," *Toxicology and Applied Pharmacology*, vol. 206, no. 2, pp. 198–206, 2005.

[8] S. Capewell, E. S. Ford, J. B. Croft, J. A. Critchley, K. J. Greenlund, and D. R. Labarthe, "Cardiovascular risk factor trends and potential for reducing coronary heart disease mortality in the United States of America," *Bulletin of the World Health Organization*, vol. 88, pp. 120–130, 2010.

[9] P. M. Kearney, M. Whelton, K. Reynolds, P. Muntner, P. K. Whelton, and J. He, "Global burden of hypertension: analysis of worldwide data," *The Lancet*, vol. 365, no. 9455, pp. 217–223, 2005.

[10] C. J. Chen, S. L. Wang, J. M. Chiou et al., "Arsenic and diabetes and hypertension in human populations: a review," *Toxicology and Applied Pharmacology*, vol. 222, no. 3, pp. 298–304, 2007.

[11] S. Greenland, "Quantitative methods in the review of epidemiologic literature," *Epidemiologic Reviews*, vol. 9, no. 1, pp. 1–30, 1987.

[12] R. DerSimonian and N. Laird, "Meta-analysis in clinical trials," *Controlled Clinical Trials*, vol. 7, no. 3, pp. 177–188, 1986.

[13] J. P. Higgins, S. G. Thompson, J. J. Deeks, and D. G. Altman, "Measuring inconsistency in meta-analyses," *The British Medical Journal*, vol. 327, no. 7414, pp. 557–560, 2003.

[14] M. Egger, G. D. Smith, M. Schneider, and C. Minder, "Bias in meta-analysis detected by a simple, graphical test," *The British Medical Journal*, vol. 315, no. 7109, pp. 629–634, 1997.

[15] C. B. Begg and M. Mazumdar, "Operating characteristics of a rank correlation test for publication bias," *Biometrics*, vol. 50, no. 4, pp. 1088–1101, 1994.

[16] S. G. Thompson and S. J. Sharp, "Explaining heterogeneity in meta-analysis: a comparison of methods," *Statistics in Medicine*, vol. 18, no. 20, pp. 2693–2708, 1999.

[17] S. G. Thompson and J. P. T. Higgins, "How should meta-regression analyses be undertaken and interpreted?" *Statistics in Medicine*, vol. 21, no. 11, pp. 1559–1573, 2002.

[18] K. M. Zierold, L. Knobeloch, and H. Anderson, "Prevalence of chronic diseases in adults exposed to arsenic-contaminated drinking water," *The American Journal of Public Health*, vol. 94, no. 11, pp. 1936–1937, 2004.

[19] C. J. Chen, Y. M. Hsueh, M. S. Lai et al., "Increased prevalence of hypertension and long-term arsenic exposure," *Hypertension*, vol. 25, no. 1, pp. 53–60, 1995.

[20] Y. K. Huang, C. H. Tseng, Y. L. Huang, M. H. Yang, C. J. Chen, and Y. M. Hsueh, "Arsenic methylation capability and hypertension risk in subjects living in arseniasis-hyperendemic areas in southwestern Taiwan," *Toxicology and Applied Pharmacology*, vol. 218, no. 2, pp. 135–142, 2007.

[21] M. Rahman, M. Tondel, S. A. Ahmad, I. A. Chowdhury, M. H. Faruquee, and O. Axelson, "Hypertension and arsenic exposure in Bangladesh," *Hypertension*, vol. 33, no. 1 I, pp. 74–78, 1999.

[22] M. R. Jones, M. Tellez-Plaza, A. R. Sharrett, E. Guallar, and A. Navas-Acien, "Urine arsenic and hypertension in US adults: the 2003–2008 national health and nutrition examination survey," *Epidemiology*, vol. 22, no. 2, pp. 153–161, 2011.

[23] S. Dastgiri, M. Mosaferi, M. Fizi et al., "Chronic arsenic exposure and dermatological lesions, hypertension and chromosomal abnormalities: an Epidemiological Study," *Epidemiology*, vol. 19, no. 6, p. S244, 2008.

[24] M. H. Khan, S. Sarkar, N. Khan, and S. A. Ahmad, "Assessment of ankle brachial systolic pressure index among arsenic exposed and nonexposed populations: a pilot study," in *Proceedings of the International Workshop on Arsenic and Humic Substances in Groundwater and Their Health Effects*, Tainan City, Taiwan, May 2009.

[25] Y. Chen, *Dietary Factors, Arsenic Exposure, and Risk of High Blood Pressure in Bangladesh*, Columbia University UMI, 2005.

8

Are Cosmetics Used in Developing Countries Safe? Use and Dermal Irritation of Body Care Products in Jimma Town, Southwestern Ethiopia

Wayessa Amasa,[1] Dante Santiago,[2] Seblework Mekonen,[2] and Argaw Ambelu[2,3]

[1] *Department of Eco-Bology, Addis Ababa Science and Technology University, P.O. Box 16417, Addis Ababa, Ethiopia*
[2] *Department of Environmental Health Sciences and Technology, College of Public Health and Medical Sciences, Jimma University, P.O. Box 378, Jimma, Ethiopia*
[3] *Department of Environmental Health Sciences and Technology, College of Public Health and Medical Sciences, Jimma University, P.O. Box 807, Jimma, Ethiopia*

· Correspondence should be addressed to Argaw Ambelu, aambelu@yahoo.com

Academic Editor: Lucio Guido Costa

Background. Rabbit skin model was used to test skin irritation of the most commonly used cosmetic products in Jimma town, southwestern Ethiopia. The most commonly used cosmetics were Dove, Glysolid, College, Top Society, Fair and Lovely, Nivea, Lux, Magic fruit world, Solea, Body talk, Kris, Holly, Victoria, and Sweet Heart. *Methods.* Intact and abraded rabbit skins were tested for erythema and edema under shade and under sun exposure. Draize Primary Irritation Index (PII) was used to calculate skin irritation of each cosmetic. Cosmetic ingredients were analyzed from the labels. *Results and Discussion.* Only Dove cream caused no skin irritation except for an abraded skin under sun exposure for five consecutive days. It has been identified that application of cosmetics on abraded skin under sunny condition worsens the irritation. Cosmetic labels revealed that most ingredients used in all products were those restricted chemicals due to their adverse health effects. *Conclusion.* This study has concluded that use of cosmetics under sunshine and also on abraded skin increases skin irritation. Hence, those users who have abraded skin are advised not to apply those cosmetics on continuous basis specifically under sun exposure.

1. Introduction

Cosmetics refer to all of the products used to care for and clean the human skin and make it more beautiful. The intentions of using cosmetic products is to maintain the body in a good condition, protect it from the effects of the environment and aging processes, change the appearance, and make the body smell nicer. Cosmetic products are widely used by every socioeconomic class of human beings to cleanse, perfume, protect, and change the appearance of skin [1].

Public observations and reviewing of the relevant literatures indicated that most of the cosmetic users were not seriously concerned about the effect of usage of products to their skin and focus on the short term result of skin appearance rather than the long-term effects to the whole body. Generally, consumers assume that cosmetic products are safer and pose no risk to the human health [2]. Some consumers did not read the label to identify the ingredients and other useful information of the cosmetic products before they decide to use them. The cosmetics sector grows tremendously, driven by demands from consumers but some users are not very concerned about the implications of cosmetics to their healthy body such as skin and physical outlook [2, 3].

In Ethiopia, cosmetics do not need marketing authorization unlike that of medicinal products which can only be marketed if marketing authorization is granted. DACA do not spend little or no time to protect the public against the harmful effects emanating from these products as it is true also in many other countries [4–7]. It is the companies' responsibility to check the safety of the cosmetic products and these firms are business oriented and give little or no attention to the cosmetics safety because of many reasons. Some of them are the requirement to change test methods, formulations, packaging, and advertising could increase costs for the sector [8].

Therefore there could be inadequacies and inconsistencies in container label disclosure by manufacturers [9]. These things create a gap in the event of defective product release in to the market [10]. Labeling is required for all cosmetic products and safety information must appear on cosmetic containers or packaging. According to Health Science Authority, labels on cosmetics should contain the function of the cosmetic product, instruction for use, list of all ingredients, country of manufacture, content (weight/volume), batch number, and manufacturing and expiry dates [11]. Cosmetics and personal-care products may contain ingredients whose safety is unclear or which are known to pose health risks. Adverse reactions to cosmetics are the commonest single reason for hospital referrals with allergic contact dermatitis [12, 13].

Most chemicals are added to cosmetic product in the form of preservatives and fragrances to increase the shelf life of the product and to have a good odor and appearance to the users [14]. These additive chemicals are the most common cause of skin problems such as skin irritation, photo toxicity, contact allergy, and other dermatological problems [15–17]. Documents indicate that in the previous times extracts of natural materials were used but currently synthetic ingredients are often used in the cosmetic products [18]. Some of these synthetic additives could be dangerous for the consumers' health. Estrogenic chemicals of body care cosmetics to the underarm and breast area are being investigated as a possible cause of breast cancer [19]. Literatures indicate that the concentration of lead in the candy lipstick cosmetic product is 2.8 times higher than the American FDA recommended concentration of lead [20].

Another problem associated with cosmetic use is the clarity of the labels on the cosmetic containers. The Tanzanian Food and Drug Authority have found that every container of any product shall be affixed with a label bearing legible and indelible letters in Kiswahili or Kiswahili and English: name of a cosmetic; form of a cosmetic; intended use; instructions on use of the cosmetic; net content given by weight or volume, in metric system; name and address of the manufacturer, including country of origin; dates of manufacture and expiry of a cosmetic in clear terms; list of ingredients in alphabetical order; batch or lot number; precautions and warnings; storage conditions where applicable [21]. Studies conducted somewhere else by the Environmental Defense in Canada have identified, using laboratory analysis, that heavy metals such as lead, arsenic, and antimony were found as ingredients which were not listed on the product label [22]. A similar study done has identified high levels of mercury in cream cosmetics [23]. Endocrine-disrupting chemicals were also identified in cosmetic products [24]. A study done in Nigeria also found an elevated level of lead in facial talcum powders and other metals in personal care products [25, 26].

Table 1: United States Testing Company (USTC) erythematic and edema evaluation scale [31].

Erythema	Scale	Edema	Scale
No erythema	0	No edema	0
Very slight erythema (barely perceptible)	1	Very slight edema (barely perceptible)	1
Well-defined erythema	2	Slight edema (edges of area well defined by definite raising)	2
Moderate to severe erythema	3	Moderate edema (raised approximately 1 millimeter)	3
Severe erythema (beef redness) to eschar formation preventing grading of erythema	4	Severe edema (raised more than 1 millimeter and extending beyond the area exposed).	4

A number of chemicals are usually added to cosmetics product as preservatives and fragrances. Many of them are toxic and prohibited from usage as ingredients because they can cause cancer, mutation, reproductive toxicity, and endocrine disruption. Preservatives added to skin cream products have been found above the maximum allowed concentration and do not comply with European Cosmetics Directives [27].

Cosmetics used for body care should be evaluated for irritancy potential to human skin of any chemical or formulation is a necessity. The most commonly used test is the rabbit skin irritation test as described in the OECD test guideline 404 and in the European Chemicals Bureau [28–30].

The nonmedicated cosmetics in Ethiopia are used without passing through structured safety evaluation and laboratory assessments. This might possibly lead to the presence and use of unsafe cosmetic products which could pose public health risk to the consumers. Hence, this study has been conducted to identify the safety of cosmetic products commonly used in urban communities considering Jimma as the case in point. This study helps the Federal Government of Ethiopia to formulate rules over the cosmetic products to protect the public safety and aware consumers.

Therefore the main aim of this study was to assess the skin irritation of cosmetics most commonly used in Jimma town using rabbit as a test animal whose result can be directly predicted for human skin irritation for both erythema and edema.

2. Materials and Methods

2.1. Study Area and Period. The study was conducted in Jimma town southwest Ethiopia from April to June, 2011. According to the Central Statistics Agency the current estimated population of the town is about 650,000 [32]. Jimma has many shops in which cosmetics could be sold. According to the town Trade and Industry office, there are above 350 shops in which cosmetics are being sold. However, the popular shops in which majority of the consumers could buy cosmetics are about 15. For the purpose of this study, shops keepers from these shops were interviewed to identify the most commonly used cosmetic products. In addition, one working day (Saturday) onsite observation was done at each shop to verify consumer preferences to cosmetics and interview them for labeling and content of the product. Saturday was preferred because it is major shopping day in Ethiopia and therefore many consumers could be surveyed. For comparative purpose, the Ethiopian-made products, Kris (*Kri*) and Victoria (*Vic*) lotions, and one face make-up called Sweet Heart (*Swe*) were selected to be included in the study.

2.2. Test Rabbit. Six New Zealand white rabbits were bought from Ethiopian Health and Nutrition Research Institute in Addis Ababa. The rabbits were acclimatized to the laboratory environment prior to the experiment for a period of five days to normalize the animal's physiological status during transportation and adopt them to the environment. Each rabbit was given a number unique within the study written with a black indelible marker pen on the inner surface of the ear and on the cage label. The animals were individually housed in cages and kept at ambient temperature and relative humidity.

2.3. Dermal Irritation Test Procedure. The selected cosmetics were tested for *skin irritation* using rabbits as test animals. Rabbit is a suitable model for this test of study since the results can be of value in predicting the likely skin irritancy potential of the test material to human [33].

One day before the test, six quadrants, 2.5 cm × 2.5 cm in dimension of each rabbit skin was clipped free of fur from the dorsal and flank area using shaving machines on five places for the selected cosmetics and one for the untreated control which was treated with distilled water. Only animals with healthy intact epidermis by gross observation were used for the study, and three rabbits were used per test.

2.3.1. Toxicity Test on Intact Skin. A quantity of 0.5 g test material, moistened with 0.5 mL of physiological saline, was put onto a piece of cotton gauze patch and placed in position on the assigned quadrant on shorn skin. 0.5 mL physiological saline was mixed with the test material so as to make the product moistened and to be attached well to the rabbit skin. The patches were secured in position with a strip of surgical adhesive tape. To prevent the rabbit removing the patches, the trunk of each rabbit was wrapped in a corset, and the animals were kept in individual cages for the duration of the exposure period. Four hours after application, the corset and patches were removed from each animal and any residual test material, gently swabbed away with cotton wool soaked in distilled water. The test quadrants were examined for evidence of primary irritation both erythema (redness) and edema (swelling) at 24, 48, and 72 hours after removal of the cosmetic material. The standard procedure of the United States Testing Company, OECD, and European Chemicals Bureau for the Cosmetic Product uses similar procedures as it has been initially described by Draize and his colleagues in 1944 [31, 34]. Table 1 indicates erythema and edema scale based on United States Testing Company (USTC) scale.

2.3.2. Toxicity Test on Abraded Skin. This test simulated the condition where the skin bears wound such as pimples and scratches. The same procedure as for the intact skin was used except that the shaved skin was rubbed with a fine abrasive paper five times.

2.3.3. Daily Applications on Sun-Exposed Intact Skin. The intention of this test was to determine the effect of sun light on cosmetic products whether the sun light can activate the chemical species present in the products and cause irritation effect on the skin. This test is similar to Test 1 except that the cosmetics were applied on the bare rabbit skin for five consecutive days, and the rabbits were exposed to the sun or kept under shade for four hour per day.

2.4. Determination of Primary Irritation Index. The duration of observation was three days for single topical application on intact and abraded skin but up to five days for repeated application. The primary irritation index (PII) for each treatment was calculated using the following formula:

$$\text{PII} = \frac{\Sigma \text{ erythema grade at 24, 48 and 72 hr} + \Sigma \text{ edema grade at 24, 48 and 72 hr}}{\text{total number of observations}}. \quad (1)$$

2.5. Interpretation of Results. The scores for erythema and edema at 24, 48, and 72 hours readings were totaled for the three test rabbits after the patch is removed and then divided by 18 to obtain the primary irritation index of the test material. The denominator 18 represents the number of rabbits used (three) multiplied by two types of observations (erythema and edema) multiplied by the three observation times (24, 48, and 72 hr), and the result was interpreted against the skin irritation category. According to Draize (1959), if the calculated PII is 0–0.4, 0.5–1.9, 2.0–4.9, and 5.0–8.0, the irritation category is, respectively, negligible, slight irritation, moderate irritation, and severe irritation [35].

3. Results

3.1. Cosmetics Survey. The cosmetic products identified in the survey as the most commonly bought by 433 consumers are given in Table 2. Top five cream cosmetic products most commonly used in Jimma town were Dove (*Dov*), Glysolid (*Gly*), College (*Col*), Top Society (*Top*), and Fair & Lovely (*Fai*) while the top five hand and body lotions were Body Talk

TABLE 2: Most commonly used cosmetic products by consumers and preference ranks given by shopkeepers in Jimma town, May, 2011. Cosmetics are listed using their abbreviations used in the result section.

Rank	Cosmetics	Country of origin	Percentage of consumer preference
1	*Dov*	India	86.7
2	*Gly*	Germany	73.3
3	*Bod*	S. Africa	66.7
4	*Col*	S. Africa	60
5	*Top*	India	53.3
6	*Fai*	India	53.3
7	*Niv*	Germany	53.3
8	*Sol*	Germany	53.3
9	*Lux*	S. Africa	46.7
10	*Mag*	China	40
11	*Hol*	Indonesia	40
12	*Vic*	Ethiopia	33.3
13	*Kri*	Ethiopia	20

Because of multiple responses, the sum of the percentages is above 100.

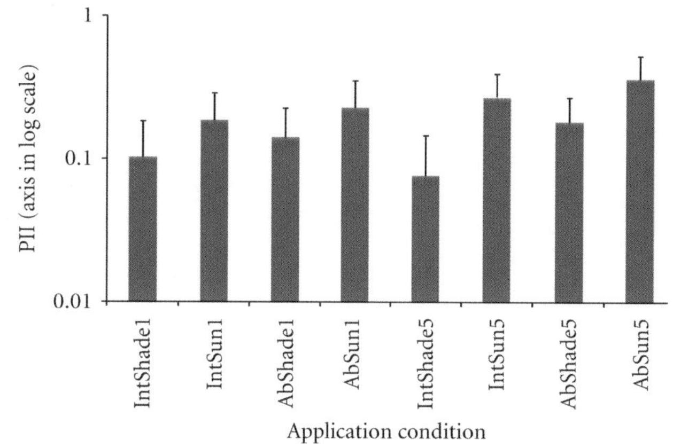

FIGURE 1: The average PII and standard deviation (error bar) of the cosmetics applied once and five consecutive days on a rabbit skin at different condition. IntShade1: applied once on intact skin under shade, IntSun1: applied once on intact skin under sun, AbShade1: applied once on abraded skin under shade, AbSun1: applied once on abraded skin under sun, IntShade5: applied five consecutive days on intact skin under shade, IntSun5: applied five consecutive days on intact skin under sun, AbShade5: applied five consecutive days on abraded skin under shade, AbSun5: applied five consecutive days on abraded skin under sun.

(*Bod*), Nivea (*Niv*), Solea (*Sol*), Lux (*Lux*), and Magic Fruit World (*Mag*).

Consumers were asked whether they read the label on the container while buying the cosmetic product from the source (wholesalers) and nearly all of them (99.2%) do not pay attention to what is written on the labels of cosmetic products. However, about 98% of the consumers interviewed were aware and curious about the expiry date but other label information such as ingredients from which the product is made was not considered. Many consumers (78%) do not like to buy the Chinese, Indonesian, Indian, and Ethiopian products because they were not sure about the quality of the product and might not be safe to human health. In addition, most consumers (81%) do not trust products imported from china as well.

We have identified that the main criteria that the shopkeepers were bringing the cosmetic products to sale were only based on customer preferences and the shelf life marked on the label.

3.2. Product Ingredients. Based on the investigation made on the product labels, the different ingredients were identified. Most of the products those are commonly sold in Jimma town cosmetic shops contain prohibited ingredients due to their possible health effects. The ingredients were parabens, linalool, limonene, disodium EDTA, sodium lauryl sulphate, and triethanolamine (Table 5).

No ingredient label was found on *Swe* and *Vic*. For some of the products, such as *Col*, *Niv*, *Mag*, and *Kri*, no expiry dates were mentioned.

3.3. Rabbit Model Experimental Result

3.3.1. Single Application of Creams and Lotions on Intact and Abraded Rabbit Skin. After a single application on intact and abraded rabbit skin, Dov did not show any skin edema or erythema as the calculated PII score was zero under shade or under sun conditions. All creams except *Gly* and all lotions and creams showed higher PII when the cosmetics are applied under sun exposed skin (Table 3). Mann-Whitney *U* test indicated no significant difference between the creams applied once on intact and abraded skin ($P = 0.71$). For all creams, except Dove, the erythema appeared after 24 h and disappeared after 72 h. The untreated control group showed no erythema and edema.

Regarding the lotions, *Bod* and Holly (*Hol*) caused PII of 0.06 on intact and PII of 0.1 to 0.17 on abraded skin. Magic Fruit showed the higher PII (0.47) among the lotions. PII of lotions significantly differed between applications on intact and abraded skin ($P = 0.0021$). However, no significant difference was observed between the PII under shade and under sun.

3.3.2. Effect of Five Day Application of Cosmetics on Rabbit Skin. This test was conducted to determine any adverse skin reaction to creams when used continuously for five days with or without exposure to direct sunlight. The results showed that all creams tested caused a maximum PII of 0.17 without direct sunlight exposure and PII of 0.45 under direct sunlight. Dov could not show any sign of irritation when applied for five consecutive days except for abraded skin under sunlight. Among lotions, the application of *Sol* for five days resulted in the maximum PII of 0.7. In general maximum PII was observed for cosmetics applied on abraded skin under direct sunlight (Figure 1). Statistically significant difference has been observed between PII of abraded skin and intact skin ($P = 0.012$). Strong significant difference of PII was observed for cosmetics applied under

TABLE 3: Primary irritation index (PII) of creams, lotions and make-ups applied once on intact and abraded rabbit skin, calculated from combined erythema and edema ratings for three rabbits at three observation periods (24, 48, and 72 h), Jimma, 2011.

Cosmeti group	Brand	PII Under shade Intac skin	PII Under shade Abrade skin	PII Under sun Intac skin	PII Under sun Abrade skin
Creams	*Dov*	0	0	0	0
	Gly	0	0.06	0.12	0.18
	Col	0.06	0.1	0.1	0.18
	Top	0.1	0.1	0.1	0.1
	Fai	0.1	0.1	0.1	0.1
Lotions,	*Bod*	0	0.06	0.12	0.18
	Lux	0.06	0.17	0.28	0.39
	Sol	0.1	0.17	0.24	0.31
	Niv	0.17	0.19	0.21	0.23
	Mag	0.17	0.27	0.37	0.47
	Hol	0.06	0.1	0.14	0.18
	Kri	0.17	0.2	0.23	0.26
Make-ups	*Swe*	0.28	0.3	0.32	0.34
	Vic	0.17	0.17	0.27	0.28
Control		0	0	0	0

TABLE 4: Primary irritation index (PII) of creams, lotions, and make-ups applied on rabbit skin for five consecutive days, under shade and under sun, Jimma town, 2011. The results were calculated from combined erythema and edema ratings for three rabbits at five observation days.

Cosmetic groups	Brands	PII Under shade Intact skin	PII Under shade Abraded skin	PII Under sun Intact skin	PII Under sun Abraded skin
Creams	*Dov*	0	0	0	0.1
	Gly	0	0.11	0.2	0.36
	Fai	0.03	0.09	0.13	0.21
	Col	0.07	0.13	0.19	0.25
	Top	0.03	0.17	0.31	0.45
Lotions	*Niv*	0.13	0.21	0.29	0.37
	Lux	0	0.34	0.48	0.6
	Mag	0.07	0.13	0.19	0.25
	Sol	0.10	0.30	0.50	0.70
	Bod	0.20	0.21	0.21	0.23
	Kri	0.10	0.24	0.38	0.45
	Hol	0.03	0.17	0.31	0.45
Make-ups	*Vic*	0.14	0.22	0.31	0.4
	Swe	0.17	0.23	0.29	0.35
Control		0	0	0	0

shade and under direct sunlight ($P = 0.000$). Table 4 shows PII results of different cosmetics applied under different skin conditions.

Post hoc analysis was made to compare the irritation index between cosmetics applied between intact and abraded skin under shade or sun-exposed conditions. Irritation index was higher for the cosmetics applied on abraded skin under sun exposed (AbSun) than the rest of the applications. Figure 2 compares the four groups of cosmetic applications using PII of 95% confidence interval. PII resulted

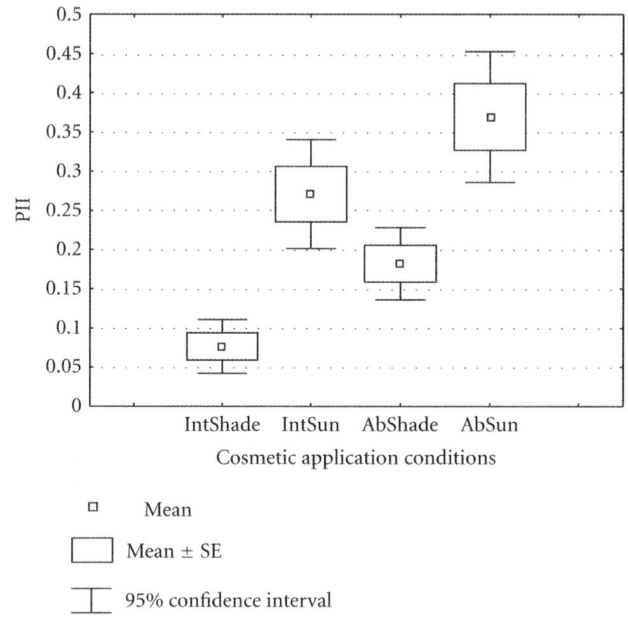

FIGURE 2: Box plot of primary irritation index (PII) of cosmetics applied under different environmental conditions on a rabbit skin. IntShad: intact skin under shade, IntSun: intact skin under sun, AbShade: abraded skin under shade, and AbSun: abraded skin under sun.

from application of cosmetics on intact skin under shade (IntShade) was significantly ($P < 0.0001$) lower than PII of cosmetics applied on both intact and abraded skin under sun exposed conditions. No significant difference ($P = 0.08$) was observed between PII of cosmetics applied on intact skin under shade (IntSun) and abraded skin under shade (IntShade).

According to the Mann-Whitney U Test, the PII calculated from cosmetics applied just once significantly differed from the application of five consecutive days (P value = 0.038). With similar statistical test, the PII calculated under shade significantly differed from the PII under sun (P = 0.000). Significant difference of PII also observed between intact and abraded skin (P = 0.006). Figure 1 explains the PII under different application conditions.

4. Discussion

Cosmetics and personal care products should be nontoxic, nonirritating, and must be safe for the consumers. The people use these products every day without knowing or being aware of the side effects of cosmetic products specifically in countries like Ethiopia where the literacy rate is very low. Therefore, in this study, an effort had been made to assess the possible *skin irritation* (dermal reaction), using rabbit as a model animal, that may result from the daily usage of these products in order to protect the consumers by educating the community and if necessary to call the attention of government about the need to regulate production and import of cosmetic products in the country. Our study has identified most cosmetics used by communities in Jimma town were unsafe for daily use. The absence strict safety regulation governing nonmedicated cosmetics by DACA most probably has lead to the presence of unsafe cosmetic products in shops. But some African countries like Tanzania have their own cosmetics directives similar to the European and Australian cosmetics directives [21].

Among the 14 cosmetic products selected, those who have no expiry date (*Col, Niv, Mag,* and *Kri*) could pose public health risk as consumers could use them at any time due to absence of shelf life. In developed countries, such as developed EC member countries, these products could not be sold for public use. The European Directive for Cosmetics (directive number 76/768/EEC) insists that products should have a clear label specifying the ingredient composition, country of manufacture, and expiry date of the products.

Almost all of the products commonly used by consumers in Jimma town contain at least two ingredients that were prohibited from usage [36, 37]. Almost all of the examined cosmetics in our study contain paraben or parabenzoic acid (methyl paraben, propyl paraben) which is suspected of causing endocrine disruption and breast cancer [19, 38]. Darbre and Harvey (2008) in their review of resent studies have confirmed that parabens were found in urine after topical application of skin care products on healthy human skin [38]. Therefore, those products identified in our study may not be safe for human health. A similarly study conducted by EWG (2009) indicated that 833 name-brand sunscreens were found unsafe due to unhealthy ingredients [6].

Another risk identified in our study was the absence of list of ingredients on *Swe* and *Vic* which makes someone to suspect that there might be some toxic chemical component. These products do not meet the safety requirements for cosmetics and should not be allowed for public marketing. High level of mercury was found in cream cosmetics which have no product label [39]. Table 5 explains the ingredients and the possible health effects along with each cosmetic product.

Regarding the erythema and edema, creams showed the least PII compared to other cosmetics for both single- and five-day application. Among creams, Dov was found to be the safest which has no skin irritation except for five-day application on abraded skin under sun exposure. This also could indicate that the product may have no skin irritating chemicals in the products formula, and the manufacturing company could have been complied with the USFDA standards which urge that cosmetic products should be nonirritating. However, the harmful ingredient found in Dov (Table 5) has to be replaced by safest ones.

The other cream cosmetics, *Col, Top,* and *Fai,* produce erythema and edema which were rated as PII of 0.06 to 0.18 for a single application. These products have negligible skin irritation and could be safe to be used by consumers as the PII ranges between 0–0.4 provided that the ingredients are also safe [34]. However, *Top* may not be safe on repeated application when used on abraded skin under sun exposure as the PII score was found to be greater than 0.4.

The PII of *Niv, Lux, Mag, Sol,* and *Bod* lotions was between 0.0 and 0.27 with single application under shade,

TABLE 5: Prohibited ingredients identified due to their health effects among the cosmetics commonly used in Jimma town [36, 37].

Products	Prohibited ingredients	Possible health risk
All creams and *Mag*	Sodium methylparabens and propylparabens*	Can have endocrine-disrupting action, breast cancer
Dov, Gly, Fai, and *Lux*	Linalool	Causes CNS disorder
Dov, Gly, Lux	Limonene	Carcinogenic, it is an irritant and sensitizer
Dov, Fai, Lux, Mag	Disodium EDTA	Contains dangerous levels of ethylene oxide and or dixane, both potent toxins
Top, Bod	Sodium lauryl sulphate	Irritant
Dov, Col, Hol	Triethanolamine (TEA)	Induces nitrosamines, which are potent carcinogens

* propylparabens are banned for under 3 children in Denmark.

indicating that the products have negligible skin irritancy and safe to use as topical application. However, based on single application under sun exposure, Magic Fruit may not be safe when used on abraded skin. On the basis of five-day application, *Lux, Sol, Kri,* and *Hol* may not be safe to human skin when used continuously under sun exposure, and the effect could be worse when used on abraded skin. This study has revealed that continuous application of those cosmetics on abraded skin under sun exposure could be dangerous for skin health. Hence individuals with abraded skin better not to use cosmetic products unless otherwise advised by their physicians.

This study has identified that the cosmetics used may not be safe for topical application on human skin due to the ingredients found in them, absence of expiry date, and the skin irritation posed by them. Hence consumers have to be very curious and clearly know what they are using for their skin care. We have identified cosmetics containing chemical ingredients that could cause public health problem such as cancer, endocrine disruption, or low sperm count in males [36, 37]. Similarly, study done in Denmark has indicated that the prevalence of allergic contact sensitization to cosmetic haptens among younger adults in the general population was a public health problem [39].

Strategic followup and screening of body care products that are imported from abroad and produced in Ethiopia could help to partly safeguard consumers' health. At least each product should have labels, and the ingredients should not have a suspected effect on human health. In addition, public health personnel should work on awareness creation related to use of body care products.

5. Conclusions

Cosmetics and personal care products should be nontoxic and should pose no risk under normal use. All The products tested for their skin reaction showed negligible skin irritancy but Dove had zero irritancy under the entire test conducted. But, there are prohibited ingredients in all of the products tested which made the products unsafe for the intended use. Some products have no appropriate label claims according to legislation set by USFDCA as well as the European cosmetic directives, and the products sold openly on the market are misbranded. This could expose consumers for public health risk. Therefore, consumers have to be aware about the side effects related to cosmetic products, and they should be informed to read the labels on the products' container. The consumers should avoid an attitude that cosmetic products are safe. Similarly, cosmetic industries, importers, distributors, and retailers should consider whether the product they sale to the consumer meets appropriate label requested by the DACA or not. Further study is suggested to know the chronic effect of those cosmetics in this study as well as laboratory analysis of the ingredients to identify mainly heavy metals.

Conflict of Interests

The authors declared no potential conflict of interests with respect to the research, authorship, and/or publication of this paper.

Acknowledgments

The authors are very grateful to Jimma University Research and Graduate Study Coordinating Office for supporting the study. They are also thankful to College of Agriculture and Veterinary Medicine for providing place and care to the test rabbits.

References

[1] S. Kapoor and S. Saraf, "Risk analysis tools for toxicological profile of cosmetics," *The Internet Journal of Toxicology*, vol. 5, no. 2, 2008.

[2] C. S. Cortez-Pereira, A. R. Baby, and M. V. R. Velasco, "Fragrance technology for the dermatologist—a review and practical application," *Journal of Cosmetic Dermatology*, vol. 9, no. 3, pp. 230–241, 2010.

[3] M. Norudin, E. Desnika, and R. Mohd, "Cosmetic usage in Malaysia: understanding of the major determinants affecting the users," *International Journal of Business and Social Science*, vol. 1, pp. 273–281, 2010.

[4] L. Marie, U. Louise, and S. Jørgen, "Changes in European legislation make it timely to introduce a transparent market surveillance system for cosmetics," *Acta Dermato-Venereologica*, vol. 87, no. 6, pp. 485–492, 2007.

[5] L. Tim, L. Sanford, and L. Pamela, "Hidden liabilities, market risk and drivers of change in the cosmetics and personal care products industry," *Beneath the Skin, Investor in Environmental Health Network*, pp. 1–38, 2007.

[6] EWG, "Campaign for Safe Cosmetics Report: toxic chemicals found in kid's bath products," Environmental Working Group, 2009, http://www.ewg.org/report/toxic-tub/31209.

[7] J. Frasca, "Cosmetics testing ensures safety for the public," 2010, http://www.prlog.org/10558136-cosmetics-testing-ensures-safety-for-the-public.html.

[8] RPA, *Study on Cosmetics Legislation in the EU and Other Principal Markets with Special Attention to So-Called Borderline Products*, Risk & Policy Analysts Limited, London, UK, 2004.

[9] L. Tim, L. Sanford, and L. Pamela, "Hidden liabilities, market risk and drivers of change in the cosmetics and personal care products industry," *Beneath the Skin, Investor in Environmental Health Network*, pp. 1–38, 2007.

[10] G. Hugbo, O. Anthony, L. Onyekwe, and I. Ijoma, "Microbial contamination and preservative capacity of some brands of cosmetic creams," *Tropical Journal of Pharmaceutical Research*, vol. 2, pp. 229–234, 2003.

[11] HAS, *On the Control of Cosmetic Products*, Health Sciences Authority, Singapore, 2007.

[12] A. C. De Groot, "Labelling cosmetics with their ingredients," *BMJ*, vol. 300, no. 6740, pp. 1636–1638, 1990.

[13] P. Nigam, "Adverse reactions to cosmetics and methods of testing," *Indian Journal of Dermatology, Venereology and Leprology*, vol. 75, no. 1, pp. 10–19, 2009.

[14] S. Wolfgang, "Microbial quality management for the production of cosmetics and toiletries," *Cosmetic Science and Technology*, pp. 189–195, 2005.

[15] H. J. Eiermann, W. Larsen, and H. I. Maibach, "Prospective study of cosmetic reactions: 1977–1980," *Journal of the American Academy of Dermatology*, vol. 6, no. 5, pp. 909–917, 1982.

[16] A. C. de Groot and P. J. Frosch, "Fragrances as a cause of contact dermatitis in cosmetics: clinical aspects and epidemiological data," in *Fragrances, Benificial and Adverse Effects*, P. J. Frosch, J. D. Johansen, and I. R. White, Eds., pp. 66–75, Springer, Berlin, Germany, 1998.

[17] L. Magnus, T. Monica, B. Asa et al., "Are adverse skin reactions to cosmetics underestimated in the clinical assessment of contact dermatitis? A prospective study among 1075 patients attending swedish patch test clinics," *Acta Dermato-Venereologica*, vol. 84, pp. 291–295, 2004.

[18] RIFM, *Fragrance and Cosmetic-Sharing Strategies*, vol. 121, Research Institute for Fragrance Materials, Cosmetic and Toiletries Magazine, 2006.

[19] P. D. Darbre, "Environmental oestrogens, cosmetics and breast cancer," *Best Practice and Research*, vol. 20, no. 1, pp. 121–143, 2006.

[20] I. C. Nnorom, J. C. Igwe, and C. G. Oji-Nnorom, "Trace metal contents of facial (make-up) cosmetics commonly used in Nigeria," *African Journal of Biotechnology*, vol. 4, no. 10, pp. 1133–1138, 2005.

[21] TFDA, *Guidelines for Registration of Cosmetic Productsedition*, Tanzania Food and Drugs Authority, Dar es Salaam, Tanzania, 1st edition, 2008.

[22] Environmental Defense, *Heavy Metal Hazard: the Health Risks of Hidden Heavy Metals in Face Makeup*, Environmental Defense, Ontario, Canada, 2011, http://www.greenbiz.com/sites/default/files/HeavyMetalHazard_May16_0.pdf.

[23] K. W. Sin and H. F. Tsang, "Large-scale mercury exposure due to a cream cosmetic: community-wide case series," *Hong Kong Medical Journal*, vol. 9, no. 5, pp. 329–334, 2003.

[24] J. K. Hyun and M. L. Byung, "Estimated exposure to phthalates in cosmetics and risk assessment," *Journal of Toxicology and Environmental Health—Part A*, vol. 67, no. 23-24, pp. 1901–1914, 2004.

[25] J. G. Ayenimo, A. M. Yusuf, W. O. Doherty, and O. A. Ogunkunle, "Iron, lead, and nickel in selected consumer products in Nigeria: a potential public health concern," *Toxicological and Environmental Chemistry*, vol. 92, no. 1, pp. 51–59, 2010.

[26] I. C. Nnorom, "Trace metals in cosmetic facial talcum powders marketed in Nigeria," *Toxicological and Environmental Chemistry*, vol. 93, no. 6, pp. 1135–1148, 2011.

[27] S. C. Rastogi, G. H. Jensen, M. R. Petersen, I. M. Worsøe, and C. Christoffersen, "Preservatives in skin creams. Analytical Chemical Control of Chemical Substances and Chemical Preparations," NERI Technical Report 297, National Environmental Research Institute, Aarhus, Denmark, 1999.

[28] OECD, "Acute dermal irritation/corrosion," OECD Guidelines for the Testing of Chemicals 404, OECD, Paris, France, 2002.

[29] European Commission, "Commission Directive 2004/73/EC of 29 April 2004 adapting to technical progress for the 29th time Council Directive 67/548/EEC on the approximation of laws, regulations and administrative provisions relating to the classification, packaging and labelling of dangerous substances," *Official Journal of the European Union*, vol. L152, pp. 1–316, 2004.

[30] K. Arun, A. K. Mishra, A. Mishra, A. K. Ghosh, and P. Chattopadhyay, "Evaluation of skin irritation of herbal O/W sunscreen cream on rabbit model," *Journal of Pharmaceutics & Cosmetology*, vol. 1, pp. 44–49, 2011.

[31] USTC, *Report of Testing. Biological Services Division*, United States Testing Company, Los Angeles, Calif, USA, 1973.

[32] C. S. A. (Central Statistical Agency), *Summary and Statistical Report of the Population and Housing Census Results*, Federal Democratic Republic of Ethiopia, Population Census Commission, Addis Ababa, Ethiopia, 2007.

[33] A. Sanders, "Acute dermal irritation in the rabbit," *Harlan*, pp. 1–14, 2007.

[34] J. H. Draize, G. Woodard, and H. Calvery, "Methods for the study of irritation and toxicity of substances applied topically to the skin and mucous membrane," *Journal of Pharmacology and Experimental Therapeutics*, vol. 82, pp. 377–390, 1944.

[35] J. H. Draize, *Dermal Toxicity Appraisal of the Safety of Chemicals in Foods, Drugs and Cosmetics*, Association of Food and Drug Officials of the United States, Austin, Tex, USA, 1959.

[36] M. Pauwels and V. Rogiers, "EU legislations affecting safety data availability of cosmetic ingredients," *Regulatory Toxicology and Pharmacology*, vol. 49, no. 3, pp. 308–315, 2007.

[37] NPA, "Standard and Certification for Personal Care Products," *Natural Product Association, the Natural Standard*, pp. 1–9, 2010.

[38] P. D. Darbre and P. W. Harvey, "Paraben esters: review of recent studies of endocrine toxicity, absorption, esterase and human exposure, and discussion of potential human health risks," *Journal of Applied Toxicology*, vol. 28, no. 5, pp. 561–578, 2008.

[39] N. Henrik, A. Linneberg, T. Menné et al., "Allergic contact sensitization in an adult Danish population: two cross-sectional surveys eight years apart (The Copenhagen Allergy Study)," *Acta Dermato-Venereologica*, vol. 81, no. 1, pp. 31–34, 2001.

9

Oxidative Stress and the ER Stress Response in a Murine Model for Early-Stage Alcoholic Liver Disease

James J. Galligan,[1] Rebecca L. Smathers,[2] Colin T. Shearn,[2] Kristofer S. Fritz,[2] Donald S. Backos,[2] Hua Jiang,[3] Christopher C. Franklin,[2] David J. Orlicky,[4] Kenneth N. MacLean,[3] and Dennis R. Petersen[2]

[1] *Department of Pharmacology, University of Colorado Anschutz Medical Campus, Aurora, CO 80045, USA*
[2] *Department of Pharmaceutical Sciences, University of Colorado Anschutz Medical Campus, Aurora, CO 80045, USA*
[3] *Department of Pediatrics, University of Colorado Anschutz Medical Campus, Aurora, CO 80045, USA*
[4] *Department of Pathology, University of Colorado Anschutz Medical Campus, Aurora, CO 80045, USA*

Correspondence should be addressed to Dennis R. Petersen, dennis.petersen@ucdenver.edu

Academic Editor: J. J. Stegeman

Alcoholic liver disease (ALD) is a primary cause of morbidity and mortality in the United States and constitutes a significant socioeconomic burden. Previous work has implicated oxidative stress and endoplasmic reticulum (ER) stress in the etiology of ALD; however, the complex and interrelated nature of these cellular responses presently confounds our understanding of ethanol-induced hepatopathy. In this paper, we assessed the pathological contribution of oxidative stress and ER stress in a time-course mouse model of early-stage ALD. Ethanol-treated mice exhibited significant hepatic panlobular steatosis and elevated plasma ALT values compared to isocaloric controls. Oxidative stress was observed in the ethanol-treated animals through a significant increase in hepatic TBARS and immunohistochemical staining of 4-HNE-modified proteins. Hepatic glutathione (GSH) levels were significantly decreased as a consequence of decreased CBS activity, increased GSH utilization, and increased protein glutathionylation. At the same time, immunoblot analysis of the PERK, IRE1α, ATF6, and SREBP pathways reveals no significant role for these UPR pathways in the etiology of hepatic steatosis associated with early-stage ALD. Collectively, our results indicate a primary pathogenic role for oxidative stress in the early initiating stages of ALD that precedes the involvement of the ER stress response.

1. Introduction

As the predominant cause of liver injury, alcoholic liver disease (ALD) remains a major cause of both morbidity and mortality in the Western world. Alcohol consumption in developing countries is increasing significantly and ALD is becoming a major socioeconomic burden. In 2003, it was estimated that alcohol was responsible for 44% of all deaths from liver disease [1]. Despite its overwhelming prevalence, only 10–15% of alcoholics ever develop hepatitis and cirrhosis [2]. As a result, it is crucial to intervene therapeutically during the early initiating stages of the disease where recovery is possible. ALD is a multifactorial disease, resulting from numerous cellular derangements, creating difficulties when trying to develop a targeted therapy [3]. One of the major confounding factors in our understanding of the pathogenesis of ALD is the generation of reactive oxygen species (ROS) resulting from the oxidative metabolism of ethanol.

A well-documented consequence of ethanol ingestion is the induction of cytochrome P450s, specifically CYP2E1, and depletion of cellular antioxidants leading to a prooxidative state [4]. While enhanced generation of ROS is likely to occur through multiple mechanisms, CYP2E1 and NADPH oxidase (Nox) are thought to be major sources [2, 4, 5]. Sustained exposure to ROS leads to prolonged oxidative stress, which promotes lipid peroxidation and generation of reactive aldehydes, such as 4-hydroxy-2-nonenal (4-HNE). This highly reactive aldehyde has been shown to covalently modify numerous cellular proteins, often resulting in alterations in protein structure, localization, function, and/or activity [6].

Protein folding is a critical function of the hepatic ER, yet despite the presence of a large number of chaperone proteins in the ER, an estimated 30% of nascent proteins fail to reach their properly folded state [7, 8]. Given this high frequency of improper folding, the ER incorporates a quality control system known as ER-associated degradation (ERAD), which eliminates unwanted proteins through ubiquitination and subsequent proteasomal degradation [9]. Under situations of sustained stress, where ERAD processes cannot eliminate all unfolded/misfolded proteins, the cell undergoes a series of adaptive signaling events termed the unfolded protein response (UPR). The overall goal of UPR signaling is to selectively increase the transcription of chaperones and increase ERAD processes, while decreasing overall translation [10]. UPR signaling is also known to induce selective signaling associated with both lipid and cholesterol homeostasis through activation of the sterol regulatory element-binding proteins (SREBPs) [11, 12]. These transcription factors tightly regulate fatty acid synthesis (SREBP-1) and cholesterol synthesis (SREBP-2). Previous studies by Ji et al. have implicated a role for the UPR in a rodent model of ALD [13, 14]. Although the proposed mechanism of this ALD-associated UPR induction is through increased plasma homocysteine, others have suggested a prominent role for oxidative stress in the activation of the UPR [8, 15–17]. In addition, sustained UPR activation has been shown to lead to enhanced ROS generation resulting in oxidative stress through activation of the ER oxidoreductases (Ero1) and NAD(P)H oxidase 4 (Nox4) [17, 18].

Altered redox control in the ER is linked to numerous hepatic disease states, including ALD [15, 19]. The transition from steatosis to steatohepatitis is considered to be the critical pathogenic determinant in ALD, furthering a need for therapeutic intervention during the early initiating steatotic stages of disease progression [20]. The mechanisms behind this transition remain elusive, and research on ALD is rarely focused on this stage. In this paper, we demonstrate a clear role for oxidative stress in the initiation of ALD that precedes the involvement of the UPR. These findings show, for the first time, a clear dissociation between oxidative stress and UPR signaling in the initiation of ALD.

2. Experimental Procedures

2.1. Animal Model. All procedures involving animals were approved by the Institutional Animal Care and Use Committee of the University of Colorado and were performed in accordance with published National Institutes of Health guidelines. Male C57/BL6J mice (12 per group) were utilized for the analysis and characterization of ethanol-mediated liver damage. Briefly, mice were fed a modified Lieber-DeCarli liquid-based diet (Bio-Serv, Frenchtown, NJ) for a period of 6 wk. The diet consisted of 44% fat-derived calories and 16% protein-derived calories, and the remaining balance was comprised of either maltose-dextrin or ethanol-derived calories. Ethanol-fed mice began the study on a diet consisting of 2% (v/v) ethanol, with the ethanol-derived calories increasing on a weekly basis until sacrifice; week 6 consisted of 6% ethanol (v/v) or 31.8% ethanol-derived calories. Pair-fed control animals received the remaining caloric intake from carbohydrate source (the caloric content of the diet used for the ethanol administration paradigm is presented in Table 1). Food consumption was monitored daily, and body weights were measured once per week. Upon completion of the study, animals were anesthetized via intraperitoneal injection with sodium pentobarbital and euthanized by exsanguination. Blood was collected from the inferior vena cava, and plasma was separated through centrifugation and assayed for alanine aminotransferase (ALT) activity (Diagnostic Chemicals Limited, Oxford, CT). Livers were excised, weighed, and frozen for biochemical characterization or subjected to differential centrifugation for subcellular fractionation as previously described [21].

As a positive control, endoplasmic reticulum stress was induced in C57BL/6J mice (7–11 wks) by a single IP injection with tunicamycin (Tm) at 0.5 mg/kg body weight [22]. Liver tissue was harvested 72 hours after injection.

2.2. Biochemical Analysis. Liver triglycerides were measured using a 2 : 1 chloroform : methanol extraction from liver homogenates using a kit from Diagnostic Chemicals Limited. Protein concentrations were determined using a BCA Protein Assay from Pierce (Rockford, IL) or a modified Lowry Protein Assay from Bio-Rad (Hercules, CA). Thiobarbituric acid reactive substances (TBARSs) were measured in whole liver homogenates (500 μg) by incubating samples in thiobarbituric acid reagent (15% w/v trichloroacetic acid, 0.375% w/v thiobarbituric acid, and 0.25 N HCl). Samples were boiled at 100°C for 15 min, cooled to room temperature, and then centrifuged at 10,000 rpm. Absorbance of the cleared supernatant was read spectrophotometrically on a microplate reader at 535 nm, and the concentration of malondialdehyde (MDA) was calculated from the extinction coefficient, $\varepsilon = 156,000\ M^{-1}\ cm^{-1}$. The activity of glutathione reductase (GR) was determined in cytosolic fractions according to Babu et al. [23] Glutathione S-transferase (GST) activity was measured in whole liver homogenates according to Rinaldi et al. [24]. Glutathione peroxidase (GPx) activity was determined in whole liver homogenates using a commercially available kit (Cayman Chemical, Ann Arbor, MI). The enzymatic activity of glutaredoxin (GRx) was determined using the HEDS assay according to Mesecke et al. [25].

2.3. Quantification of Blood Ethanol Concentration (BEC). BEC was determined as previously described [26]. Briefly, blood was collected on a weekly basis from the submandibular area of the mouse and placed in a heparinized tube; 0.6 M perchloric acid was added to each tube to precipitate protein. Samples were then centrifuged at 20,000 ×g for 10 minutes, and isopropanol was added to each tube as the internal standard. Samples were capped with air-tight rubber septums and heated for 15 min at 60°C. Head space gas was withdrawn (0.2 mL) and injected with a gas-tight syringe into a Hewlett-Packard 5710A gas chromatograph (injection port: 150°C, detector: 250°C, oven: 85°C). Separation of ethanol and isopropanol was performed on a 6 ft column

Table 1: Composition of ethanol and isocaloric diets. Values are presented as a percentage of the total caloric intake.

Parameter	Week 1		Week 3		Week 6	
	Control	Ethanol	Control	Ethanol	Control	Ethanol
Fat-derived calories (%)	45.0	45.0	45.0	45.0	45.0	45.0
Protein-derived calories (%)	15.0	15.0	15.0	15.0	15.0	15.0
Maltose-dextrin-derived calories (%)	40.0	29.2	40.0	18.5	40.0	8.2
Ethanol-derived calories (%)	N/A	10.8	N/A	21.5	N/A	31.8

packed with 60/80 Carbopack B (Supelco, Inc., Bellefonte, PA). Nitrogen was used as the carrier gas (flow rate = 40 mL/min). Ethanol concentrations were quantified against a standard curve using isopropanol as an internal standard to control for injection volume variation.

2.4. Cystathionine β-Synthase (CBS), Cystathionine γ-Lyase (CGL), and Glutamate-Cysteine Ligase (GCL) Measurements. Mouse livers were homogenized in buffer containing 100 mM potassium phosphate, pH 7.4, 1 mM EDTA, and 1 : 50 (v/v) protease inhibitor cocktail (Sigma Aldrich). The ratio of liver tissue to lysis buffer was 1 : 5. The homogenate was subsequently centrifuged at 4°C at 20,000 ×g for 20 min. The resultant supernatant was used as a crude extract. Protein concentration of the crude extract was determined by the Bradford method using bovine serum albumin as a standard. CBS activity assays were carried out using modifications to the method of Kashiwamata and Greenberg with a ninhydrin reagent specifically targeting cystathionine as described by Villanueva et al. [27, 28]. Briefly, 700 μg of crude liver extract protein was incubated in assay buffer containing 100 mM Tris-HCl, pH 8.6, 10 mM L-serine, 1 mM pyridoxal 5-phosphate, and 2 mM DL-propargylglycine at 37°C for 5 min. L-homocysteine was then added to a final concentration of 26 mM and a final volume of 50 μL to start the reaction at 37°C for 1 h. The reaction was stopped by the addition of 50 μL of 10% trichloroacetic acid (TCA). Samples were subsequently centrifuged at 20,000 ×g for 5 min, and a 50 μL sample of the supernatant was taken for cystathionine quantification as described previously [27]. Duplicate reactions were run in the absence of 10 mM L-serine as a negative control for each sample. CGL activity assays were performed using an enzyme-coupled assay with lactic dehydrogenase (LDH) as described previously [29]. Assay reactions were preincubated at 37°C and contained 100 mM potassium phosphate, pH 8.0, 2 mM L-cystathionine, 175 mM NADH, and five units of LDH. Reactions were started by the addition of 25 μg of crude liver extract to give a final reaction volume of 100 μL. The oxidation rate of NADH was monitored at 340 nm for 2 min at 37°C as an index of CGL activity. GCL activity was assayed from 1.0 mg of whole liver extract utilizing previously described protocols [30].

2.5. Measurement of Reduced and Oxidized Glutathione. Glutathione measurements were performed using a modified method from Reed et al. [31]. Briefly, fresh liver tissue was homogenized in 0.1 N perchloric acid using a sonicator and centrifuged at 13,000 rpm for 15 min, and the cleared supernatant was further neutralized with sodium bicarbonate and treated with 1 : 10 iodoacetic acid (IAA) (14.9 mg/mL) in the dark for 45 min at room temperature. Samples were then derivatized (1 : 1) with Sanger's reagent (1.5% 1-fluoro-2,4-dinitrobenzene (DFNB) in absolute ethanol) overnight in the dark at room temperature. Derivatized samples were stored at 4°C in the dark until analyzed by HPLC. Samples were applied (50 μL injection) to a Supelco LC-NH_2 5 μm, 25 cm × 4.1 mm column (Sigma Aldrich, St. Louis, MO) separated with a gradient mobile phase system. Solvent A (80% methanol) and Solvent B (80% Solvent B, 20% acetic acid/ammonium acetate solution (756 mL glacial acetic acid, 244 mL water, and 308 g of ammonium acetate)) were used for the separation of derivatized reduced (GSH) and oxidized (GSSG) glutathione using a Shimadzu LC-10AD dual pump system (flow rate of 1.0 mL/min) coupled to a Shimadzu SPD-M10AV diode array detector (Kyoto, Japan) set to 350 nm. HPLC running conditions were as follows: isocratic period of 50% solvent B for 10 min, followed by a linear gradient from 50% solvent B to 95% solvent B for 15 min, for a total run time of 35 min. Typical elution times were 11.55 min for GSH and 17.05 min for GSSG. Nanomolar concentrations of GSH and GSSG were calculated against a standard curve of 7 points for each molecule.

2.6. Western Blotting. Proteins from either whole liver extracts or subcellular fractions were subjected to standard SDS-PAGE or native PAGE. Native PAGE was employed to analyze the relative levels of monomeric GCLC and GCL holoenzyme. Native samples were mixed with loading buffer lacking 2-mercaptoethanol and were not boiled prior to loading on 8% polyacrylamide gels without a stacking gel or SDS. All gels were transferred to a Hybond-P membrane (GE Healthcare, Buckinghamshire, UK) and then blocked for 30 min with a tris-buffered saline solution containing 1% Tween-20 (TBST) and 5% nonfat dry milk (NFDM). Membranes were probed with primary antibodies directed against inositol-requiring enzyme 1 (IRE-1) and its phosphorylated form (p-IRE1), eukaryotic translation initiating factor 2α (eIF2α), growth-arrest-and-DNA-damage-inducible gene 153 (GADD153, also known as CHOP), SREBP1, SREBP2, Nox-4, Lamin B1, activating transcription factor 6 (ATF6) (Abcam, Cambridge, MA), KDEL (GRP78 and GRP94) (Stressgen, Ann Arbor, MI), Ero1α and Ero1β (ProteinTech Group, Chicago, IL), p-eIF2α (Epitomics, Burlingame, CA), β-actin (Sigma), and GCLC and GCLM (antibodies were generously provided by Dr. Terrance Kavanagh, University of Washington, Seattle, WA). A horseradish peroxidase conjugated secondary (Jackson Labs, Bar Harbor, ME) was then applied and membranes were developed using ECL-Plus Reagent from GE Healthcare. Chemiluminescence was visualized using a Storm 860 scanner from Molecular Dynamics (Sunnyvale, CA).

2.7. Immunohistochemistry. Following excision, livers were sectioned and placed in 10% neutral buffered formalin for 8 h. Samples were processed, imbedded in paraffin, and mounted on slides by Colorado HistoPrep (Fort Collins, CO). One pair of slides was stained with hematoxylin and eosin (H&E) for histological characterization while the remaining slides were subject to deparaffinization and rehydration for immunohistochemical characterization using either custom antibodies generated in our laboratory directed against 4-HNE modified proteins, anti-CYP2E1 (Calbiochem, San Diego, CA), or anti-protein-SSG (ViroGen, Watertown, MA).

2.8. Measurement of Proteasome Activity. Liver samples from control and ethanol-treated mice were homogenized in 0.1 M Tris-HCl and 0.25 M sucrose. Homogenates were centrifuged at 105,000 ×g for 1 h, and the resulting supernatant (cytosolic fraction) was assayed for chymotrypsin-like activity utilizing a commercially available kit (BioVision, San Francisco, CA). Values were calculated against a standard curve and are reported as a % of control-fed mice.

2.9. Image Analysis. Images of H&E or immunohistochemically stained liver sections were captured on an Olympus BX51 microscope equipped with a four-megapixel Macrofire digital camera (Optronics, Goleta, CA) using the Picture-Frame Application 2.3 (Optronics, Goleta, CA). All images were processed by Photoshop (Adobe Systems Inc. Mountain View, CA).

2.10. Statistical Analysis. Statistical analysis and generation of graphs were performed using GraphPad Prism 4.02 (GraphPad Software, San Diego, CA). Differences between control and ethanol-fed mice were assessed using a paired Student's t-test. Differences were considered significant if $P < 0.05$.

3. Results

3.1. Biochemical Characterization of Early-Stage ALD. As shown in Table 1, compared to their isocaloric controls, ethanol-fed mice displayed a decrease in overall body weight at each time point with the ethanol-treated mice weighing 16% less ($P < 0.001$) at the conclusion of the study (6 weeks). As outlined, the ethanol concentration was increased incrementally throughout the course of the study. Blood ethanol concentration (BEC) was monitored and displayed a consistent increase at each time point, with maximum concentrations observed at week 6 (245.383 mg/dL ± 33.747). Consistent with early-stage ALD, a significant increase in liver/body weight ratio was observed (Table 2). This phenomenon was observed as early as 3 weeks, with the largest difference observed following 6 weeks. To assess liver damage, plasma ALT values were determined at each time point; ethanol-fed mice displayed greater than a two-fold increase in plasma ALT levels by week 6, with no significant difference being observed at weeks 1 and 3. Given these parameters, it was determined that mice treated for 6 weeks with ethanol displayed the earliest significant signs of ethanol-induced liver injury, demonstrating pathologies consistent with early-stage ALD.

3.2. Continuous Ethanol Ingestion Results in Steatosis and Lipid Peroxidation. Hepatic steatosis is among the most prevalent and predictable outcomes of chronic ethanol consumption [3]. As shown in Figure 1(a), an increase in lipid was observed histologically as early as week 3 (here seen as very small lipid vesicles in zone 2), with a marked accumulation in lipid seen at week 6 (here involving both zones 1 and 2). Triglyceride content was also quantified at each time point; as shown in Figure 1(b), only the week 6 ethanol-fed-mice displayed a significant increase in hepatic triglycerides.

The increased accumulation of lipid observed in ALD provides the ideal environment for the generation of lipid aldehydes resulting from oxidative stress [32, 33]. As shown in Figure 1(c), immunohistochemical analysis reveals a substantial increase in hepatic staining of 4-HNE-modified proteins in as little as 3 weeks of feeding. The largest difference in staining, however, appeared following 6 weeks of ethanol ingestion with heavily stained hepatocytes localized predominately to zones 1 and 2. To validate this observation, hepatic TBARS was also quantified and is presented in Figure 1(d). Agreeing with the immunohistochemical staining in Figure 1(c), a significant increase in TBARS was observed at the week 6 time point, displaying nearly a two-fold increase. Collectively, these parameters indicate pathologies consistent with early-stage ALD, demonstrating a significant increase in hepatic lipid content and oxidative stress indices.

3.3. Effects of Ethanol Ingestion on GSH Synthesis and Utilization. As noted, decreased antioxidant capacity has been proposed to play a major role in the unbalanced generation of reactive aldehydes during ALD [6]. In line with this proposed mechanism, we sought to investigate the effects of ethanol consumption on hepatic GSH content and biosynthesis. As shown in Table 3, a significant depletion in reduced GSH was observed in mice treated for 6 weeks with ethanol compared to their respective isocaloric controls, indicating a decrease in the total antioxidant capacity of the liver at this time point. Oxidized GSH (GSSG) was also measured, observing no significant alterations at all time points analyzed. The reduction of GSSG to GSH is catalyzed by glutathione reductase (GR) and is thought to be the predominant mechanism for GSH cycling [34]. As shown in Table 3, GR activity was found to be significantly increased at the week 6 time point, with no variation observed at week 1 or week 3. This phenomenon has been observed in other

Table 2: Significant signs of alcohol-mediated liver injury are achieved following 6 weeks of ethanol ingestion. Blood ethanol concentration (BEC) is reported as mg/dL; ethanol ingestion results in a significant increase in liver-body weight ratio as early as 3 weeks; plasma ALT activity is significantly elevated after week 6. Values represent the average ± standard error of the mean ($n = 12$, $^{*}P < 0.05$, $^{**}P < 0.01$, $^{***}P < 0.001$).

Parameter	Week 1		Week 3		Week 6	
	Control	Ethanol	Control	Ethanol	Control	Ethanol
Food Consumption/day (mL/Day)	15.031 ± 0.263	16.510 ± 0.302***	15.151 ± 0.181	16.389 ± 0.183***	16.994 ± 0.205	17.778 ± 0.326**
BEC (mg/dL)	N/A	20.848 ± 0.367	N/A	32.577 ± 6.293	N/A	245.383 ± 33.747
Body weight (g)	25.667 ± 0.607	25.000 ± 0.663	26.900 ± 0.688	26.392 ± 0.601	31.017 ± 0.752	25.783 ± 0.647***
Liver weight (g)	1.102 ± 0.036	1.113 ± 0.031	1.086 ± 0.035	1.190 ± 0.034	1.148 ± 0.038	1.123 ± 0.036
Liver/body weight	0.043 ± 0.001	0.045 ± 0.000	0.040 ± 0.000	0.045 ± 0.001**	0.038 ± 0.001	0.044 ± 0.001***
Serum ALT activity (U/L)	15.698 ± 1.076	14.744 ± 0.803	11.332 ± 1.175	10.090 ± 0.808	18.411 ± 4.612	42.985 ± 4.523**

Table 3: Ethanol ingestion leads to decreased GSH and altered GSH metabolism. Reduced GSH is significantly decreased following ethanol consumption; the activities of GSH cycling and metabolizing enzymes show significant fluctuations, consistent with sustained oxidative stress ($n = 6$; $^{*}P < 0.05$, $^{**}P < 0.01$, $^{***}P < 0.001$).

Parameter	Week 1		Week 3		Week 6	
	Control	Ethanol	Control	Ethanol	Control	Ethanol
GSH (μmol/g tissue)	2.667 ± 0.145	2.421 ± 0.134	2.283 ± 0.065	2.046 ± 0.185	3.367 ± 0.239	2.516 ± 0.157*
GSSG (μmol/g tissue)	0.238 ± 0.012	0.169 ± 0.006	0.100 ± 0.008	0.118 ± 0.012	0.173 ± 0.006	0.155 ± 0.008
GR activity (U/mg protein)	0.981 ± 0.019	0.958 ± 0.027	0.890 ± 0.040	0.850 ± 0.020	0.879 ± 0.028	1.149 ± 0.047**
GCL activity (U/mg protein)	0.899 ± 0.042	1.230 ± 0.025***	1.008 ± 0.032	1.154 ± 0.063	1.029 ± 0.052	1.449 ± 0.083***
CBS activity (U/mg protein)	10.335 ± 1.285	8.459 ± 0.648	9.136 ± 0.873	9.415 ± 0.554	4.931 ± 0.224	3.549 ± 0.0812***

models for oxidative stress and has been proposed to be a compensatory mechanism [28].

We and others have shown that oxidative stress and products of lipid peroxidation can also alter GSH biosynthesis via actions on GCL. This has been shown to occur through posttranslational modification of preexisting protein and/or changes in the relative levels of GCL holoenzyme, which has a significantly greater specific activity than monomeric GCLC [30, 35]. As shown in Table 3, the activity of GCL was significantly increased following 1 and 6 weeks of ethanol consumption. Standard immunoblotting revealed that ethanol ingestion had no significant effect on GCLC or GCLM expression (data not shown). Analysis of GCL holoenzyme formation by native gel electrophoresis and immunoblotting revealed no significant effect of ethanol ingestion on the relative levels of GCL holoenzyme compared to monomeric GCLC (data not shown). While these findings suggest that ethanol-induced oxidative stress increases hepatic GCL activity, it should be noted that these GCL activity measurements were performed under saturating substrate concentrations and thus reflect optimal GCL enzymatic activity. Importantly, such measurements do not take into account the potential contribution of altered substrate availability.

Indeed, cysteine availability is often the rate-limiting factor in GSH biosynthesis. To assess endogenous cysteine synthesis and its effects on GSH biosynthesis, the transsulfuration pathway was investigated, specifically cystathionine beta synthase (CBS). As shown in Table 3, a significant decrease in CBS activity was observed at the week 6 time point ($P < 0.001$). This is likely a result of a significant decrease in protein expression (~30%, $P < 0.05$, data not shown) as a result of ethanol ingestion. The activity and expression of the transsulfuration enzyme cystathionine γ-lyase was also assessed and displayed no significant alterations in either parameter. Collectively, these data suggest that not only alcohol consumption leads to the increased utilization of GSH as an antioxidant but also the endogenous synthesis of the GSH precursor cysteine is significantly altered, providing a dual mechanism for the observed decrease in GSH.

3.4. Ethanol Ingestion Leads to Increased Protein Glutathionylation. The binding of GSSG to protein thiols is referred to as protein glutathionylation (protein-SSG) and has been linked to numerous disease states associated with oxidative stress [36]. We, therefore, sought to investigate this phenomenon in our model for ALD. As shown in Figure 2(a), immunohistochemical staining for protein-SSG reveals a marked increase in zone 3 hepatocyte staining. Although the impact of this modification is unknown, current theories propose protein-SSG to be a protective mechanism, shielding critical cysteine residues from more permanent oxidative modifications, that is, 4-HNE [37].

Mechanisms behind protein-SSG remain unknown; however, recent reports have proposed a role for the glutathione s-transferase (GST) and glutaredoxin (GRx)

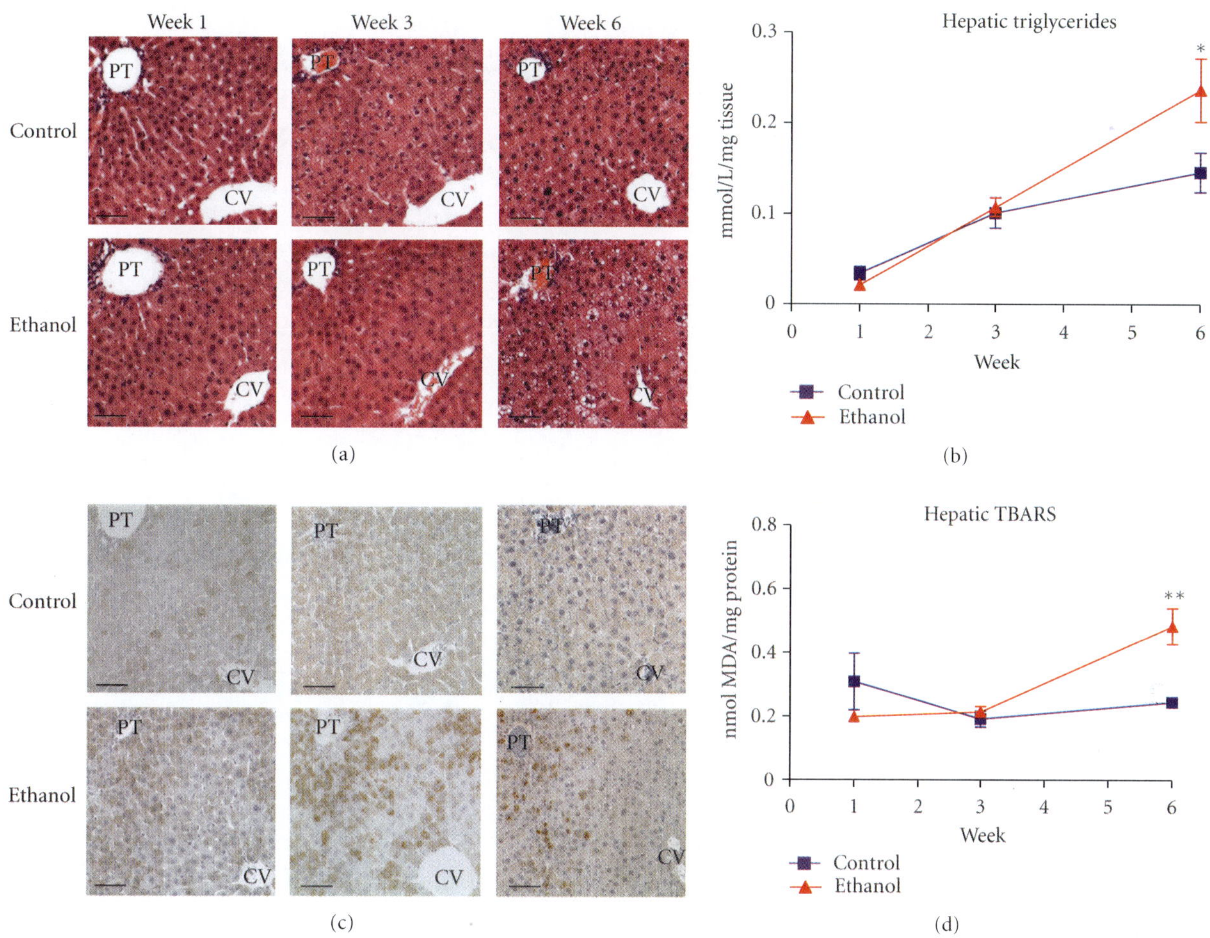

FIGURE 1: Chronic ethanol ingestion leads to increased hepatic lipid accumulation and lipid peroxidation. (a) H&E staining reveals marked pan-lobular lipid accumulation following 6 weeks of ethanol consumption. (b) Liver triglycerides are significantly increased following 6 weeks of ethanol ingestion. (c) Immunohistochemical analysis with 4-HNE antibodies reveals increased staining in ethanol-fed mice throughout zones 1 and 2 as early as week 3. (d) Hepatic TBARSs are significantly elevated following 6 weeks of ethanol ingestion. Magnification: 400x. Scale bar represents approximately 50 μm. PT: portal triad; CV: central vein ($n = 12$, $^*P < 0.05$, $^{**}P < 0.01$).

family of enzymes [38, 39]. We, therefore, measured these enzymes in our disease model. As shown in Figures 2(b) and 2(c), a significant increase in pan-GST and GRx activities was observed in the ethanol-fed mice following 6 weeks, while no significant difference was observed at weeks 1 or 3. The expression of these enzymes was also assessed via immunoblotting, revealing no significant differences in protein expression (data not shown). These data demonstrate, for the first time, protein-SSG as a consequence of sustained ethanol ingestion and provide novel avenues for research in the field of ALD.

3.5. Ethanol Ingestion Leads to Increased Protein Ubiquitination. The effects of ethanol consumption and 4-HNE on proteasome activity have been previously documented [40, 41]. Immunohistochemical staining presented in Figure 1(c) reveals a significant increase in 4-HNE protein adducts, suggesting a mechanism for altered protein folding following sustained ethanol consumption. To investigate the impact of sustained oxidative stress on protein folding in this model, immunohistochemical staining was performed using antiubiquitin antibodies to target misfolded proteins targeted for degradation. As shown in Figure 3(a), marked accumulation of ubiquitinated proteins was found throughout zones 2 and 3 in ethanol-consuming mice following 6 weeks. These data suggest an increase in protein misfolding and/or erred protein load as noted by an increasing need for protein disposal. Given the large increase in protein ubiquitination at the week 6 time point, proteasome activity was quantified to determine if the effects on protein ubiquitination were due to altered disposal or increased protein misfolding. As shown in Figure 3(b), no significant alterations in proteasome activity were found between the week 6 control and ethanol-fed mice. These data collectively suggest an increase in protein misfolding following ethanol ingestion, with large quantities of tagged protein being observed during pathologic situations. Given these observations, it was our goal to investigate the role of the UPR in our model for early-stage ALD.

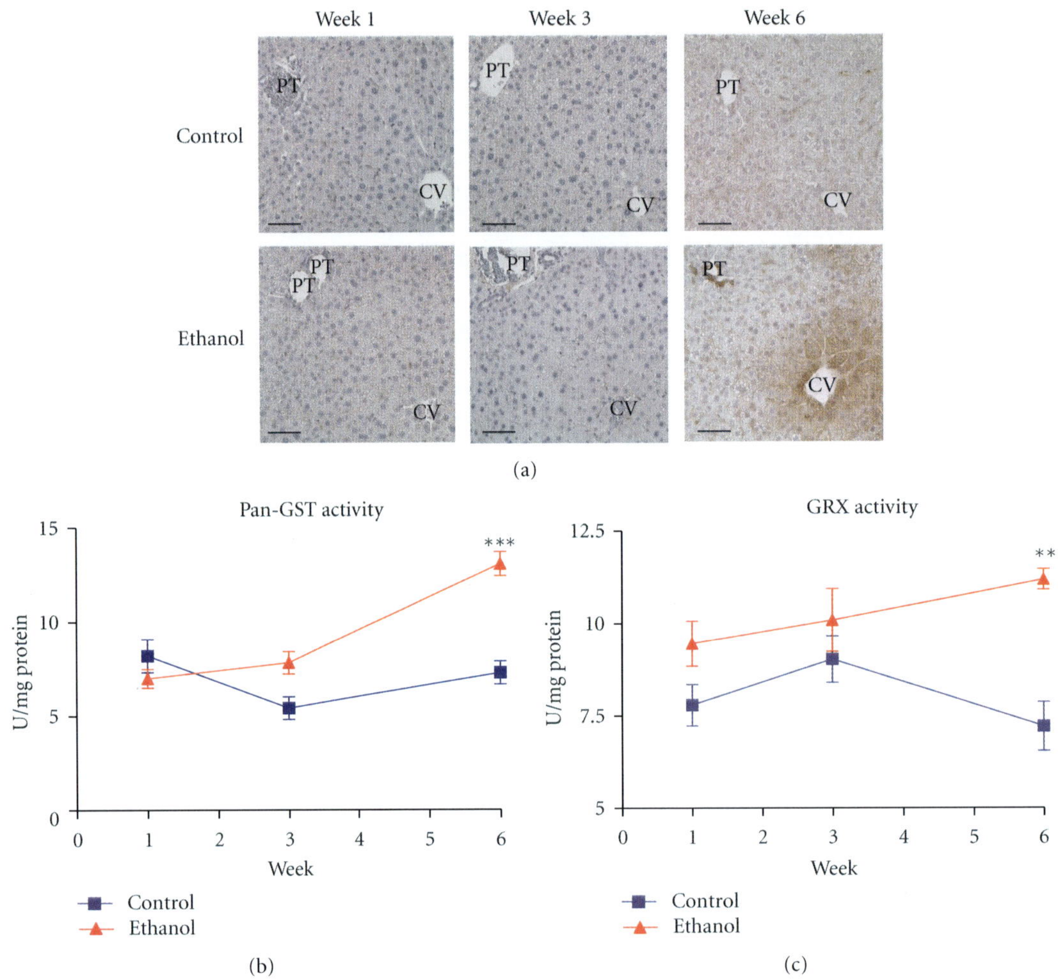

FIGURE 2: Ethanol ingestion results in increased protein-SSG. (a) Immunohistochemical staining with antibodies directed against protein-SSG reveals a marked increase in the zone 3 staining in the week 6 ethanol-fed mice. (b) pan-GST activity and (c) GRx activity significantly elevated at week 6. Magnification: 400x. Scale bar represents approximately 50 μm. PT: portal triad: CV: central vein ($n = 6$, $^{**}P < 0.01$, $^{***}P < 0.001$).

3.6. No Evidence for UPR Activation in Early-Stage ALD. UPR signaling is not only limited to protein expression, as these pathways remain extremely complex and reliant on protein localization and posttranslational modifications [42]. To assess these parameters, immunoblotting was conducted to evaluate UPR protein expression, localization and phosphorylation status. As a positive control, a liver homogenate was utilized from a mouse, which received an intraperitoneal injection of tunicamycin (Tm). As shown in Figure 4(a), the expression of the hallmark indicator for the UPR, glucose regulated protein 78kDa (Grp78), showed no change in expression at any time point. The activation of IRE1α, as measured by the relative expression level of its phosphorylated form (p-IRE1α), was also observed indicating no major role for this pathway following ethanol ingestion. To investigate the PERK pathway, both total eIF2α and activated eIF2α (p-eIF2α) were assessed. No significant activation of this pathway was observed (Figure 4(a)). Finally, nuclear localization of ATF6 (nATF6) is the major indicator for the activation of this pathway following initiation of UPR signaling. As shown in Figure 4(a), no change in nATF6 was observed between control and ethanol-fed mice, despite a potent activation of this protein following Tm injection.

The ER stress response has been shown to lead to a host of cellular responses, including steatosis [43, 44]. Relevant to the pathologies associated with early-stage ALD, lipogenic mediators initiated by UPR signaling were investigated (Figure 4(a)). No significant change in the nuclear localization of SREBP1 (nSREBP1) or nSREBP2 was observed between control and ethanol-fed mice at any time point. Although a trending increase in SREBP1 activation was observed, blot densitometry revealed no significant difference among treatment groups (data not shown).

Previous reports have shown a clear association between the ER stress response and oxidative stress. This link is thought to occur through the induction of the Ero1 proteins (Ero1α and Ero1β) and Nox4. To investigate a possible separation between these responses, the expression of Ero1α, Ero1β and Nox4 was assessed via immunoblotting. As shown in Figure 4(b), no significant change in expression

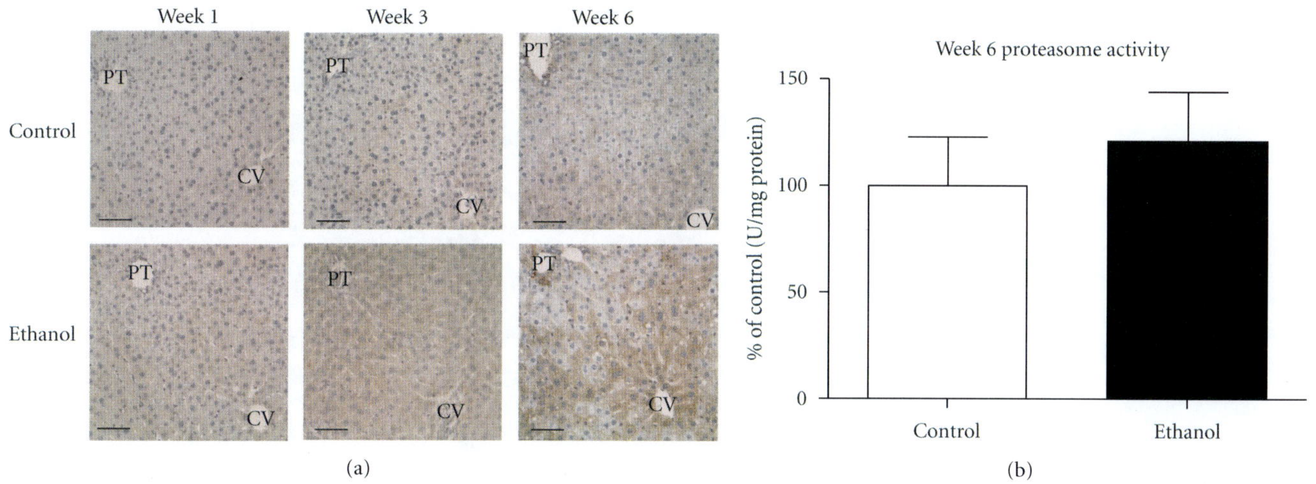

FIGURE 3: Early-Stage ALD leads to a significant increase in protein ubiquitination. (a) Immunohistochemical analysis reveals marked staining of ubiquitinated proteins in zone 3 and zone 2 of ethanol-fed mice following 6-week ingestion. PT: portal triad; CV: central vein. ($n = 4$ pairs; $^{**}P < 0.01$). Magnification, 400x; Scale bar represents approximately 50 μm. (b) Hepatic proteasome activity revealed no change at the week 6 time point ($n = 6$ pairs; $P =$ n.s.).

was observed, indicating that the observed oxidative stress associated with early-stage ALD precedes the involvement of UPR signaling.

4. Discussion

Previous work has supported roles for oxidative stress and ER stress in the etiology of ALD [4, 5, 8, 13, 14, 45, 46]. These pathological processes are intrinsically linked, with each capable of activating the other [16]. In order to elucidate the mechanisms involved in the initiation of ALD hepatopathy, our aim was to focus on the earliest initiating stages of the disease where therapeutic intervention is typically most effective. This 6-week Lieber-DeCarli model for early-state ALD represents the earliest initiating stages of disease progression as shown through the documented sustained ingestion of substantial quantities of alcohol resulting in significant elevations in plasma ALT, liver triglycerides and increased liver : body weight ratio. Histological analyses revealed a marked increase in pan-lobular hepatic lipid accumulation consistent with the early signs of steatosis. Collectively, these data demonstrate a reliable model for early-stage ALD, which allowed for further investigation into the parameters associated with the initiating stages of disease progression.

Oxidative stress is a well-recognized outcome of chronic ethanol ingestion and is likely to play a major role in ethanol-mediated liver damage [4, 5, 8]. Previous works utilizing N-acetylcysteine have demonstrated a protective role for antioxidant therapies in ethanol-mediated liver injury [47, 48]. These studies revealed a significant decrease in ALT measurements, steatosis, and TBARS content. While these data do not definitively prove that oxidative stress is responsible for the early-initiating stages of disease development, a strong correlation can be established. Data presented here reveals a significant decrease in GSH following 6 weeks of ethanol consumption, indicating a decrease in the overall antioxidant capacity of the liver at this time point. Further, a significant decrease in the activity of CBS was observed at the week 6 time point, demonstrating a potential decrease in the GSH precursor cysteine. Previous work conducted on CBS has shown a decrease in enzymatic activity following other hepatic insults such as a methionine-choline-deficient diet and other cellular stresses [49, 50]. We postulate that the effects on CBS activity in the control animals may be due to the high fat content in the control diet. More importantly, the effects of this diet on CBS activity appear to be exacerbated following ethanol consumption. The availability of cysteine is often the rate-limiting determinant in GSH biosynthesis, and these effects on CBS activity offer a potential novel mechanism for the observed decrease in GSH following sustained ethanol ingestion.

The decrease in GSH was consistent with an increase in lipid peroxidation, as demonstrated by increased staining of 4-HNE modified proteins in the livers of ethanol-fed mice. Previous reports by Backos et al. have highlighted the effects of 4-HNE on the activity of GCL utilizing cultured cells; GCL activity was found to be significantly increased following treatment with 4-HNE, despite a significant depletion of cellular GSH [30]. Our findings revealed a similar result, where GCL activity was found to be significantly increased despite no change in the overall expression of the enzyme. Although the effects of 4-HNE on GCL activity are noted, the precise role of aldehyde adduction in the alcoholic liver remains to be fully characterized.

Following 6 weeks of ethanol ingestion, hepatic pan-lobular steatosis is observed, with larger lipid droplets present throughout zones 1 and 2. These macrosteatotic vesicles are likely contributing to the increased lipid peroxidation observed, as demonstrated by staining with 4-HNE throughout these zones. It should be noted as well that

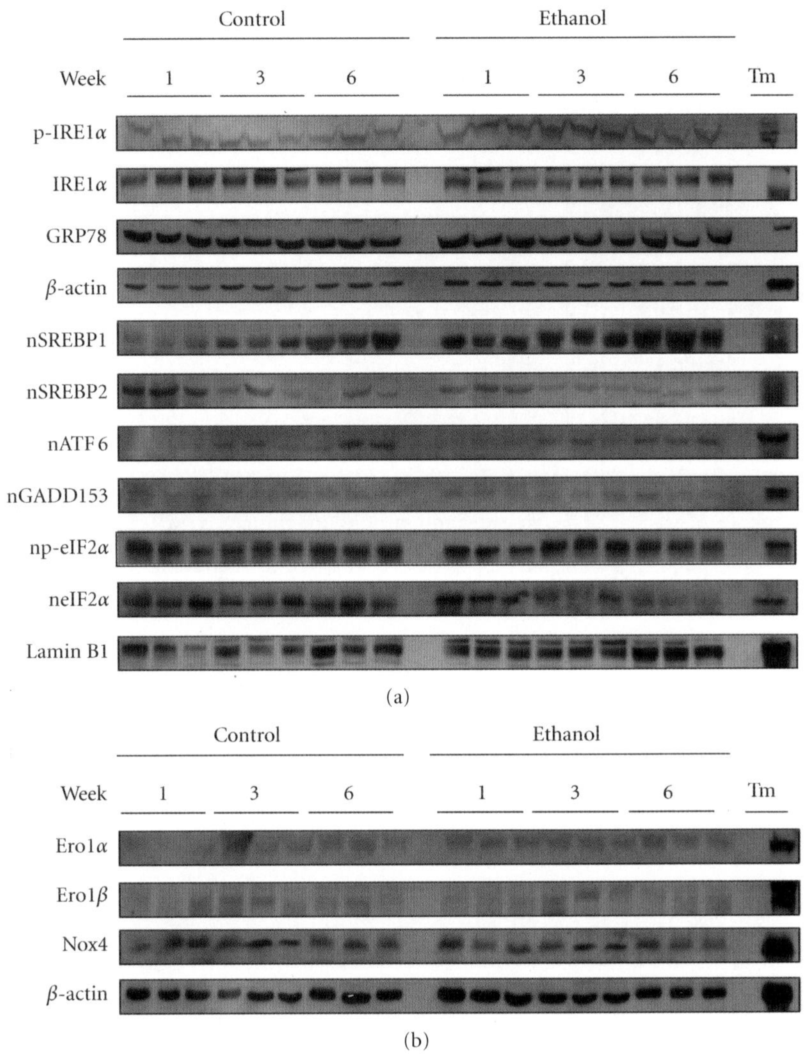

FIGURE 4: Western blotting reveals a disconnect between the UPR and oxidative stress in the pathogenesis of ALD. (a) Standard western blotting shows a lack of activation in classical UPR signaling cascades at any time point. (b) No induction of the Ero1 proteins or Nox4 was observed, confirming a lack of UPR-induced oxidative stress. β-actin was utilized as a loading control for total liver extracts while Lamin B1 was used as a nuclear loading control.

CYP2E1 is found almost exclusively throughout zone 3 and is completely absent in zones 1 and 2. This may, in part, provide a likely explanation for the observed increase in zone 3 staining of protein-SSG, whereby these modifications act to protect critical thiol residues. Oxidative stress occurring in zone 3 has been documented by numerous other groups; however, the staining of ubiquitinated proteins in this region remains a novel finding. It is conceivable that the increased oxidative stress in zone 3 is resulting in other damaging oxidative modifications stemming from CYP2E1-mediated free radical generation. At the current time, the precise mechanisms and rationale behind the increased ubiquitin staining in zone 3 are unknown. Reports from our laboratory utilizing the Lieber-DeCarli model in rats, however, have identified the ER-resident protein disulfide isomerase (PDI) to be a target for modification by 4-HNE *in vivo*; this leads to a decrease in enzymatic activity and impaired protein folding [51]. Collectively, these data suggest a potential mechanism for oxidative-stress-induced UPR signaling in rodent models for ALD [51, 52].

In the past decade, ER stress has been associated with an increasing number of hepatic disease states, most notably ALD [10, 53]. Previous research in mice by Ji et al. has suggested a role for ER stress in an intragastric model of ALD [13, 14, 45]. However, the intragastric model represents a model for more severe pathologies of ALD, as shown by a roughly 8-fold increase in serum ALT (versus an approximate doubling here) and a significant increase in inflammation (inflammation was not seen in our model). The transition from steatosis to steatohepatitis is considered to be the critical pathogenic determinant in ALD furthering a need for therapeutic intervention during the initiating stages of disease progression [20]. Recent reports have suggested an association between the inflammatory response and

UPR signaling, outlining a mechanism similar to that with oxidative stress [54–57]. Consistent with early-stage ALD, our data demonstrate clearly that the inflammatory response does not precede disease pathogenesis and UPR induction in this model.

To further understand the mechanisms behind ALD progression, our research focused on the relative pathogenic contributions of ER stress and oxidative stress during the initiating stages of the disease. Previous work in rodent models of ALD has hypothesized a role for the ER stress response in the activation of lipogenic pathways. This was shown to occur through SREBP1 activation and this mechanism was thought to be a major contributor to the observed hepatic steatosis [13, 45]. To investigate these reports, our studies utilized the Lieber-DeCarli model for ALD. Immunoblotting for both hallmark and lipogenic UPR signaling cascades revealed no significant activation during our time course model for ALD despite the generation of significant pathologies, such as increased lipid accumulation and serum ALT levels. Taken together, these data validate a minimal role for the UPR during the development of ethanol-induced steatosis in a murine model for early-stage ALD.

Oxidative stress has gained considerable attention as a possible mechanism for the induction of various cellular responses, including the ER stress response [8, 15–19, 58]. Additionally, UPR signaling has been shown to lead to induction of the Ero1 proteins and Nox4, furthering the oxidative stress burden in the cell. This oxidative protein folding relay has been estimated by Tu and Weissman to account for up to 25% of total cellular ROS [59]. This creates a vicious cycle of cellular derangements, where each response propagates the other. Regarding the alcoholic liver, UPR signaling and oxidative stress have been intimately associated with the progression of ALD. To date, these responses have not been investigated in relation to the initiation of ALD and therefore the relative role each has during early-stage ALD is not understood.

Our data demonstrate a clear delineation between the ER stress response and oxidative stress in early-stage ALD, indicating that oxidative stress is a primary initiating factor responsible for the progression of ALD. The observed increase in protein glutathionylation demonstrates a potential involvement for this posttranslational modification following increased oxidative stress and provides interesting avenues for research in this field. The effects of oxidative stress in our model were determined to be independent of UPR induction, indicating that the ER stress response may play a pivotal role during more advanced stages of disease progression.

Abbreviations

ALD:	Alcoholic liver disease
CYP2E1:	Cytochrome P450 2E1
ROS:	Reactive oxygen species
Nox:	NAD(P)H oxidase
4-HNE:	4-Hydroxy-2-nonenal
PDI:	Protein disulfide isomerase
ERAD:	ER-associated degradation
UPR:	Unfolded protein response
SREBP:	Sterol regulatory element-binding protein
GADD153/CHOP:	Growth arrest and DNA damage 153
Grp78/94:	Glucose regulated protein 78/94
Ero1:	ER oxidoreductase 1
ALT:	Alanine aminotransferase
TBARS:	Thiobarbituric acid reactive substances
MDA:	Malondialdehyde
GR:	Glutathione reductase
GST:	Glutathione S-transferase
GPx:	Glutathione peroxidase
GSH:	Glutathione
CBS:	Cystathionine β-synthase
GCL:	Glutamate-cysteine ligase
H&E:	Hematoxylin & eosin
GR:	Glutathione reductase
Protein-SSG:	Protein glutathionylation.

Acknowledgment

Studies were supported by the National Institutes of Health/National Institutes of Alcoholism and Alcohol Abuse under Grant nos. R37AA09300 (to D. R. Petersen), R01DK074487-01 (to D. R. Petersen), and F31AA018606-01 (to J. J. Galligan).

References

[1] R. S. Oshea, S. Dasarathy, and A. J. McCullough, "Alcoholic liver disease," *American Journal of Gastroenterology*, vol. 105, no. 1, pp. 14–32, 2010.

[2] S. Zakhari and T. K. Li, "Determinants of alcohol use and abuse: impact of quantity and frequency patterns on liver disease," *Hepatology*, vol. 46, no. 6, pp. 2032–2039, 2007.

[3] G. Arteel, L. Marsano, C. Mendez, F. Bentley, and C. J. McClain, "Advances in alcoholic liver disease," *Bailliere's Best Practice and Research in Clinical Gastroenterology*, vol. 17, no. 4, pp. 625–647, 2003.

[4] A. I. Cederbaum, Y. Lu, and D. Wu, "Role of oxidative stress in alcohol-induced liver injury," *Archives of Toxicology*, vol. 83, no. 6, pp. 519–548, 2009.

[5] S. De Minicis and D. A. Brenner, "Oxidative stress in alcoholic liver disease: role of NADPH oxidase complex," *Journal of Gastroenterology and Hepatology*, vol. 23, no. 1, supplement, pp. S98–S103, 2008.

[6] G. Poli, R. J. Schaur, W. G. Siems, and G. Leonarduzzi, "4-Hydroxynonenal: a membrane lipid oxidation product of medicinal interest," *Medicinal Research Reviews*, vol. 28, no. 4, pp. 569–631, 2008.

[7] C. Ji, "Dissection of endoplasmic reticulum stress signaling in alcoholic and non-alcoholic liver injury," *Journal of Gastroenterology and Hepatology*, vol. 23, no. 1, supplement, pp. S16–S24, 2008.

[8] M. Marí, A. Colell, A. Morales, C. Von Montfort, C. Garcia-Ruiz, and J. C. Fernández-Checa, "Redox control of liver function in health and disease," *Antioxidants and Redox Signaling*, vol. 12, no. 11, pp. 1295–1331, 2010.

[9] A. Görlach, P. Klappa, and T. Kietzmann, "The endoplasmic reticulum: folding, calcium homeostasis, signaling, and redox

control," *Antioxidants and Redox Signaling*, vol. 8, no. 9-10, pp. 1391–1418, 2006.

[10] H. Yoshida, "ER stress and diseases," *FEBS Journal*, vol. 274, no. 3, pp. 630–658, 2007.

[11] N. Kaplowitz and C. Ji, "Unfolding new mechanisms of alcoholic liver disease in the endoplasmic reticulum," *Journal of Gastroenterology and Hepatology*, vol. 21, no. 3, supplement, pp. S7–S9, 2006.

[12] M. Sozio and D. W. Crabb, "Alcohol and lipid metabolism," *American Journal of Physiology*, vol. 295, no. 1, pp. E10–E16, 2008.

[13] C. Ji, C. Chan, and N. Kaplowitz, "Predominant role of sterol response element binding proteins (SREBP) lipogenic pathways in hepatic steatosis in the murine intragastric ethanol feeding model," *Journal of Hepatology*, vol. 45, no. 5, pp. 717–724, 2006.

[14] C. Ji and N. Kaplowitz, "Betaine decreases hyperhomocysteinemia, endoplasmic reticulum stress, and liver injury in alcohol-fed mice," *Gastroenterology*, vol. 124, no. 5, pp. 1488–1499, 2003.

[15] M. Csala, É. Margittai, and G. Bánhegyi, "Redox control of endoplasmic reticulum function," *Antioxidants and Redox Signaling*, vol. 13, no. 1, pp. 77–108, 2010.

[16] J. D. Malhotra and R. J. Kaufman, "Endoplasmic reticulum stress and oxidative stress: a vicious cycle or a double-edged sword?" *Antioxidants and Redox Signaling*, vol. 9, no. 12, pp. 2277–2293, 2007.

[17] C. X. Santos, L. Y. Tanaka, J. Wosniak, and F. R. Laurindo, "Mechanisms and implications of reactive oxygen species generation during the unfolded protein response: roles of endoplasmic reticulum oxidoreductases, mitochondrial electron transport, and NADPH oxidase," *Antioxidants & Redox Signaling*, vol. 11, no. 10, pp. 2409–2427, 2009.

[18] E. Pedruzzi, C. Guichard, V. Ollivier et al., "NAD(P)H oxidase Nox-4 mediates 7-ketocholesterol-induced endoplasmic reticulum stress and apoptosis in human aortic smooth muscle cells," *Molecular and Cellular Biology*, vol. 24, no. 24, pp. 10703–10717, 2004.

[19] R. C. Austin, "The unfolded protein response in health and disease," *Antioxidants and Redox Signaling*, vol. 11, no. 9, pp. 2279–2287, 2009.

[20] A. M. Diehl, "Liver disease in alcohol abusers: clinical perspective," *Alcohol*, vol. 27, no. 1, pp. 7–11, 2002.

[21] J. R. Roede, B. J. Stewart, and D. R. Petersen, "Decreased expression of peroxiredoxin 6 in a mouse model of ethanol consumption," *Free Radical Biology and Medicine*, vol. 45, no. 11, pp. 1551–1558, 2008.

[22] J. W. Finnie and J. D. O'Shea, "Acute hepatotoxicity with resultant pulmonary and cerebral embolism in guinea pigs given tunicamycin," *Pathology*, vol. 21, no. 3, pp. 194–199, 1989.

[23] G. N. Babu, A. Kumar, R. Chandra et al., "Oxidant-antioxidant imbalance in the erythrocytes of sporadic amyotrophic lateral sclerosis patients correlates with the progression of disease," *Neurochemistry International*, vol. 52, no. 6, pp. 1284–1289, 2008.

[24] R. Rinaldi, Y. Aniya, R. Svensson et al., "NADPH dependent activation of microsomal glutathione transferase 1," *Chemico-Biological Interactions*, vol. 147, no. 2, pp. 163–172, 2004.

[25] N. Mesecke, A. Spang, M. Deponte, and J. M. Herrmann, "A novel group of glutaredoxins in the cis-Golgi critical for oxidative stress resistance," *Molecular Biology of the Cell*, vol. 19, no. 6, pp. 2673–2680, 2008.

[26] D. P. Hartley and D. R. Petersen, "Co-metabolism of ethanol, ethanol-derived acetaldehyde, and 4- hydroxynonenal in isolated rat hepatocytes," *Alcoholism*, vol. 21, no. 2, pp. 298–304, 1997.

[27] S. Kashiwamata and D. M. Greenberg, "Studies on cystathionine synthase of rat liver properties of the highly purified enzyme," *Biochimica et Biophysica Acta*, vol. 212, no. 3, pp. 488–500, 1970.

[28] J. A. Villanueva, F. Esfandiari, D. H. Wong et al., "Abnormal transsulfuration and glutathione metabolism in the micropig model of alcoholic liver disease," *Alcoholism*, vol. 30, no. 7, pp. 1262–1270, 2006.

[29] M. H. Stipanuk, "Effect of excess dietary methionine on the catabolism of cysteine in rats," *Journal of Nutrition*, vol. 109, no. 12, pp. 2126–2139, 1979.

[30] D. S. Backos, K. S. Fritz, J. R. Roede, D. R. Petersen, and C. C. Franklin, "Posttranslational modification and regulation of glutamate-cysteine ligase by the α,β-unsaturated aldehyde 4-hydroxy-2-nonenal," *Free Radical Biology and Medicine*, vol. 50, no. 1, pp. 14–26, 2011.

[31] D. J. Reed, J. R. Babson, and P. W. Beatty, "High-performance liquid chromatography analysis of nanomole levels of glutathione, glutathione disulfide, and related thiol and disulfides," *Analytical Biochemistry*, vol. 106, no. 1, pp. 55–62, 1980.

[32] E. Albano, "Alcohol, oxidative stress and free radical damage," *Proceedings of the Nutrition Society*, vol. 65, no. 3, pp. 278–290, 2006.

[33] S. K. Ramaiah, C. Rivera, and G. E. Arteel, "Early-phase alcoholic liver disease: an update on animal models, pathology, and pathogenesis," *International Journal of Toxicology*, vol. 23, no. 4, pp. 217–231, 2004.

[34] S. C. Lu, "Regulation of hepatic glutathione synthesis: current concepts and controversies," *FASEB Journal*, vol. 13, no. 10, pp. 1169–1183, 1999.

[35] C. M. Krejsa, C. C. Franklin, C. C. White, J. A. Ledbetter, G. L. Schieven, and T. J. Kavanagh, "Rapid activation of glutamate cysteine ligase following oxidative stress," *The Journal of Biological Chemistry*, vol. 285, no. 21, pp. 16116–16124, 2010.

[36] J. J. Mieyal, M. M. Gallogly, S. Qanungo, E. A. Sabens, and M. D. Shelton, "Molecular mechanisms and clinical implications of reversible protein S-glutathionylation," *Antioxidants and Redox Signaling*, vol. 10, no. 11, pp. 1941–1988, 2008.

[37] D. Giustarini, R. Rossi, A. Milzani, R. Colombo, and I. Dalle-Donne, "S-glutathionylation: from redox regulation of protein functions to human diseases," *Journal of Cellular and Molecular Medicine*, vol. 8, no. 2, pp. 201–212, 2004.

[38] J. Garcia, D. Han, H. Sancheti, L. P. Yap, N. Kaplowitz, and E. Cadenas, "Regulation of mitochondrial glutathione redox status and protein glutathionylation by respiratory substrates," *The Journal of Biological Chemistry*, vol. 285, no. 51, pp. 39646–39654, 2010.

[39] M. M. Gallogly and J. J. Mieyal, "Mechanisms of reversible protein glutathionylation in redox signaling and oxidative stress," *Current Opinion in Pharmacology*, vol. 7, no. 4, pp. 381–391, 2007.

[40] F. Bardag-Gorce, "Effects of ethanol on the proteasome interacting proteins," *World Journal of Gastroenterology*, vol. 16, no. 11, pp. 1349–1357, 2010.

[41] F. Bardag-Gorce, J. Li, B. A. French, and S. W. French, "The effect of ethanol-induced CYP2E1 on proteasome activity: the role of 4-hydroxynonenal," *Experimental and Molecular Pathology*, vol. 78, no. 2, pp. 109–115, 2005.

[42] P. Walter and D. Ron, "The unfolded protein response: from stress pathway to homeostatic regulation," *Science*, vol. 334, pp. 1081–1086, 2011.

[43] A. H. Lee and L. H. Glimcher, "Intersection of the unfolded protein response and hepatic lipid metabolism," *Cellular and Molecular Life Sciences*, vol. 66, no. 17, pp. 2835–2850, 2009.

[44] J. D. Malhotra and R. J. Kaufman, "The endoplasmic reticulum and the unfolded protein response," *Seminars in Cell and Developmental Biology*, vol. 18, no. 6, pp. 716–731, 2007.

[45] C. Ji, R. Mehrian-Shai, C. Chan, Y. H. Hsu, and N. Kaplowitz, "Role of CHOP in hepatic apoptosis in the murine model of intragastric ethanol feeding," *Alcoholism*, vol. 29, no. 8, pp. 1496–1503, 2005.

[46] M. R. Lucey, P. Mathurin, and T. R. Morgan, "Alcoholic hepatitis," *The New England Journal of Medicine*, vol. 360, no. 26, pp. 2704–2769, 2009.

[47] M. J. J. Ronis, L. Hennings, B. Stewart et al., "Effects of long-term ethanol administration in a rat total enteral nutrition model of alcoholic liver disease," *American Journal of Physiology*, vol. 300, no. 1, pp. G109–G119, 2011.

[48] R. Ozaras, V. Tahan, S. Aydin, H. Uzun, S. Kaya, and H. Senturk, "N-acetylcysteine attenuates alcohol-induced oxidative stress in the rat," *World Journal of Gastroenterology*, vol. 9, no. 1, pp. 125–128, 2003.

[49] K. N. Maclean, M. Janok, E. Kraus et al., "Cystathionine β-synthase is coordinately regulated with proliferation through a redox-sensitive mechanism in cultured human cells and *Saccharomyces cerevisiae*," *Journal of Cellular Physiology*, vol. 192, no. 1, pp. 81–92, 2002.

[50] B. Tang, A. Mustafa, S. Gupta, S. Melnyk, S. J. James, and W. D. Kruger, "Methionine-deficient diet induces post-transcriptional downregulation of cystathionine β-synthase," *Nutrition*, vol. 26, no. 11-12, pp. 1170–1175, 2010.

[51] D. L. Carbone, J. A. Doorn, Z. Kiebler, and D. R. Petersen, "Cysteine modification by lipid peroxidation products inhibits protein disulfide isomerase," *Chemical Research in Toxicology*, vol. 18, no. 8, pp. 1324–1331, 2005.

[52] P. Haberzettl, E. Vladykovskaya, S. Srivastava, and A. Bhatnagar, "Role of endoplasmic reticulum stress in acrolein-induced endothelial activation," *Toxicology and Applied Pharmacology*, vol. 234, no. 1, pp. 14–24, 2009.

[53] N. Kaplowitz, T. A. Than, M. Shinohara, and C. Ji, "Endoplasmic reticulum stress and liver injury," *Seminars in Liver Disease*, vol. 27, no. 4, pp. 367–377, 2007.

[54] I. De Domenico and J. Kaplan, "A new wrinkle in the fold: hepcidin links inflammation to the unfolded protein respons," *Cell Metabolism*, vol. 10, no. 4, pp. 245–246, 2009.

[55] G. S. Hotamisligil, "Endoplasmic Reticulum Stress and the Inflammatory Basis of Metabolic Disease," *Cell*, vol. 140, no. 6, pp. 900–917, 2010.

[56] K. Zhang, X. Shen, J. Wu et al., "Endoplasmic reticulum stress activates cleavage of CREBH to induce a systemic inflammatory response," *Cell*, vol. 124, no. 3, pp. 587–599, 2006.

[57] K. Zhang and R. J. Kaufman, "From endoplasmic-reticulum stress to the inflammatory response," *Nature*, vol. 454, no. 7203, pp. 455–462, 2008.

[58] J. D. Malhotra, H. Miao, K. Zhang et al., "Antioxidants reduce endoplasmic reticulum stress and improve protein secretion," *Proceedings of the National Academy of Sciences of the United States of America*, vol. 105, no. 47, pp. 18525–18530, 2008.

[59] B. P. Tu and J. S. Weissman, "Oxidative protein folding in eukaryotes: mechanisms and consequences," *Journal of Cell Biology*, vol. 164, no. 3, pp. 341–346, 2004.

10

Application of Neurochemical Markers for Assessing Health Effects after Developmental Methylmercury and PCB Coexposure

E. Roda,[1] L. Manzo,[1,2] and T. Coccini[1]

[1] *Laboratory of Clinical Toxicology, Salvatore Maugeri Foundation IRCCS, Institute of Pavia, 27100 Pavia, Italy*
[2] *Department of Internal Medicine and Therapeutics, Division of Toxicology, University of Pavia, 27100 Pavia, Italy*

Correspondence should be addressed to E. Roda, elisa.roda@fsm.it

Academic Editor: Yasir Hasan Siddique

Cholinergic muscarinic receptors (MRs) and monoamine oxidase activity (MAO-B), expressed both in brain and blood cells, were investigated in animals and exposed subjects to assess (i) MeHg (0.5–1 mg/kg/day GD7-PD7) and/or PCB153 (20 mg/kg/day GD10–GD16) effects on cerebellar MAO-B and MRs, and lymphocyte MRs, in dams and offspring 21 days postpartum; (ii) MAO-B in platelets and MRs in lymphocytes of a Faroese 7-year-old children cohort, prenatally exposed to MeHg/PCBs. *Animal Data.* MAO-B was altered in male cerebellum by MeHg, PCB153, and their combination (35%, 45%, and 25% decrease, resp.). Cerebellar MRs were enhanced by MeHg alone in dams (87%) and male pups (27%). PCB153 alone and in mixture did not modify cerebellar MRs. Similarly to brain, lymphocyte MRs were enhanced in both dams and offspring by MeHg alone. All changes were caused by 1 MeHg mg/kg/day, the lower dose was ineffective. *Human Data.* Both biomarkers showed homogeneous distributions within the cohort (MRs, range 0.1–36.78 fmol/million cells; MAO-B, 0.95–14.95 nmol/mg protein/h). No correlation was found between the two biomarkers and neurotoxicant concentrations in blood (pre- and postnatally).

1. Introduction

In the last few decades, the continuous exposure of humans to complex mixture of contaminating substances in food is an issue that has been giving increasing cause for concern. Clinical and experimental research has demonstrated the high vulnerability of the developing nervous system to toxic insults, leading to permanent alteration of brain functions and pathologies later in life [1, 2]. Among the neurodevelopmental toxicants that received attention in this regard, methylmercury (MeHg) and polychlorinated biphenyls (PCBs) represent a great public health concern, because low-level chronic exposure can occur at various world sites through the consumption of contaminated fish, seafood, and marine mammals meat.

The neurotoxic hazard posed by MeHg and PCBs as well as the unique susceptibility of the developing brain are well documented [3, 4] but no definitive conclusion has yet been reached about the dose-response relationship [5–7], that remain unclear, particularly in relation to concomitant exposures.

Noteworthy, several epidemiologic studies on neurobehavioural endpoints in fish-eating populations at various world sites, including the Faroe Islands [8], the Madeira Island [9], the Brazilian Amazon basin, and more recent investigations on north-american Cree Indian infants, New-Yorkers and Bostonian inhabitants, and European fish consumers, demonstrated mercury-related neuropsychological or neurophysiological adverse effects in the offspring, in the domains of language, attention and memory, as well as visuospatial and motor functions [6, 10, 11].

These effects may have been augmented by concomitant exposure to PCBs, which may affect similar neurobehavioural endpoints [12, 13].

Children exposed to PCBs and related chemicals *in utero* or through breastfeeding have an increased incidence of headaches, cognitive deficits, and significantly delayed psychomotor development [14]. In experimental animal models, a number of long-lasting impairments, for example, learning, behavioural, and neurochemical alterations have been described following maternal exposure to PCBs [15–19].

Because human populations are often exposed to mixtures, as also for MeHg and PCBs in food, raising questions about possible additive, synergistic, or antagonistic effects of the components [20], the potential of these pollutants to interact, and the valuation of their joint effects should be thoroughly investigated, even though it is extremely difficult in epidemiological studies.

To gain this goal, studies investigating biochemical parameters in easily accessible non-neural tissues, which are similar to those targeted by chemicals in the brain (see [21]), may represent a successful approach to developing markers of neurotoxicity, which could be useful in exposed people [22, 23]. In this respect, candidate non-invasive surrogate markers include neurotransmitter receptors, enzymes, and cell signalling components, which are measurable in blood, plasma, lymphocytes, and/or platelets and can be affected by neurotoxicants in these peripheral tissues with changes mirroring those occurring in the brain [21, 24–27].

Examples of these peripheral markers include the cholinergic muscarinic receptors (MRs) in lymphocytes and the enzyme activity of monoamine oxidase-B (MAO-B) in platelets [27–29].

The cholinergic system, essential for normal brain development [30], is a sensitive target for MeHg neurotoxicity [31, 32]. Both *in vitro* and *in vivo* evidences indicate that the cholinergic muscarinic system can be affected by MeHg [25, 33–40], as well as by PCBs during development [41–43]. Notably, coexposure to MeHg and either PCB153 or PCB126 had the same effect on the cerebral MRs as exposure to each compound alone [28]. It has to be considered that changes in levels and activity of MRs have been implicated in the pathophysiology of many major diseases of the CNS [44–48].

Noticeably, in mammalian species, most of the cholinergic components found in the CNS, including MRs, are also expressed in non-neuronal tissues including lymphocytes isolated from peripheral blood, thymus, lymph nodes, and spleen [49]. Accordingly, some neurotransmission parameters measured in rats, including lymphocytes MRs, after the exposure to neurotoxicants and muscarinic drugs [35, 43, 50–52], have been shown to mirror equivalent changes of these biochemical end-points in the CNS, thus providing accessible measures of the same neurochemical endpoints express in the CNS.

Both MeHg and PCBs may also affect the central monoaminergic system as well. In fact, altered dopaminergic neurotransmission has been observed following perinatal exposure to MeHg (0.5 mg/kg/day, GD7-PND7) in rats [53, 54]; moreover, MeHg can stimulate the spontaneous release of monoamines from different experimental CNS tissue preparations [55, 56]. The most consistent neurochemical effects of noncoplanar PCBs have been found to be a reduction in dopamine (DA) concentrations besides an increase in DA concentration both in cells and striatal tissue cultures [57–59] as well as in laboratory animals brains after developmental or adult exposure (for a review, [18]), with an exacerbation of the effects of the two contaminants acting synergistically when coadministrated [58]. On the other hand, in a recent *in vivo* study, we demonstrated that perinatal exposure to MeHg (0.5 mg/kg/day) and/or PCB153 (5 mg/kg/day) given orally to rat dams, affected D1 and D2 receptors in a gender-, time-, and brain area-dependent fashion, without additive effects of the two chemical compounds when administrated in mixture [60].

Noticeably, both MeHg and PCBs may alter the activity of the enzyme monoamine oxidase (MAO), which play an important role in the degradation of monoamine neurotransmitters as well as in the neurochemical regulation of behaviour. Experimental evidences in laboratory animals showed that (i) MeHg inhibited MAO activity both *in vivo* and *in vitro* [61, 62] and (ii) prenatal exposure to PCB77 depressed postnatal development of MAO activity in whole rat brain [63]. Recently, perinatal exposure to MeHg or PCB153 in rats was shown to induce regional alterations of the central dopaminergic and serotonergic systems at weaning, but the combined treatment with both these toxicants does not exacerbate the neurochemical effects of the compounds alone [28].

In humans, the MAO-B isoenzyme is the predominant form in the brain and the sole type present in platelets. The amino acid sequences of MAO-B in both platelets and brain are identical [64], and the biochemical and pharmacological characteristics of the enzyme are also similar in the two tissues [65]. In this respect, platelet MAO has been widely used as a model of central neuronal function and a surrogate marker to investigate neurological and psychiatric disorders [66–70].

With the ultimate goal to identify potential biomarkers of CNS effects, which can be applied as accessible tools to use in environmental medicine for assessing and monitoring specific exposure scenarios, a series of *in vivo* experimental studies have been planned in our laboratory. Specifically, in the attempt to advance knowledge on these biomarkers, a first-step study has been performed in order to evaluate (i) brain and lymphocytes MRs and (ii) cerebral MAO-B activity, investigated in both dams and offspring at weaning, after perinatal exposure to MeHg (0.5 mg/kg/day or 1 mg/kg/day, from gestational day (GD)7 to postnatal day (PD)7, and PCBs (20 mg/kg/day from GD10 to GD16) alone and in combination. Then, in a second step, MRs in lymphocytes (l-MRs) and MAO-B in platelets (p-MAO-B) have been applied in a selected human population, with the aim at supporting (i) the predictive value of these biomarkers and (ii) the relevance of a translational approach in environmental medicine.

2. Experimental Protocols

2.1. Animal Studies. All experimental procedures involving animals were performed in compliance with the European Council Directive 86/609/EEC on the care and use of laboratory animals. Adult Sprague-Dawley rats (12 females and 4 males, 12 weeks old for each set of experiment) were purchased from Charles River Italia (Calco, Italy) at least 2 weeks before mating and allowed to acclimatize for 3 weeks. Throughout the experiment, animals were kept in an artificial 12 h light : 12 h dark cycle with humidity at 50 ± 10%. Animals were provided rat chow (VRF1 diet) and tap water ad libitum.

To mimic human developmental dietary exposure to this contaminant, rats were exposed to low-to-moderate doses of MeHg and PCB153 *in utero*, through maternal oral consumption.

The experimental regimen comprises 0.5 and 1 mg MeHg/kg (body weight) bw/day, administered to rat dams in the drinking water from gestational day (GD)7 to postnatal (PD)7, and/or PCB153 (20 mg/kg/day) dissolved in corn oil, administered to rats from GD10 to GD16.

The endpoints investigated in rats included total cholinergic MRs and MAO-B activity in cerebellum and total MRs in lymphocytes at weaning (i.e., PD21) both in dams and their offspring.

At the day of sacrifice, rat brains were rapidly dissected on ice to isolate cerebellum from dams and offspring and stored at -80°C until the analyses were performed. Spleens were also collected.

2.2. Human Population. The Faroese birth cohort ($n = 182$) was established in 1994–1995 and consisted of singleton term births. The studies adhered to the Declaration of Helsinki and have been performed after approval of the Faroese ethical review committee. All subjects participating in the clinical studies have been included after parental written informed consent. Of the original 182 cohort members, 177 were eligible for participation in the 7-year examinations, and 166 agreed to participate (94%). A total of 159 children (76 boys, 83 girls) completed their examinations at 7 years of age with a voluntary blood sample for the exposure analyses and for the determination of biochemical markers: MAO-B activity in platelet and MR binding in lymphocytes.

2.3. MR and MAO-B Determinations in Rat Cerebellum. (i) Total MRs in cerebellum were determined by saturation binding assays using the specific muscarinic antagonist [^{3}H]QNB, capable of labeling all subtypes of the MR family uniformly [35, 43, 52]. By these techniques, the receptor density (Bmax, expressed as femtomoles/mg protein) and affinity (defined as the reciprocal of the dissociation constant, Kd) were estimated by nonlinear regression analysis of saturation binding data.

(ii) MAO-B activity was determined radiochemically as described by Young et al., 1986 [71] using 10 μM ^{14}C-PEA as the substrate. Specific MAO-B activity was determined in the presence of 100 μM pargyline hydrochloride. The reaction was started by addition of ^{14}C-PEA to 50 μL of tissue homogenate (0.2 mL final volume) and stopped by addition of 0.1 mL citric acid 2 M after a 15-min incubation at 37°C. Deaminated reaction products were extracted into 3 mL toluene-ethylacetate (1 : 1, v/v) and the radioactivity contained in a 1-mL aliquot of the organic phase was counted in scintillation counter. The enzyme activity was expressed as nmol/mg protein/h.

2.4. MRs Determination in Lymphocytes. (i) Rat lymphocytes were obtained from the spleen of controls and differently treated animals [35]. MR density and affinity in rat lymphocytes were determined as described in [52].

(ii) Human blood was collected in EDTA tubes and immediately processed to isolate lymphocytes for MR binding as previously described [72]. The lymphocytes were resuspended in the freezing solution [90% plasma obtained from autologous blood kept on ice + 10% dimethylsulfoxide (DMSO)]. Immediately after, the cells were gradually frozen at -80°C for 24 h, and thereafter stored in liquid nitrogen.

Muscarinic receptors in humans were determined by binding assays using a single concentration (Kd) of the specific tritiated ligand antagonist [^{3}H]QNB for muscarinic receptors in lymphocytes [72]. The specific binding was measured in the presence or absence of atropine. Each sample was assayed in triplicate and data were expressed as fmol/10^6 cells.

2.5. MAO-B Determination in Human Platelet. Human blood was collected in EDTA tubes and immediately processed to isolate platelets for MAO-B activity as previously described [72]. The platelet-rich plasma (PRP) was diluted with 10% DMSO, gradually frozen at -80°C for 24 h, and thereafter stored in liquid nitrogen.

The activity of p-MAO-B was determined radiochemically in duplicate samples as described by Coccini et al., 2002 [66] using [^{14}C-PEA] as the substrate. Specific activity was determined in the presence of pargyline hydrochloride. The enzyme activity was expressed as nmol/mg protein/h.

2.6. Analytical Measurements of Total Hg Levels in Rats. Measurements of total Hg in cerebellum and blood also complemented the molecular studies to correlate neurochemical changes with the internal doses (see methods in [43, 52, 73]).

2.7. Statistical Analysis. Data are presented as the mean ± standard deviation. Data analysis was performed by one-way analysis of variance (ANOVA) followed by Fisher's posthoc test using SPSS statistical software, considering probabilities <0.05 as significant. Statistical comparison of Hg concentrations between groups (Hg versus Hg + PCB153) in brain and blood of dams and both offspring gender was performed using Student's t Test.

3. Results

The present study assessed (i) firstly, the individual and joint effect of MeHg (0.5 and 1 mg/kg/day, GD7-PD7) and PCB153 (20 mg/kg/day, GD10–GD16), given orally to rat dams, on the activity of cerebellar MAO-B and MRs as well as on lymphocytes MRs, both in dams and offspring 21 days postpartum; and then (ii) MAO-B activity and MRs in 7-year-old children from Faroese birth cohort, wherein prenatal exposure to MeHg and PCB had already been demonstrated [29, 74].

3.1. Cerebellar MAO-B Activity. Figure 1(a) shows the effects of 1 mg/kg/day MeHg (GD7-PND7) and/or 20 mg/kg/day PCB153 (GD10–GD16) maternal oral treatment on the cerebellar MAO-B activity at PD21 rats, evaluated both in dams and offspring (separately according to gender).

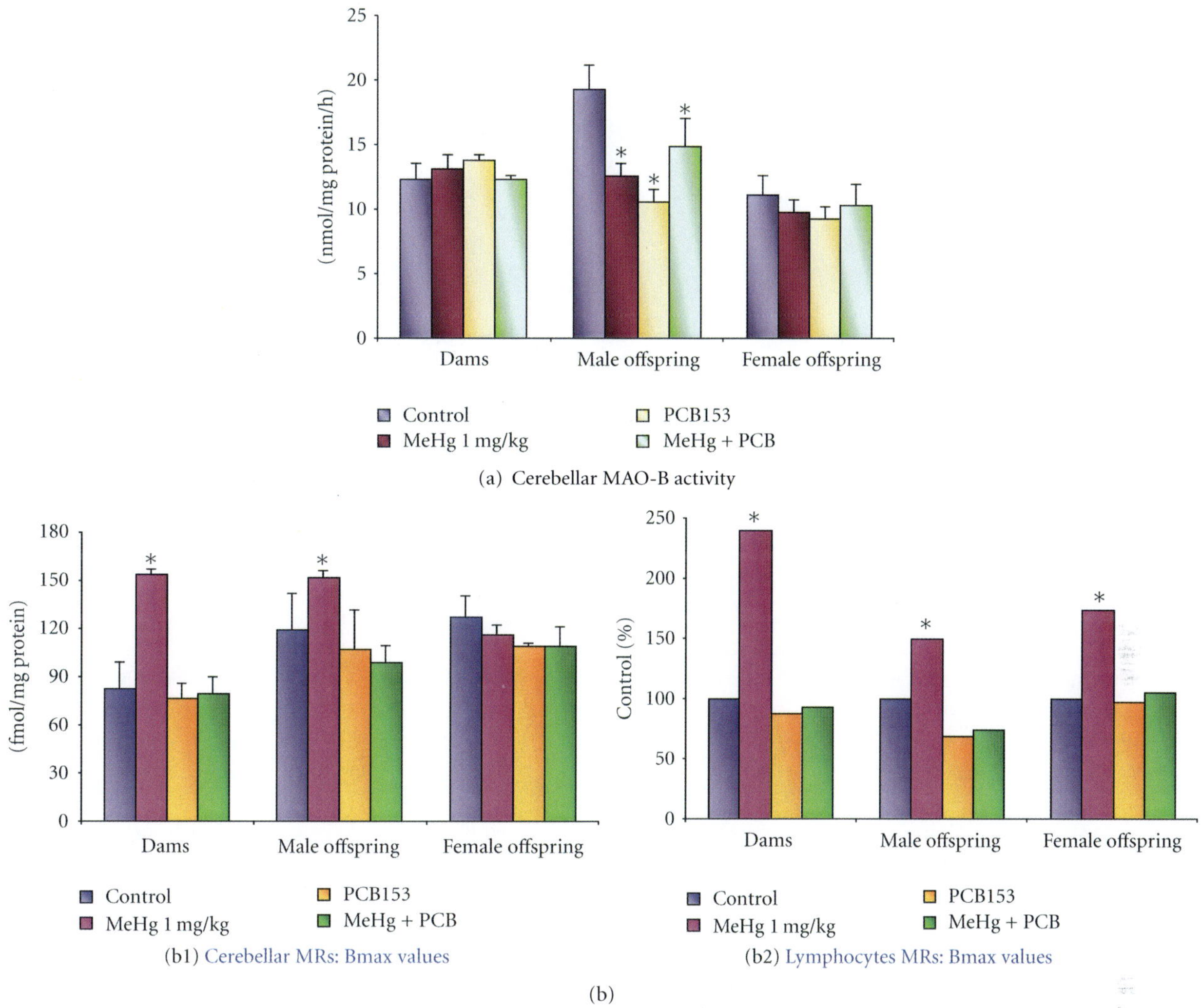

FIGURE 1: Histograms showing cerebellar MAO-B activity (a) and MRs binding in cerebellum (b1) and lymphocytes (b2) of both dams and 21-day-old male and female rats, perinatally exposed to MeHg (1 mg/kg/day, GD7-PND7) and PCB153 (20 mg/kg/day, GD10–GD16), alone or combined. Data are the mean ± SEM of $n = 3$–9 rats/treatment group/gender. *Significantly different from control group, $P < 0.05$.

The doses, timing of MeHg and PCB153 administrations, and the time-point (PD21) to determine the neurochemical endpoints were selected from previous experimental data demonstrating changes in rat cerebral MRs density, following the same regimen of perinatal exposure [42]. Furthermore, this treatment protocol neither produced any noxious effect on pregnancy, litter size at birth and ratio between male and female pups, maternal or neonatal body weight increase, nor resulted in any gross abnormality to the pups (data not shown).

In male rat cerebellum, in which the control levels of MAO-B activity (nmol/mg protein/h) were 19.26 ± 2.05, all diverse exposures caused significant changes in the enzyme activity (Figure 1(a)). Particularly, MeHg decreased MAO-B activity by 35%, PCB153 by 45%, and the combined treatment by 25%. On the contrary, in female pups, this neurochemical endpoint was not affected by any treatment (Figure 1(a)), neither was in dams.

Noticeably, no effects on MAO-B activity were observed using the lower MeHg dose (0.5 mg/kg/day from GD7 to PND7) in both male and female offspring (data not presented).

The radiochemical method, employed in the present study to determine MAO-B activity, did not allow the detection of this enzyme in rat platelets.

3.2. Cerebellar MRs Density (Bmax). In accordance to previous investigations [75], all determinations were done at the end of the lactational period (PND21), a time at which the total MR binding sites reach adult levels in rats.

Exposure to the higher dose of MeHg (1 mg/kg/day) significantly enhanced cerebellar MRs density in dams (87%), and, in the offspring, Bmax increase was observed in the male pups only (27%) (Figure 1(b1)). Differently from the response to MeHg, PCB153 did not modify cerebellar MRs density both in adult and offspring. After the concomitant

TABLE 1: Total Hg levels in blood and brain of rats perinatally treated with 1 mg MeHg/kg bw/day (GD7-PD7) and/or 20 mg PCB153/kg bw/day (GD10–GD16), alone and in combination.

	Blood Hg (μg/ml)			Brain Hg (μg/g)		
	Dams	*Offspring*		*Dams*	*Offspring*	
		Male	*Female*		*Male*	*Female*
Control	0.017 ± 0.004 $n = 3$	0.003 ± 0.001 $n = 4$	0.005 ± 0.004 $n = 4$	0.013	0.002	0.003
MeHg	11.33 ± 2.26 $n = 4$	1.35 ± 0.40 $n = 4$	1.31 ± 0.40 $n = 4$	7.53	1.67 ± 0.43 $n = 4$	1.52 ± 0.33 $n = 4$
MeHg + PCB153	10.74 ± 1.95 $n = 5$	1.33 ± 0.33 $n = 5$	1.26 ± 0.20 $n = 5$	8.78	2.80 ± 1.81 $n = 6$	1.63 ± 0.20 $n = 6$
PCB153	0.012 ± 0.001 $n = 5$	0.003 ± 0.001 $n = 4$	0.002 ± 0.001 $n = 5$	0.026	0.024 ± 0.039 $n = 4$	0.014 ± 0.024 $n = 6$

Data are the mean ± S.D.

exposure to MeHg (1 mg/kg/day) and PCB153, the MRs density was similar to that detected after the administration of PCB153 alone(Figure 1(b1)).

Noticeably, the lower dose of MeHg (0.5 mg/kg/day) either alone or in combination with PCB153 did not cause any change in MR density both in the mother and offspring cerebella (data not shown).

Cerebellar control Kd values were 0.085 ± 0.02, 0.078 ± 0.01, 0.080 ± 0.01 nM in dams, male, and female offspring, respectively. MeHg and PCB153, alone and in combination, did not affect the dissociation constant values (Kd) measured both in dams and offspring, thus suggesting that the affinity of the ligand [^{3}H]QNB for its receptor was not modified by these compounds.

3.3. Lymphocytes MRs: Animal Data. Exposure to 1 mg MeHg/kg/day during pregnancy and lactation (from GD7 to PND7) significantly enhanced lymphocyte MR density in both dams and 21 day-old rats, with a more pronounced effect in the mothers (Bmax increase of 139%) than in the male offspring (+49%) and female offspring (+73%) as compared with their respective controls (33 ± 4, 41 ± 8, and 37 ± 4 fmol/million cells, Figure 1(b2)), in accordance with the higher Hg levels detected in the adult blood (11.3 ± 2.26 mg/mL) than in pups (1.35 ± 0.4 mg/L in both genders, Table 1), and in absence of any change in their Kd values (control Kd values were 30 ± 10 nM).

Again, when the lower dose of MeHg (0.5 mg/kg/day) was administered to dams, the density of MRs of all groups did not significantly differ from that of their control groups on day 21 postpartum. This dose of MeHg was also devoid of any effect on the Kd values (data not shown).

3.4. Brain and Blood Hg Levels in Rats. Hg levels were measured in whole brains and blood of both dams and 21-day-old pups (separate accordingly to gender) treated with 1 mg MeHg/kg/day. The Hg concentrations (Table 1) in the brain were about five-fold higher in the mother than in the offspring and resulted to be not affected by the coexposure to PCB153.

Regarding the Hg retention in blood, the levels in the dams were about 10-fold higher than those found in both male and female offspring (Table 1).

3.5. Neurochemical Markers in Humans: Lymphocytes MRs and p-MAO-B. The levels of the lymphocytes MR binding ($n = 139$) and p-MAO-B activity ($n = 137$) measured in the blood of both female and male Faroese children are shown in the Figures 2(a) and 2(b). Figure 2(b) shows the single values of the MR binding in boys ($n = 73$) and girls ($n = 66$), respectively. The MR binding was similar in boys and girls and ranged from 0.1 to 36.78 fmol/million cells in boys and from 0.1 to 35.91 fmol/million cells in girls. Figure 2(a) illustrates the individual values of the MAO-B activity in both male ($n = 70$) and female ($n = 67$) children, respectively. Even for this neurochemical endpoint, the data were similar in both genders (ranges: 0.95–14.57 and 1.57–14.95 nmol/mg protein/hr for boys and girls, resp.).

No correlation (by regression analysis) was found between the two neurochemical biomarkers and neurotoxicant concentrations in blood (pre- and postnatally) [29].

4. Discussion

The present study demonstrates in laboratory animals that developmental exposure to MeHg (1 mg/kg/day, GD7-PND7) and PCB153 (20 mg/kg/day, GD10–GD16), alone and in mixture, affects selected endpoints of cholinergic and monoaminergic transmission, namely, cerebellar MAO-B activity and cerebellar and lymphocyte MRs, both in dams and weaning rats, 3 weeks after cessation of maternal dosing.

In the CNS, MAO-B activity was significantly decreased (25–45%) by all treatment types in the cerebellum of male pups only. The combined exposure to MeHg and PCB153 did not exacerbate the neurochemical effects of the individual compounds.

MRs density was significantly affected by MeHg alone both in dams and male offspring cerebella (Bmax enhancement of 87% and 27%, resp.), while, in the coexposed group, no MRs changes were observed.

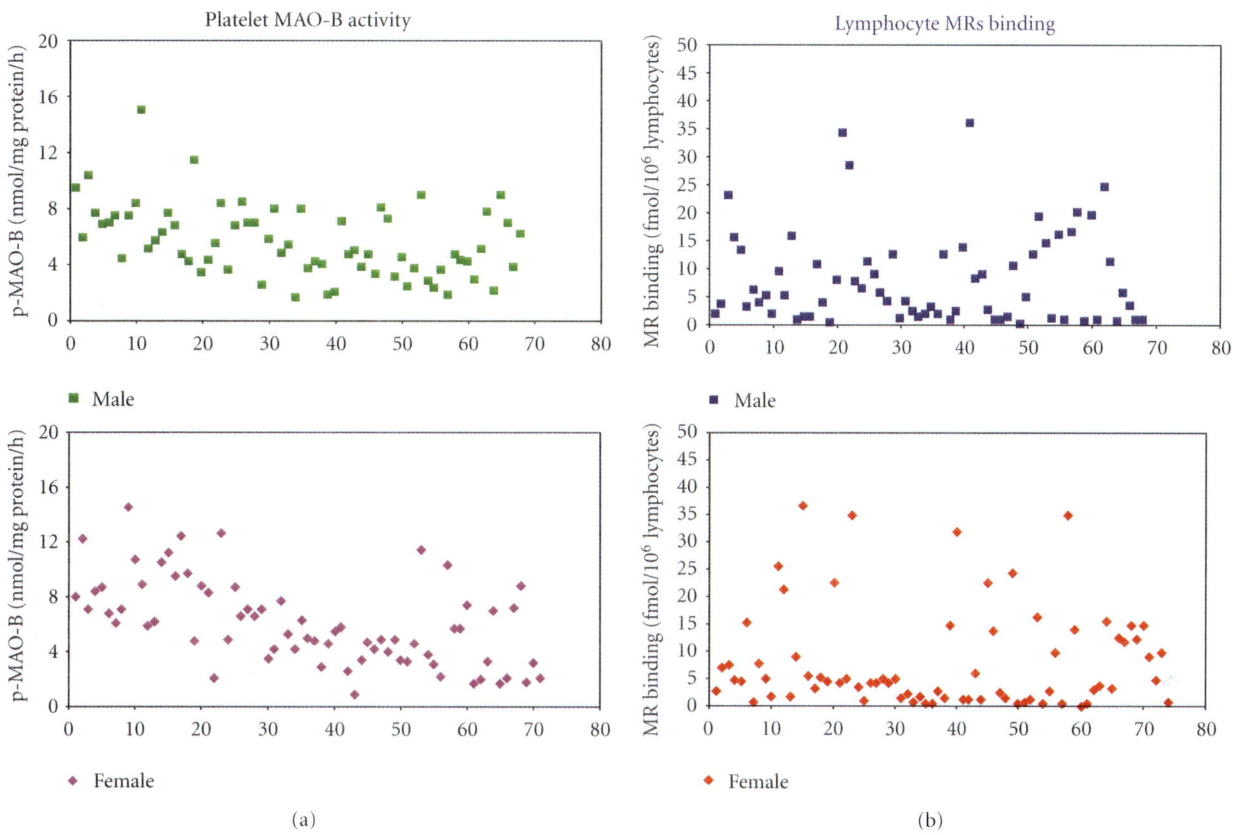

FIGURE 2: Levels of (a) p-MAO-B activity ($n = 137$) and (b) l-MR binding measured in the blood of both female and male Faroese children. (a) illustrates the individual values of the MAO-B activity in 70 boys (mean ± SD = 6.08 ± 3.12 nmol/mg protein/h, range: 0.95–14.57) and 67 girls (mean ± SD = 5.56 ± 2.55 nmol/mg protein/h, range: 1.57–14.95), respectively. (b) shows the single values of the MR binding in 73 boys (mean ± SD = 8.05 ± 9.13 fmol/10^6 cells, range: 0.1–36.78) and 66 girls (mean ± SD = 8.09 ± 8.31 fmol/10^6 cells, range: 0.1–35.91), respectively.

MRs measured in peripheral lymphocytes also displayed alterations similar to those occurring in the cerebellum, in that MeHg alone significantly enhanced MRs density both in dams and offspring, (Bmax increase of 139%, 49%, and 73% for dams, males, and females, resp.), and, when in combination with PCB153, the latter compound masked the MeHg effects.

In another set of experiments, testing the lower MeHg dose (0.5 mg/kg/day, GD7-PND21), no effects were detected for all the chosen cholinergic and monoaminergic endpoints.

Altogether the present results, obtained both in neural tissue and in peripheral cells, are in agreement with a large body of previous experimental evidence strongly supporting the notion that MR binding is modulated in a similar manner in lymphocytes and cerebral tissues. Supporting examples of this parallel modulation come from cholinergic agonist and antagonist drugs [50] as well as by environmental chemicals, such as MeHg [35] and organophosphorous insecticides [51]. Moreover, the MRs were shown to be similarly modulated in rat brain and in lymphocytes following repeated perinatal MeHg exposure [52].

Again, the present investigation demonstrates that the effects measured in lymphocytes MRs of animals coexposed to MeHg and PCB153 mirror the changes observed in cerebellum, in which the chemical mixture produced no detectable MR alterations.

Based on (i) the results obtained from this laboratory animal study (above reported), (ii) the need to identify early biomarkers of effects for delay neurological outcomes due to environmental neurotoxicants exposure, and (iii) the opportunity to measure these biochemical parameters in easily accessible non-neural tissues, we are prompted to evaluate these peripheral surrogate markers in a specific human casistic.

The human study, performed in a cohort of 7-year-old children with widely different degrees of MeHg exposure, with a built-in control group with low-level exposure, indicates that children exhibited homogeneous distributions of the two neurotoxicity biomarkers with no changes associated with increased concentrations of mercury or coexposure with PCB congeners and with no clear association with outcomes of clinical neurobehavioral testing.

These results seem to support the notion that p-MAO-B and l-MRs are not adequately sensitive markers to early detect the subclinical outcomes of MeHg and/or PCBs at low/moderate exposure doses.

Contrarily, recent investigation by Stamler et al. 2006 [68] in a Canadian fish-eating population inhabiting the St. Lawrence River (Lake St. Pierre, Quebec) demonstrated a MeHg-induced reduction in MAO-B activity, associated with blood-Hg concentrations above 3.4 μg/L.

On the other hand, in animal studies, the used perinatal dose of 1 mg MeHg/kg/day markedly affected the rat cholinergic and aminergic systems, while, contrarily, the lower dose of 0.5 mg MeHg/kg/day was totally ineffective. After the former treatment, cerebral Hg levels in weaning rats were 1.5–2.8 ppm and blood Hg levels were $1.3 \pm 0.4\,\mu$g/mL (in both pup genders). These latter data are clearly much higher (250 to 40 times) compared to humans blood Hg levels, for instance, 1300 ppb (in rat blood at PD21) versus 27.6 and 5.27 ppb in cord blood and 7-year-old children blood of the present cohort, respectively [29]. These observations put forward that MeHg-exposure levels may affect the alterations in neurotransmission pathways and, consequently, the changes in both central and peripheral markers. Furthermore, other confounding factors, such as genetic variables, may also be to taken into consideration for their potential impact on the background levels of these biomarkers [76–79].

Moreover, since the precise time point at which these peripheral biomarkers become predictive of neuropsychological outcomes (noticeable later in life) has not been yet clarified, this should be investigated correlating these parameters (neurochemical and neuropsychological) in an early (e.g., cord blood) and late time point manner within the same subject. In this way, one could try to minimize the influence of the blood cell turnover on the levels of these cell-coupled surrogate markers, in that, because of this mechanism, the response to a moderate environmental toxicant exposure may not reflect the possible effect at vulnerable time windows (e.g., *in utero* period) that may cause permanent changes in neuropsychological outcomes.

Nevertheless, a great body of epidemiological evidence indicated the suitability of these biomarkers when employed as peripheral indicators of abnormal behaviour/personality or changes in response to a diagnosed pathological conditions [80–82], and drug dependence [66, 83–85].

Therefore, even though all these above-reported findings and the available bulk of literature seem to be sometimes and somewhere controversial, integrated approaches combining biochemical markers in combination with neurophysiological and behavioral assays could represent a valuable methodological approach by which human neurotoxicity assessment may become more focused.

Conflict of Interests

The authors declare that there is no conflict of interests.

Acknowledgments

The present study was supported by the EU Grants ANEMONE (Quality of Life and Management of Living Re-sources Programme QLK4-CT-2001-00186) and the Italian Ministry of Health. The authors wish to thank Mr. Davide Acerbi for his excellent technical assistance.

References

[1] D. C. Rice and S. Barone Jr., "Critical periods of vulnerability for the developing nervous system: evidence from humans and animal models," *Environmental Health Perspectives*, vol. 108, no. 3, pp. 511–531, 2000.

[2] L. G. Costa, M. Aschner, A. Vitalone, T. Syversen, and O. P. Soldin, "Developmental neuropathology of environmental agents," *Annual Review of Pharmacology and Toxicology*, vol. 44, pp. 87–110, 2004.

[3] M. C. Newland and E. M. Paletz, "Animal studies of methylmercury and PCBs: what do they tell us about expected effects in humans?" *NeuroToxicology*, vol. 21, no. 6, pp. 1003–1027, 2000.

[4] S. L. Schantz and J. J. Widholm, "Cognitive effects of endocrine-disrupting chemicals in animals," *Environmental Health Perspectives*, vol. 109, no. 12, pp. 1197–1206, 2001.

[5] R. A. Lincoln, J. P. Shine, E. J. Chesney, D. J. Vorhees, P. Grandjean, and D. B. Senna, "Fish consumption and mercury exposure among louisiana recreational anglers," *Environmental Health Perspectives*, vol. 119, pp. 245–251, 2011.

[6] P. Grandjean and K. T. Herz, "Methylmercury and brain development: imprecision and underestimation of developmental neurotoxicity in humans," *Mount Sinai Journal of Medicine*, vol. 78, pp. 107–118, 2011.

[7] L. Needham, P. Grandjean, B. Heinzow et al., "Partition of environmental chemicals between maternal and fetal blood and tissues," *Environmental Science & Technology*, vol. 45, pp. 1121–1126, 2011.

[8] P. Grandjean, P. Weihe, R. F. White et al., "Cognitive deficit in 7-year-old children with prenatal exposure to methylmercury," *Neurotoxicology and Teratology*, vol. 19, no. 6, pp. 417–428, 1997.

[9] K. Murata, P. Weihe, A. Renzoni et al., "Delayed evoked potentials in children exposed to methylmercury from seafood," *Neurotoxicology and Teratology*, vol. 21, no. 4, pp. 343–348, 1999.

[10] P. Grandjean and P. Landrigan, "Developmental neurotoxicity of industrial chemicals," *The Lancet*, vol. 368, no. 9553, pp. 2167–2178, 2006.

[11] S. Ceccatelli, E. Daré, and M. Moors, "Methylmercury-induced neurotoxicity and apoptosis," *Chemico-Biological Interactions*, vol. 188, no. 2, pp. 301–308, 2010.

[12] P. Grandjean, P. Weihe, V. W. Burse et al., "Neurobehavioral deficits associated with PCB in 7-year-old children prenatally exposed to seafood neurotoxicants," *Neurotoxicology and Teratology*, vol. 23, no. 4, pp. 305–317, 2001.

[13] P. W. Stewart, J. Reihman, E. I. Lonky, and T. J. Darvill, "Cognitive development in preschool children prenatally exposed to PCBs and MeHg," *Neurotoxicology and Teratology*, vol. 25, no. 1, pp. 11–22, 2003.

[14] J. L. Jacobson and S. W. Jacobson, "Intellectual impairment in children exposed to polychlorinated biphenyls in utero," *The New England Journal of Medicine*, vol. 335, no. 11, pp. 783–789, 1996.

[15] E. Holene, I. Nafstad, J. U. Skaare, and T. Sagvolden, "Behavioural hyperactivity in rats following postnatal exposure to sub- toxic doses of polychlorinated biphenyl congeners 153 and 126," *Behavioural Brain Research*, vol. 94, no. 1, pp. 213–224, 1998.

[16] A. Roth-Haerer, H. Lilienthal, M. Bubser et al., "Neurotransmitter concentrations and binding at dopamine receptors in rats after maternal exposure to 3,4,30,40,-tetrachlorobiphenyl:

the role of reduced thyroid hormone concentrations," *Environmental Toxicology and Pharmacology*, vol. 9, no. 3, pp. 103–115, 2001.

[17] S. L. Schantz, J. Moshtaghian, and D. K. Ness, "Spatial learning deficits in adult rats exposed to ortho-substituted PCB congeners during gestation and lactation," *Fundamental and Applied Toxicology*, vol. 26, no. 1, pp. 117–126, 1995.

[18] H. A. Tilson and P. R. S. Kodavanti, "Neurochemical effects of polychlorinated biphenyls: an overview and identification of research needs," *NeuroToxicology*, vol. 18, no. 3, pp. 727–744, 1997.

[19] C. S. Roegge, V. C. Wang, B. E. Powers et al., "Motor impairment in rats exposed to PCBs and methylmercury during early development," *Toxicological Sciences*, vol. 77, no. 2, pp. 315–324, 2004.

[20] D. A. Cory-Slechta, "Studying toxicants as single chemicals: does this strategy adequately identify neurotoxic risk?" *NeuroToxicology*, vol. 26, no. 4, pp. 491–510, 2005.

[21] L. Manzo, F. Artigas, E. Martine et al., "Biochemical markers of neurotoxicity. A review of mechanistic studies and applications," *Human & Experimental Toxicology*, vol. 15, supplement 1, pp. S20–S35, 1996.

[22] L. Manzo, A. F. Castoldi, T. Coccini, A. D. Rossi, P. L. Nicotera, and L. G. Costa, "Mechanisms of neurotoxicity: applications to human biomonitoring," *Toxicology Letters*, vol. 77, pp. 63–72, 1995.

[23] E. K. Silbergeld and D. L. Davis, "Role of biomarkers in identifying and understanding environmentally induced disease," *Clinical Chemistry*, vol. 40, no. 7, pp. 1363–1367, 1994.

[24] A. F. Castoldi, T. Coccini, A. Rossi et al., "Biomarkers in environmental medicine: alterations of cell signalling as early indicators of neurotoxicity," *Functional Neurology*, vol. 9, no. 2, pp. 101–109, 1994.

[25] A. F. Castoldi, S. M. Candura, P. Costa, L. Manzo, and L. G. Costa, "Interaction of mercury compounds with muscarinic receptor subtypes in the rat brain," *NeuroToxicology*, vol. 17, no. 3-4, pp. 735–742, 1996.

[26] L. G. Costa, "Biomarker research in neurotoxicology: the role of mechanistic studies to bridge the gap between the laboratory and epidemiological investigations," *Environmental Health Perspectives*, vol. 104, no. 1, pp. 55–67, 1996.

[27] L. Manzo, A. F. Castoldi, T. Coccini, and L. D. Prockop, "Assessing effects of neurotoxic pollutants by biochemical markers," *Environmental Research Section A*, vol. 85, no. 1, pp. 31–36, 2001.

[28] A. F. Castoldi, F. Blandini, G. Randine, A. Samuele, L. Manzo, and T. Coccini, "Brain monoaminergic neurotransmission parameters in weanling rats after perinatal exposure to methylmercury and 2,2′,4,4′,5,5′-hexachlorobiphenyl (PCB153)," *Brain Research*, vol. 1112, no. 1, pp. 91–98, 2006.

[29] T. Coccini, L. Manzo, F. Debes, U. Steuerwald, P. Weihe, and P. Grandjean, "No changes in lymphocyte muscarinic receptors and platelet monoamine oxidase-B examined as surrogate central nervous system biomarkers in a Faroese children cohort prenatally exposed to methylmercury and polychlorinated biphenyls," *Biomarkers*, vol. 14, no. 2, pp. 67–76, 2009.

[30] C. F. Hohmann and J. Berger-Sweeney, "Cholinergic regulation of cortical development and plasticity: new twists to an old story," *Perspectives on Developmental Neurobiology*, vol. 5, no. 4, pp. 401–425, 1998.

[31] Y. Yuan and W. D. Atchison, "Disruption by methylmercury of membrane excitability and synaptic transmission of CA1 neurons in hippocampal slices of the rat," *Toxicology and Applied Pharmacology*, vol. 120, no. 2, pp. 203–215, 1993.

[32] T. L. Limke, S. R. Heidemann, and W. D. Atchison, "Disruption of intraneuronal divalent cation regulation by methylmercury: are specific targets involved in altered neuronal development and cytotoxicity in methylmercury poisoning?" *NeuroToxicology*, vol. 25, no. 5, pp. 741–760, 2004.

[33] N. Basu, C. J. Stamler, K. M. Loua, and H. M. Chan, "An interspecies comparison of mercury inhibition on muscarinic acetylcholine receptor binding in the cerebral cortex and cerebellum," *Toxicology and Applied Pharmacology*, vol. 205, no. 1, pp. 71–76, 2005.

[34] A. F. Castoldi, T. Coccini, S. Ceccatelli, and L. Manzo, "Neurotoxicity and molecular effects of methylmercury," *Brain Research Bulletin*, vol. 55, no. 2, pp. 197–203, 2001.

[35] T. Coccini, G. Randine, S. M. Candura, R. E. Nappi, L. D. Prockop, and L. Manzo, "Low-level exposure to methylmercury modifies muscarinic cholinergic receptor binding characteristics in rat brain and lymphocytes: physiologic implications and new opportunities in biologic monitoring," *Environmental Health Perspectives*, vol. 108, no. 1, pp. 29–33, 2000.

[36] M. E. Eldefrawi, N. A. Mansour, and A. T. Eldefrawi, "Interactions of acetylcholine receptors with organic mercury compounds," *Advances in Experimental Medicine and Biology*, vol. 84, pp. 449–463, 1977.

[37] P. D. Hrdina, D. A. V. Peters, and R. L. Singhal, "Effects of chronic exposure to cadmium, lead and mercury on brain biogenic amines in the rat," *Research Communications in Chemical Pathology & Pharmacology*, vol. 15, no. 3, pp. 483–493, 1976.

[38] H. Kobayashi, A. Yuyama, N. Matsusaka, K. Takeno, and I. Yanagiya, "Effects of methylmercury chloride on various cholinergic parameters in vitro," *Journal of Toxicological Sciences*, vol. 4, no. 4, pp. 351–362, 1979.

[39] Y. Tsuzuki, "Effect of chronic methylmercury exposure on activities of neurotransmitter enzymes in rat cerebellum," *Toxicology and Applied Pharmacology*, vol. 60, no. 2, pp. 379–381, 1981.

[40] R. Von Burg, F. K. Northington, and A. Shamoo, "Methylmercury inhibition of rat brain muscarinic receptors," *Toxicology and Applied Pharmacology*, vol. 53, no. 2, pp. 285–292, 1980.

[41] P. Eriksson, U. Lundkvist, and A. Frederiksson, "Neonatal exposure to 3,30,40-tetrachlorobiphenyl: changes in spontaneous behaviour and cholinergic muscarinic receptors in the adult mouse," *Toxicology*, vol. 69, no. 1, pp. 27–34, 1991.

[42] T. Coccini, G. Randine, A. F. Castoldi et al., "Effects of developmental co-exposure to methylmercury and 2,29,4,49,5,59-hexachlorobiphenyl (PCB153) on cholinergic muscarinic receptors in rat brain," *NeuroToxicology*, vol. 27, no. 4, pp. 468–477, 2006.

[43] T. Coccini, E. Roda, A. F. Castoldi et al., "Perinatal co-exposure to methylmercury and PCB153 or PCB126 in rats alters the cerebral cholinergic muscarinic receptors at weaning and puberty," *Toxicology*, vol. 238, no. 1, pp. 34–48, 2007.

[44] K. Masuyama, K. Uno, R. Minoda, M. Eura, Y. Samejima, and T. Ishikawa, "Muscarinic acetylcholine receptors on human lymphocytes in patients with Meniere's disease," *Acta Oto-Laryngologica*, vol. 116, no. 3, pp. 369–373, 1996.

[45] C. C. Felder, F. P. Bymaster, J. Ward, and N. DeLapp, "Therapeutic opportunities for muscarinic receptors in the central nervous system," *Journal of Medicinal Chemistry*, vol. 43, no. 23, pp. 4333–4353, 2000.

[46] R. M. Eglen, A. Choppin, and N. Watson, "Therapeutic opportunities from muscarinic receptor research," *Trends in Pharmacological Sciences*, vol. 22, no. 8, pp. 409–414, 2001.

[47] J. Wess, "Muscarinic acetylcholine receptor knockout mice: novel phenotypes and clinical implications," *Annual Review of Pharmacology and Toxicology*, vol. 44, pp. 423–450, 2004.

[48] R. M. Eglen, "Muscarinic receptor subtype pharmacology and physiology," *Progress in Medicinal Chemistry*, vol. 43, pp. 105–136, 2005.

[49] K. Kawashima and T. Fujii, "The lymphocytic cholinergic system and its contribution to the regulation of immune activity," *Life Sciences*, vol. 74, no. 6, pp. 675–696, 2003.

[50] L. G. Costa, G. Kaylor, and S. D. Murphy, "In vitro and in vivo modulation of cholinergic muscarinic receptors in rat lymphocytes and brain by cholinergic agents," *International Journal of Immunopharmacology*, vol. 12, no. 1, pp. 67–75, 1990.

[51] B. B. Fitzgerald and L. G. Costa, "Modulation of muscarinic receptors and acetylcholinesterase activity in lymphocytes and in brain areas following repeated organophosphate exposure in rats," *Fundamental and Applied Toxicology*, vol. 20, no. 2, pp. 210–216, 1993.

[52] T. Coccini, G. Randine, A. F. Castoldi, D. Acerbi, and L. Manzo, "Methylmercury interaction with lymphocyte cholinergic muscarinic receptors in developing rats," *Environmental Research*, vol. 103, no. 2, pp. 229–237, 2007.

[53] A. D. Rossi, E. Ahlbom, S. O. Ogren, P. Nicotera, and S. Beccatelli, "Prenatal exposure to methylmercury alters locomotor activity of male but not female rats," *Experimental Brain Research*, vol. 117, no. 3, pp. 428–436, 1997.

[54] L. Gimenez-Llort, E. Ahlbom, E. Daré, M. Vahter, S. O. Ogren, and S. Ceccatelli, "Prenatal exposure to methylmercury changes dopamine-modulated motor activity during early ontogeny: age and gender-dependent effects," *Environmental Toxicology and Pharmacology*, vol. 9, no. 3, pp. 61–70, 2001.

[55] H. Komulainen and J. Tuomisto, "Interference of methyl mercury with monoamine uptake and release in rat brain synaptosomes," *Acta Pharmacologica et Toxicologica*, vol. 48, no. 3, pp. 214–222, 1981.

[56] D. J. Minnema, G. P. Cooper, and R. D. Greenland, "Effects of methylmercury on neurotransmitter release from rat brain synaptosomes," *Toxicology and Applied Pharmacology*, vol. 99, no. 3, pp. 510–521, 1989.

[57] W. Shain, B. Bush, and R. F. Seegal, "Neurotoxicity of polychlorinated biphenyls: structure-activity relationship of individual congeners," *Toxicology and Applied Pharmacology*, vol. 111, no. 1, pp. 33–42, 1991.

[58] J. C. Bemis and R. F. Seegal, "Polychlorinated biphenyls and methylmercury act synergistically to reduce rat brain dopamine content in vitro," *Environmental Health Perspectives*, vol. 107, no. 11, pp. 879–885, 1999.

[59] M. A. Chishti, J. P. Fisher, and R. F. Seegal, "Aroclors 1254 and 1260 reduce dopamine concentrations in rat striatal slices," *NeuroToxicology*, vol. 17, no. 3-4, pp. 653–660, 1996.

[60] T. Coccini, E. Roda, A. F. Castoldi et al., "Developmental exposure to methylmercury and 2,2′ ,4,4′,5,5′-hexachlorobiphenyl (PCB153) affects cerebral dopamine D1-likeand D2-like receptors of weanling and pubertal rats," *Archives of Toxicology*, vol. 85, no. 10, pp. 1281–1294, 2011.

[61] S. K. Chakrabarti, K. M. Loua, C. Bai, H. Durham, and J.-C. Panisset, "Modulation of monoamine oxidase activity in different brain regions and platelets following exposure of rats to methylmercury," *Neurotoxicology and Teratology*, vol. 20, no. 2, pp. 161–168, 1998.

[62] P. Beyrouty, C. J. Stamler, J. N. Liu, S. Kubow, and H. M. Chan, "Effects of prenatal methylmercury exposure on brain monoamine oxidase activity and neurobehaviour of rats," *Neurotoxicology and Teratology*, vol. 28, no. 2, pp. 251–259, 2006.

[63] D. R. Vincent, W. S. Bradshaw, G. M. Booth, R. E. Seegmiller, and S. D. Allen, "Effect of PCB and DES on rat monoamine oxidase, acetylcholinesterase, testosterone, and estradiol ontogeny," *Bulletin of Environmental Contamination and Toxicology*, vol. 48, no. 6, pp. 884–893, 1992.

[64] K. Chen, H. F. Wu, and J. C. Shih, "The deduced amino acid sequences of human platelet and frontal cortex monoamine oxidase B are identical," *Journal of Neurochemistry*, vol. 61, no. 1, pp. 187–190, 1993.

[65] C. H. Donnelly and D. L. Murphy, "Substrate and inhibitor related characteristics of human platelet monoamine oxidase," *Biochemical Pharmacology*, vol. 26, no. 9, pp. 853–858, 1977.

[66] T. Coccini, A. F. Castoldi, C. Gandini et al., "Platelet monoamine oxidase B activity as a state marker for alcolism: trend over time during withdrawal and influence of smoking and gender," *Alcohol and Alcoholism*, vol. 37, no. 6, pp. 566–572, 2002.

[67] C. J. Fowler and K. F. Tipton, "Deamination of 5-hydroxytryptamine by both forms of monoamine oxidase in the rat brain," *Journal of Neurochemistry*, vol. 38, no. 3, pp. 733–736, 1982.

[68] C. J. Stamler, N. Abdelouahab, C. Vanier, D. Mergler, and H. M. Chan, "Relationship between platelet monoamine oxidase-B (MAO-B) activity and mercury exposure in fish consumers from the Lake St. Pierre region of Que., Canada," *NeuroToxicology*, vol. 27, no. 3, pp. 429–436, 2006.

[69] J. B. Whitfield, D. Pang, K. K. Bucholz et al., "Monoamine oxidase: associations with alcohol dependence, smoking and other measures of psychopathology," *Psychological Medicine*, vol. 30, no. 2, pp. 443–454, 2000.

[70] R. T. Wyatt, D. L. Murphy, R. Belmaker, S. Cohen, C. H. Donnelly, and W. Pollin, "Reduced monoamine oxidase activity in platelets: a possible genetic marker for vulnerability to schizophrenia," *Science*, vol. 179, no. 4076, pp. 916–918, 1973.

[71] W. F. Young, E. R. Laws, F. W. Sharbrough, and R. M. Weinshilboum, "Human monoamine oxidase. Lack of brain and platelet correlation," *Archives of General Psychiatry*, vol. 43, no. 6, pp. 604–609, 1986.

[72] T. Coccini, G. Randine, A. F. Castoldi, L. Balloni, P. Baiardi, and L. Manzo, "Lymphocyte muscarinic receptors and platelet monoamine oxidase-B as biomarkers of CNS function: effects of age and gender in healthy humans," *Environmental Toxicology and Pharmacology*, vol. 19, no. 3, pp. 715–720, 2005.

[73] P. Grandjean, E. Budtz-Jørgensen, P. J. Jørgensen, and P. Weihe, "Umbilical cord mercury concentration as biomarker of prenatal exposure to methylmercury," *Environmental Health Perspectives*, vol. 113, no. 7, pp. 905–908, 2005.

[74] U. Steuerwald, P. Weihe, P. J. Jørgensen et al., "Maternal seafood diet, methylmercury exposure, and neonatal neurologic function," *Journal of Pediatrics*, vol. 136, no. 5, pp. 599–605, 2000.

[75] I. Aubert, D. Cécyre, S. Gauthier, and R. Quirion, "Comparative ontogenic profile of cholinergic markers, including nicotinic and muscarinic receptors, in the rat brain," *Journal of Comparative Neurology*, vol. 369, no. 1, pp. 31–55, 1996.

[76] D. M. Dick, F. Aliev, J. Kramer et al., "Association of CHRM2 with IQ: converging evidence for a gene influencing intelligence," *Behavior Genetics*, vol. 37, no. 2, pp. 265–272, 2007.

[77] M. F. Gosso, M. van Belzen, E. J. C. de Geus et al., "Association between the CHRM2 gene and intelligence in a sample of 304 Dutch families," *Genes, Brain and Behavior*, vol. 5, no. 8, pp. 577–584, 2006.

[78] L. Oreland and C. Fowler, "Brain and platelet monoamine oxidase activities in relation to central monoaminergic activity in mice and man," in *Monoamine Oxidase: Basic and Clinical Frontiers*, K. Kamijo, E. Usdin, and T. Nagatsu, Eds., pp. 312–320, Excerpta Medica, Amsterdam, The Netherlands, 1982.

[79] L. Oreland, K. Nilsson, M. Damberg, and J. Hallman, "Monoamine oxidases—activities, genotypes and the shaping of behaviour," *Journal of Neural Transmission*, vol. 114, no. 6, pp. 817–822, 2007.

[80] W. Danielczyk, M. Streifler, C. Konradi, P. Riederer, and G. Moll, "Platelet MAO-B activity and the psychopathology of Parkinson's disease, senile dementia and multi-infarct dementia," *Acta Psychiatrica Scandinavica*, vol. 78, no. 6, pp. 730–736, 1988.

[81] R. J. Perry and J. R. Hodges, "Attention and executive deficits in Alzheimer's disease: a critical review," *Brain*, vol. 122, no. 3, pp. 383–404, 1999.

[82] M. Sandler, M. A. Reveley, and V. Glover, "Human platelet monoamine oxidase activity in health and disease: a review," *Journal of Clinical Pathology*, vol. 34, no. 3, pp. 292–302, 1981.

[83] R. M. Anthenelli, T. L. Smith, C. E. Craig, B. Tabakoff, and M. A. Schuckit, "Platelet monoamine oxidase activity levels in subgroups of alcoholics: diagnostic, temporal, and clinical correlates," *Biological Psychiatry*, vol. 38, no. 6, pp. 361–368, 1995.

[84] L. D. Snell, J. Glanz, and B. Tabakoff, "Relationships between effects of smoking, gender, and alcohol dependence on platelet monoamine oxidase-B: activity, affinity labeling, and protein measurements," *Alcoholism*, vol. 26, no. 7, pp. 1105–1113, 2002.

[85] J. L. Sullivan, J. C. Baenziger, D. L. Wagner, F. P. Rauscher, J. I. Nurnberger Jr., and J. S. Holmes, "Platelet MAO in subtypes of alcoholism," *Biological Psychiatry*, vol. 27, no. 8, pp. 911–922, 1990.

Nicotine Contents in Some Commonly Used Toothpastes and Toothpowders: A Present Scenario

S. S. Agrawal and R. S. Ray

Department of Pharmacology, Delhi Institute of Pharmaceutical sciences and Research (DIPSAR), University of Delhi, Pushp Vihar, Sector 3, M.B. Road, New Delhi 110017, India

Correspondence should be addressed to R. S. Ray, pharma.ray@gmail.com

Academic Editor: Susan Sumner

The use of tobacco products as dentifrices is still prevalent in various parts of India. Tobacco use in dentifrices is a terrible scourge which motivates continued use despite its harmful effects. Indian legislation prohibits the use of nicotine in dentifrices. Nicotine is primarily injurious to people because it is responsible for tobacco addiction and is dependence forming. The present study was motivated by an interest in examining the presence of nicotine in these dentifrices. Our earlier report indicates the presence of nicotine in toothpowders. To further curb the menace of tobacco, our team again analysed the toothpowder brands of previous years and in toothpastes as well. Eight brands of commonly used toothpastes and toothpowders were evaluated by gas chromatography-mass spectroscopy. On the whole, there are a few successes but much remains to be done. Our findings indicated the presence of nicotine in two brands of *dant manjans* and four brands of toothpastes. Further our finding underscores the need for stringent regulations by the regulatory authorities for preventing the addition of nicotine in these dentifrices. Hence government policy needs to be targeted towards an effective control of tobacco in these dentifrices and should be properly addressed.

1. Introduction

Nicotine [1-methyl-2-(3-pyridyl-pyrrolidine), $C_{10}H_{14}N_2$] is the principal component of tobacco [1]. The predominant effects of nicotine include rise in blood pressure, heart rate, respiratory rate; increase in the level of catecholamines in blood; increase in level of free fatty acids, mobilization of blood sugar, and it was also found to disturb the antioxidant defense mechanisms [2–6]. There is strong evidence that smokeless tobacco use leads to oral mucosal lesions [7, 8] including oral pre-cancerous lesions, gingival recession [9], cardiovascular risk factors and disease, diabetes, reproductive health effects, and overall mortality. Nicotine rapidly crosses the placenta and has toxic effects on the foetus [10, 11]. Regular tobacco use reduces life expectancy by approximately 7 years [12].

India's share of the global burden of tobacco-induced disease and death is substantial [13]. India has one of the highest rates of oral cancers in the world; 65% of all cancers in men and 33% of all cancers in women are tobacco related. Annual incidence of oral cancer is said to be 10 per 1,00,000 per males [14].

In India, there is a widespread misconception that tobacco is good for the teeth [15]. Tobacco products are popular as a dentifrice in different parts of India and children also use such dentifrices [16]. Among female smokeless tobacco users, the dominating form is tobacco toothpowder (41.3%). Among men it was khaini (57.1%) followed by tobacco toothpowder (8.8%) [16, 17]. Many companies take advantage of this misconception and exploiting the addictive nature of nicotine by packaging and positioning their products as dental care products without explicitly stating so.

There was an amendment in Drugs & Cosmetics Act, 1940 vide notification published in the Gazette of India vide G.S.R. 443(E) and 444(E) dated 30.04.1992, mentioning that manufacture and sale of all cosmetics and all Ayurvedic drugs licensed as toothpowders/toothpastes containing tobacco have been prohibited [6, 18]. However, recent studies reported the presence of nicotine in some toothpowders [6, 18].

The present studies were motivated by an interest in examining the presence of nicotine in these dentifrices to evaluate the presence of nicotine in same brands of toothpowders (*dant manjans*) as reported in previous study. Furthermore, this year we also find it interesting to evaluate the presence of nicotine in toothpastes as well.

2. Materials and Methods

2.1. Chemicals. Eight brands of particular batches of commonly used toothpowders (*dant manjans*) and toothpastes were selected for the study from the local market. One sample from each batch was kept sealed in our laboratory as a reference sample. The toothpowders selected are coded as follows: Dabur red-M1 (8652), Vicco-M2 (008), Musaka Gul-M3 (not mentioned), Yunadent-M4 (01), Baidyanath-M5 (903), MDH-M6 (98), Gumtone-M7 (GT509), and Payokil-M8 (1503). The toothpastes selected for study were as follows: Dabur red-P1 (BD0698), Vicco-P2 (065), Arodent-P3 (64), Babool-P4 (1498), Herbodent-P5 (20), Colgate Herbal-P6 (B24CP), Ipco-P7 (not mentioned), and Dentobac-P8 (not mentioned).

Ammonia solution of extra pure quality was purchased from S.D. Fine-Chem. Ltd., Mumbai, chloroform and methanol of HPLC grade from Merck Ltd., Mumbai, and (−)-Nicotine of synthesis grade from Merck-Schuchardt, Hohebrunn, Germany. Analyses were performed with Gas chromatography Thermo Electron Corporation with MS instrument.

2.2. Extraction and Isolation of Nicotine from Toothpowders and Toothpastes. Extraction and isolation of nicotine from toothpowders were done as described by Agrawal and Rajagopal [6]. Extraction and isolation of nicotine from toothpastes were done by taking 25 g of toothpaste in a conical flask, 15 mL NH_3 (Strong) was added to completely humidify the sample followed by 250 mL chloroform, and the conical flask was closed with a cap. This is kept in mechanical shaker for about one hour. After that, 2 min hand shaking and then chloroform extract is then filtered out and dried [19]. The yield values of alkaloids obtained are 0.154, 0.44, 0.22, 0.12, 0.14, 0.24, 0.56, and 0.37, respectively.

2.3. Method for Identification and Quantification of Nicotine by GC-MSD. All mass spectra were obtained with MS, Thermo Electron Corporation. The ion source was operated in the electron ionization mode (EI; 70 eV, 150°C). Full-scan mass spectra (*m/z* 40–450) were recorded for analyte identification. Separation was achieved with a BP fused-silica capillary column with 5% diphenyl-Poly (dimethylsiloxane (BP 5), ~30 m length, 0.25 mm i.d., 1.0 μm film thickness. Samples were injected in the split mode with a split ratio of 1 : 10. The flow rate of helium as carrier gas was 1.0 mL/min. The GC operating parameters were as follows: injector temperature, 250°C; transfer line temperature, 280°C; oven temperature, programmed from 100°C (held for 3 min) at 10°C/min to 280°C (held for 3 min). The ion selected for quantification by SIM was *m/z* 162.

3. Results

The presence of nicotine in toothpowders (*dant manjans*) and toothpastes were confirmed by gas chromatography-mass spectroscopy (GC-MS) in full scan mode and selective ion mode (SIM).

3.1. Qualitative Analysis of Toothpowders and Toothpastes. Out of the eight brands of toothpowders included in the present study only, two brands were found to contain nicotine. A comparison of retention time, molecular ion peak, and base peak shows the presence of nicotine in these *dant manjans* (M2 and M3). Retention time of nicotine was found to be 17.00 min. Nicotine presence was identified by comparing the RT values of toothpowder extracts with standard nicotine. The primary target ion of nicotine has a mass of 162 *m/z* [20]. The molecular ion peak at 162 *m/z* and base peak at 84 *m/z* corresponds to the fragmentation of nicotine. The RT of M2 and M3 was found to be 16.99 and 16.94, respectively. This was further confirmed by Mass spectrum (Figures 1, 2, 3, 4, 5, and 6).

Similarly, Out of the eight brands of toothpastes analysed, four brands were found to contain nicotine. The RT of P1, P3, P7, and P8 was found to be 17.05, 17.16, 16.93, and 16.91, respectively as compared to that of nicotine standard 17.00 and was confirmed by its molecular ion peak and base peak (Figures 7, 8, 9, 10, 11, 12, 13, and 14).

3.2. Quantitative Analysis of Toothpowders and Toothpastes. The *dant manjan* extracts which indicated the presence of nicotine were also quantified with GCMS. The nicotine contents determined in GCMS of M1 and M2 were 12.95 mg/g and 216.10 mg/g respectively. Similarly, the nicotine content in toothpaste extracts of P1, P3, P7, and P8 were found to be 5.752 mg/g, 2.093 mg/g, 123.82 mg/g, and 119.13 mg/g, respectively.

4. Discussion

Abuse of tobacco, like drug and alcohol abuse, is a worldwide public health problem [21]. India's tobacco problem is more complex than probably that of any other country in the world, with a large consequential burden of tobacco-related disease and death [13]. Various tobacco products are popular as a dentifrice in different parts of India [16, 22]. Tobacco was not, perhaps, used for cleansing the teeth, but more so to get "kick" out of the contents of tobacco, and many companies exploit the addictive nature of nicotine by packaging and positioning them as dentifrice [22]. Researches comparing herbal toothpastes with conventional dentifrices, however, suggest that there is no specific advantage of herbal-based pastes over conventional pastes [23–25].

Indian legislation prohibits the use of tobacco as an ingredient in dental care products [6, 15]. After the passage of a law banning the use of tobacco in dental care products,

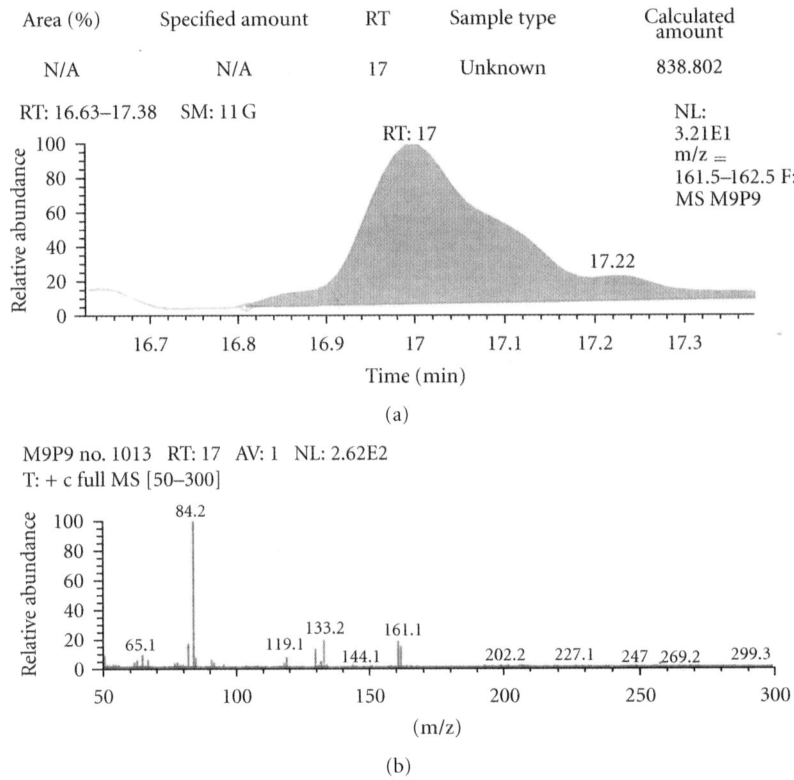

FIGURE 1: GC-MS of nicotine in full scan mode.

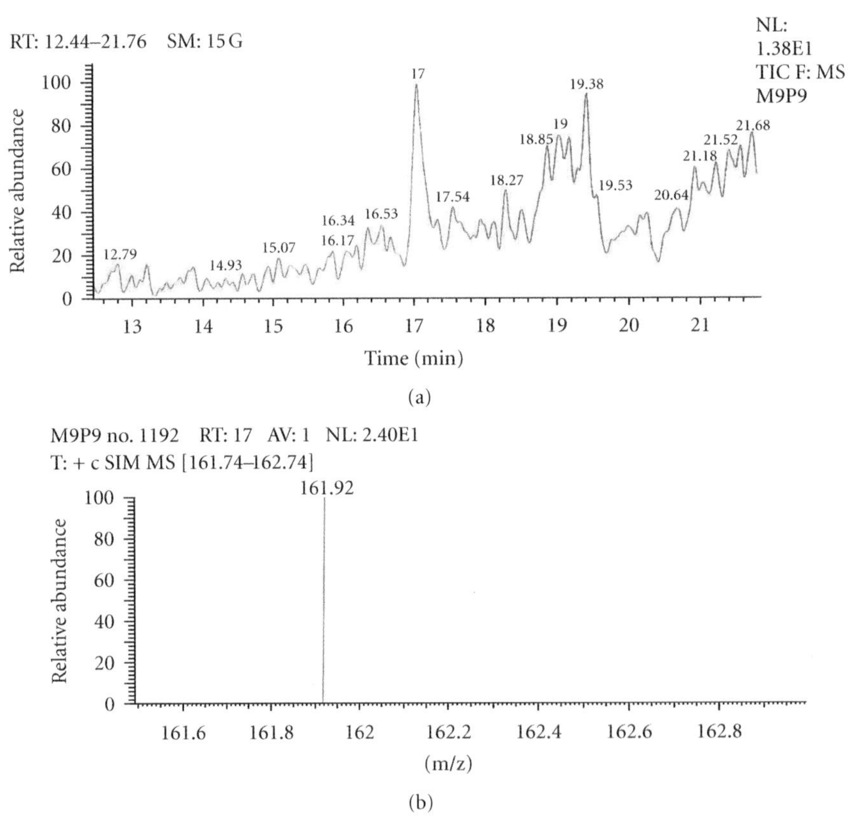

FIGURE 2: GC-MS of nicotine in SIM mode.

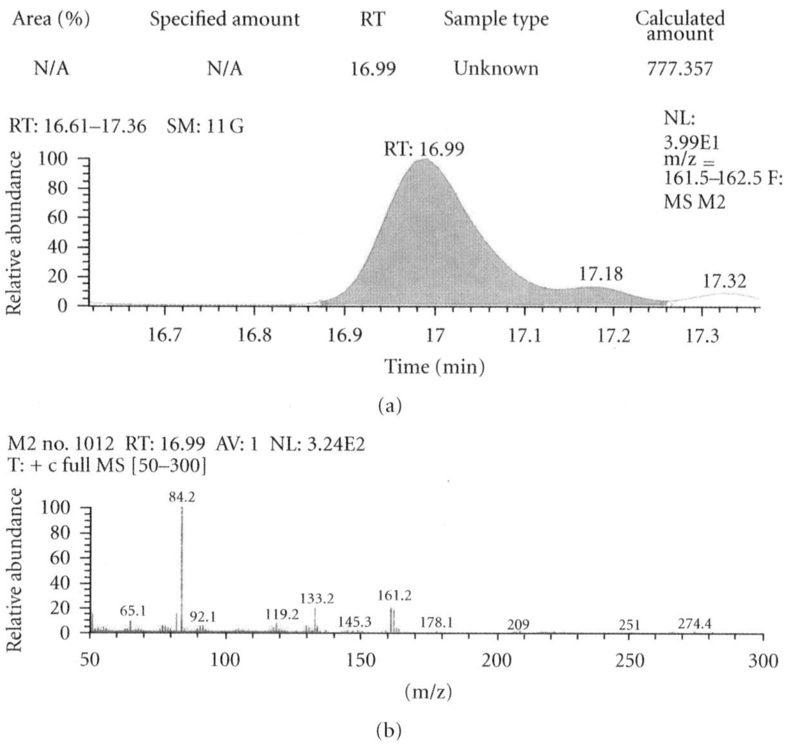

Figure 3: GC-MS of toothpowder M2 in full scan mode.

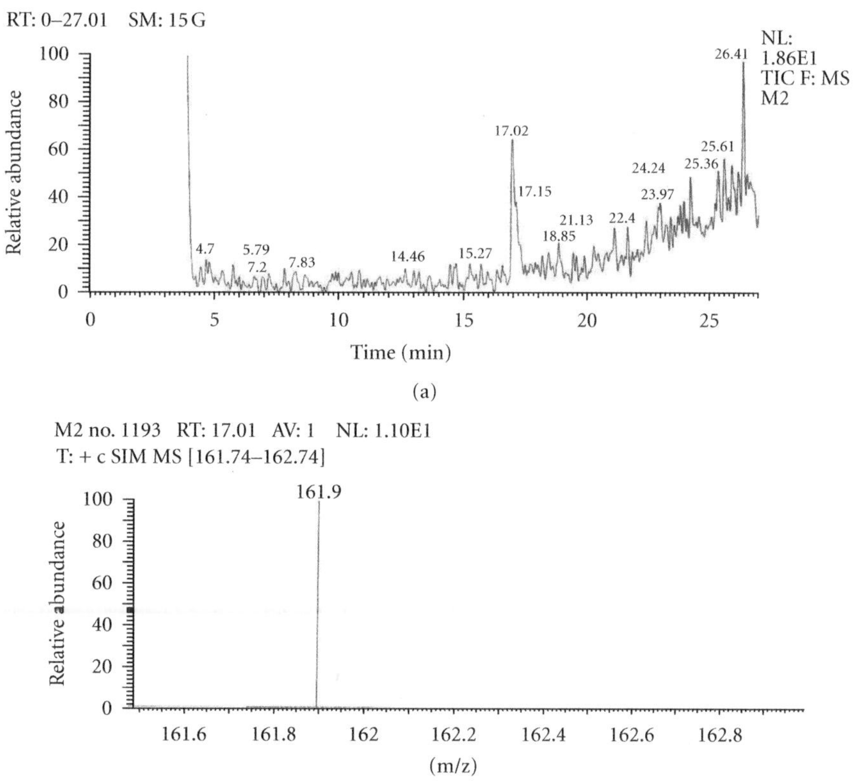

Figure 4: GC-MS of toothpowder M2 in SIM mode.

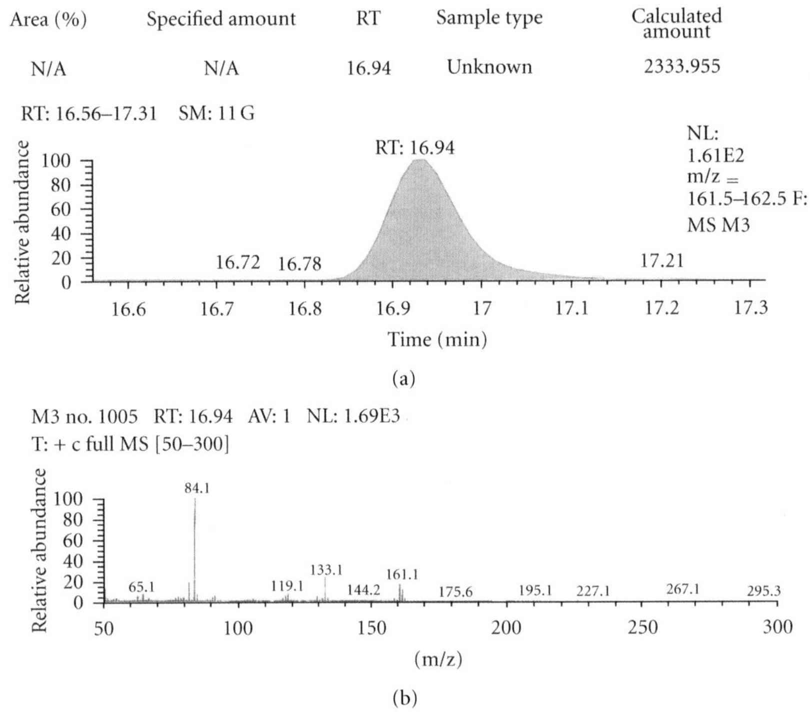

FIGURE 5: GC-MS of toothpowder M3 in full scan mode.

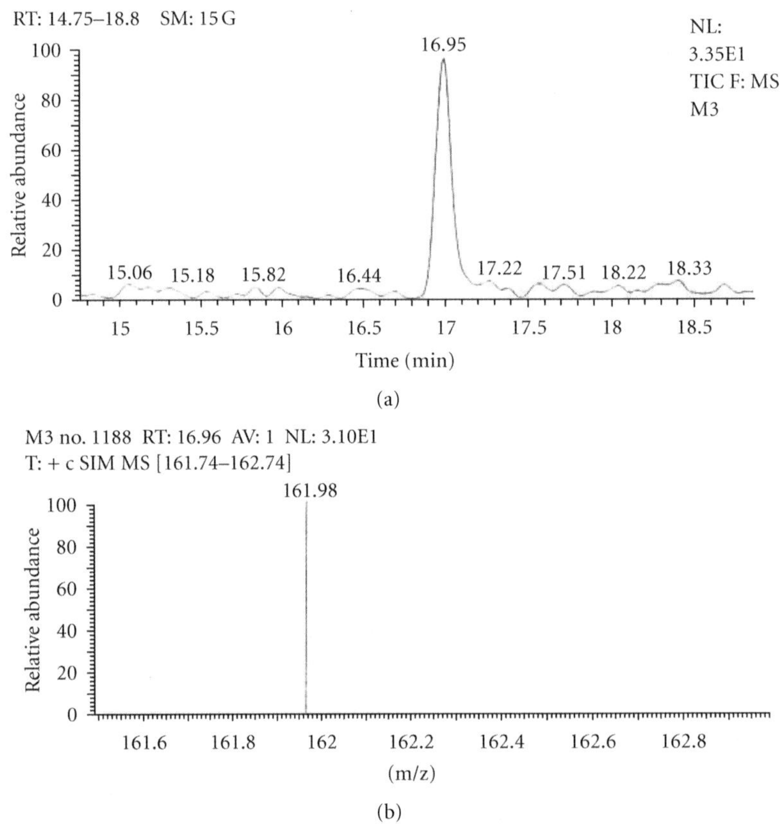

FIGURE 6: GC-MS of toothpowder M3 in SIM mode.

Area (%)	Specified amount	RT	Sample type	Calculated amount
N/A	N/A	17.05	Unknown	402.662

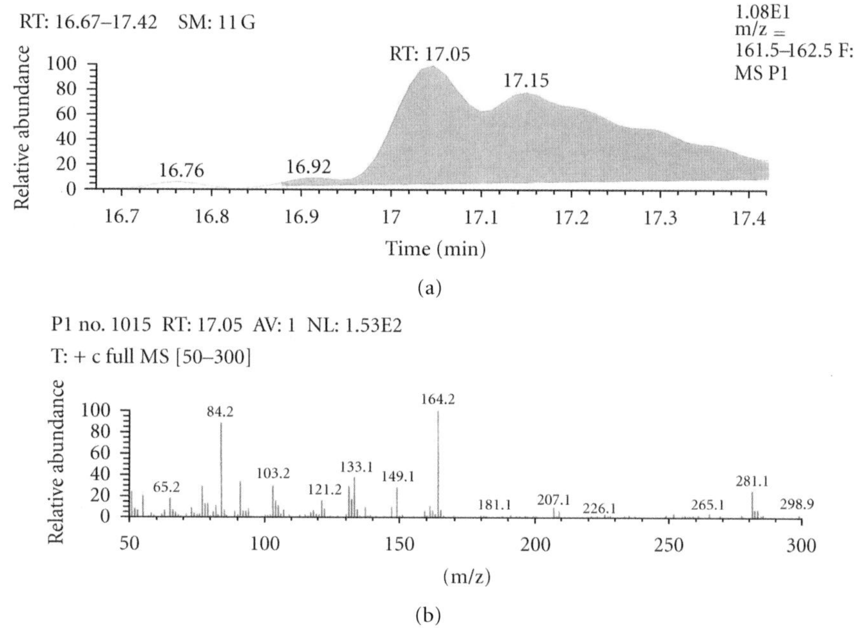

Figure 7: GC-MS of toothpaste P1 in full scan mode.

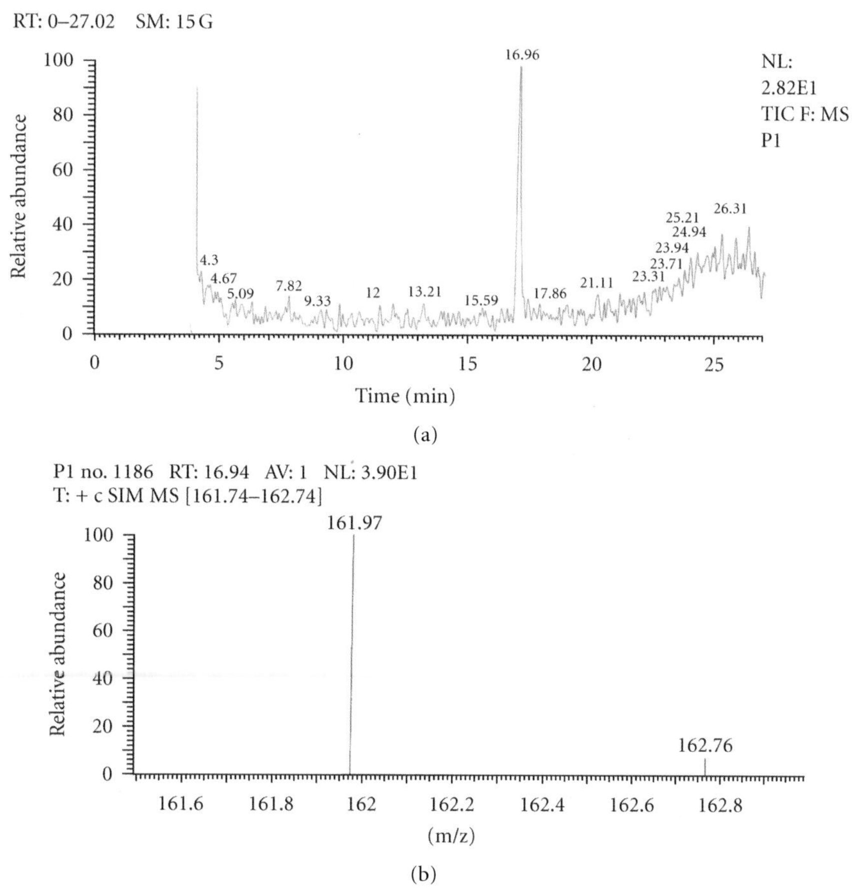

Figure 8: GC-MS of toothpaste P1 in SIM mode.

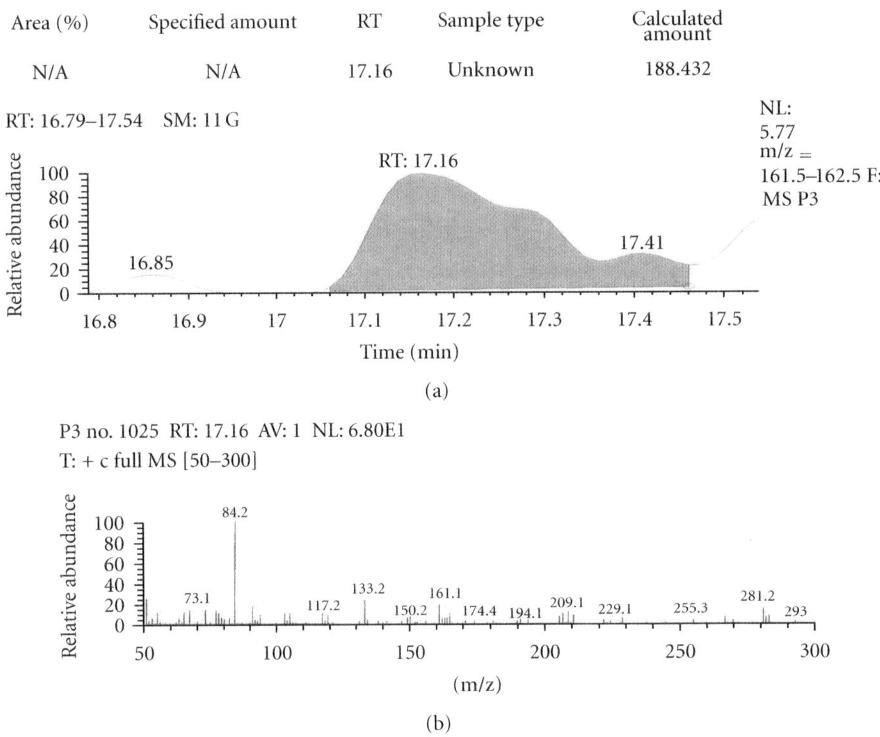

FIGURE 9: GC-MS of toothpaste P3 in full scan mode.

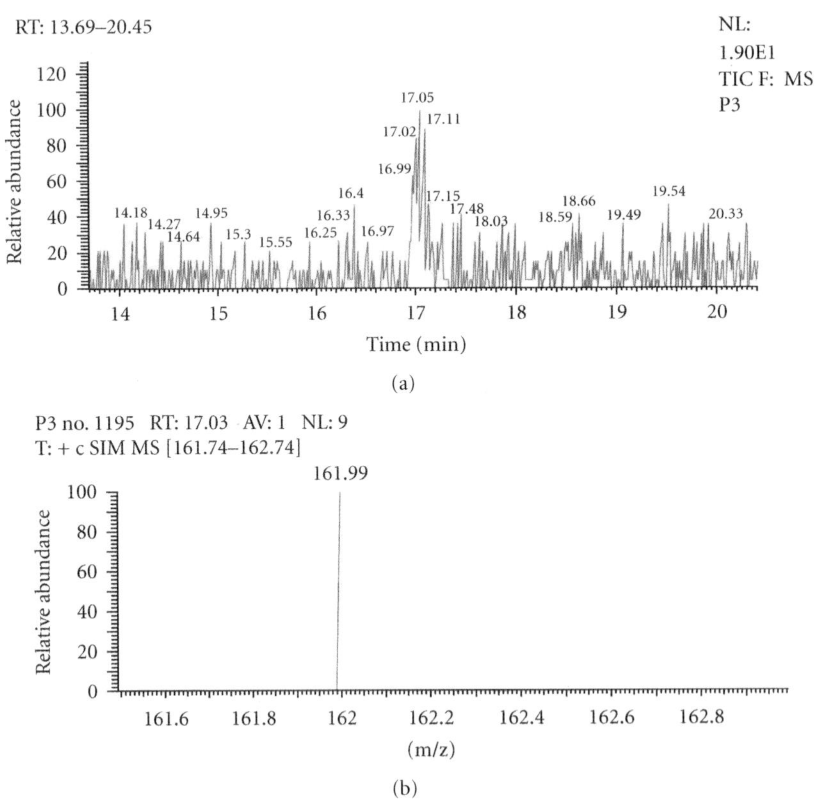

FIGURE 10: GC-MS of toothpaste P3 in SIM mode.

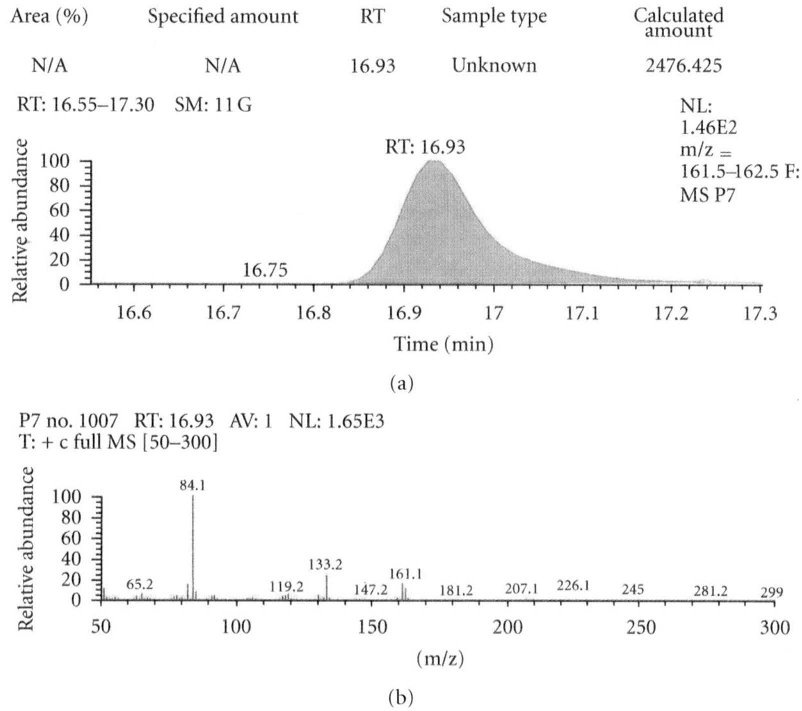

Figure 11: GC-MS of toothpaste P7 in full scan mode.

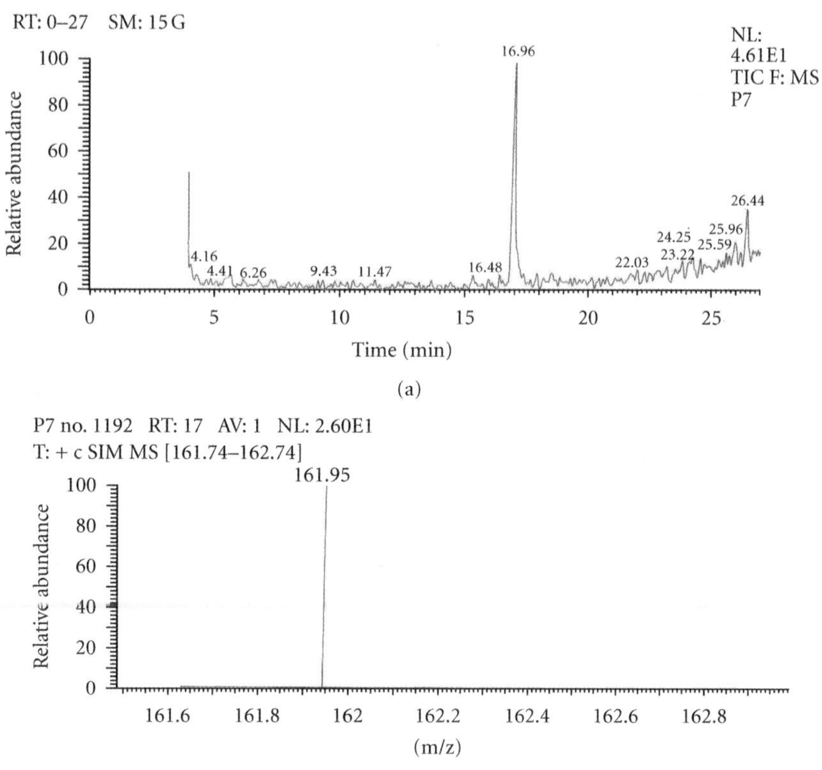

Figure 12: GC-MS of toothpaste P7 in SIM mode.

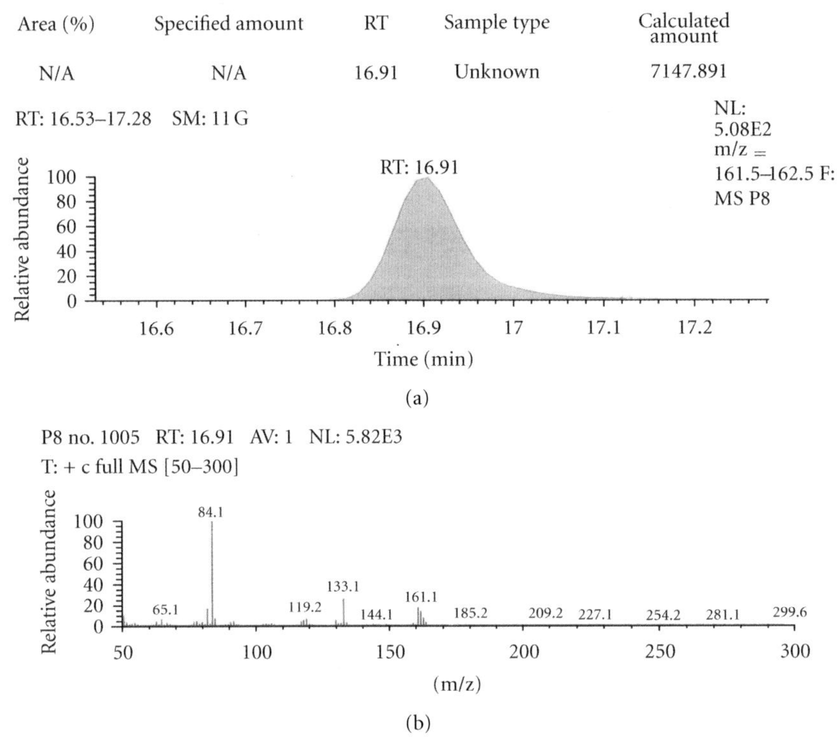

Figure 13: GC-MS of toothpaste P8 in full scan mode.

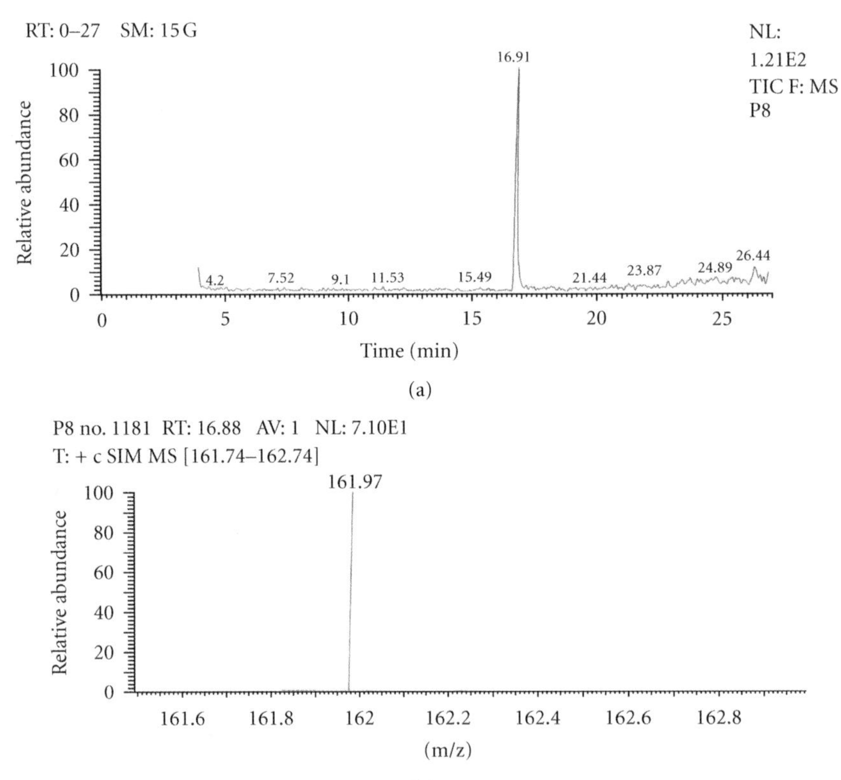

Figure 14: GC-MS of toothpaste P8 in SIM mode.

the listing of tobacco as an ingredient was stopped [26]. These products, however, continue to be available openly in the market, often without mentioning tobacco as one of the ingredient [6, 16, 17].

Nicotine is a CNS stimulant, which leads to habit formation subsequently dependence on its users. Nicotine causes withdrawal symptoms such as anger, anxiety, depressed mood, difficulty in concentration, and craving for tobacco. There is strong and compelling evidence that oral tobacco use leads to oral mucosal lesions [7] including oral precancerous lesions, gingival recession [9], oral cancer [27, 28], and overall mortality. The risk increases with the duration and frequency of the habit [29].

The present studies were motivated by an interest in examining the presence of nicotine in these dentifrices and to endow with an overview of the tobacco problem in Indian dentifrices, from public health challenges to policy responses. With this background, an attempt was made to further curb the menace of tobacco in commercially available dentifrices in India and to provide a credible basis for evolving future tobacco regulation in dentifrices. Our team again analysed the same brands as of yesteryears with an objective to review that whether the regulations with respect to tobacco/nicotine in toothpowders have been adequately implemented or not. Also it was thought to estimate nicotine in toothpastes of herbal/ayurvedic origin.

In consistent with the previous report, the presence of nicotine in four out of eight brands of *dant manjans* analysed [6], this year only two bands were found to contain nicotine and is quantified as M2 (12.95 mg/g) and M3 (216.10 mg/g), respectively. This year out of the eight most commonly available herbal toothpastes selected for the study, four brands were found to contain nicotine and was quantified as P1 (5.32 mg/g), P3 (2.093 mg/g), P7 (119.13 mg/g), and P8 (123.82 mg/g), respectively. Moreover, these nicotine-containing toothpowders (*dant manjans*) and toothpastes lack pictorial warning which implies that these manufactures are disguising it as a dentifrice.

A person on a regular oral hygiene uses 2-3 g of toothpowder/paste each day [30]. The LD50 of nicotine in mice, rats, and human is 3 mg, 50 mg, and 40–60 mg, respectively. Thus, the present study indicates that a considerable amount of nicotine (2–216 mg) could enter the oral cavity if these toothpowders and toothpastes were used. Adults remove most of the toothpowder/paste from the oral cavity by rinsing. Children may retain a much greater percentage of dentifrice than adults, because of incomplete rinsing thus resulting in ingestion [30]. Once a person is addicted to nicotine, quitting is very difficult no matter whichever form he uses it. In a survey, women were found to be addictive to tobacco paste than males [31]. Thus the presence of nicotine in these dentifrices even in low concentrations could considerably lead to addiction and oral mucosal lesions [7] due to its routine use. Hence this epidemic of addiction to nicotine among young people may have enormous implications in public health [32].

Therefore, this study underscores the importance of support of prevention of tobacco use in developing countries especially India where population is roaring; tobacco use threatens to contribute to a growing proportion of the burden of disease. Thus, even in low concentrations, one would expect tobacco to be present in these dentifrices to exert its addictive influence, which emphasizes the need for strong economic, legislative, and educational means to eradicate this menace. However, much more needs to be done including possibly enacting legislation to stop the manufacturing of such dentifrices. The findings of this study will help to design, implement, and evaluate tobacco control and prevention programmes. Thus, our study clearly confirmed the presence of nicotine in few dentifrices, and regulations have not been implemented properly even after 17 years. Such issues should be effectively addressed by the regulatory authorities in India and worldwide.

5. Conclusion

With a population of over 1 billion people, tobacco use contributes to India's and global public health threat. Our new findings substantiate the presence of nicotine in a variety of dentifrices. Thus even after 17 years of amendment of Drugs and Cosmetic Act banning tobacco toothpowders and toothpastes, nicotine is still present in some dentifrices which clearly shows that the law is not strictly enforced and implemented. Hence regulatory authorities in India and internationally should take adequate measures to stop the addition of nicotine or tobacco to the dentifrices to provide nicotine-/Tobacco-free dentifrices. However, continued surveillance of such dental products is necessary in order to better inform and educate the public regarding the risks associated with respect to this public health concern.

References

[1] H. Schievelbein, "Nicotine, resorption and fate," *Pharmacology and Therapeutics*, vol. 18, no. 2, pp. 233–248, 1982.

[2] N. L. Benowitz, "Pharmacologic aspects of cigarette smoking and nicotine addiction," *New England Journal of Medicine*, vol. 319, no. 20, pp. 1318–1330, 1988.

[3] L. Ashakumary and P. L. Vijayammal, "Lipid peroxidation in nicotine treated rats," *Journal of Ecotoxicology and Environmental Monitoring*, vol. 1, pp. 283–290, 1991.

[4] J. A. Dani and S. Heinemann, "Molecular and cellular aspects of nicotine abuse," *Neuron*, vol. 16, no. 5, pp. 905–908, 1996.

[5] H. L. Waldum, O. G. Nilsen, T. Nilsen et al., "Long-term effects of inhaled nicotine," *Life Sciences*, vol. 58, no. 16, pp. 1339–1346, 1996.

[6] S. S. Agrawal and K. Rajagopal, "Nicotine contents in various toothpowders (dant manjans): measurement and safety evaluation," *Food and Chemical Toxicology*, vol. 47, no. 3, pp. 511–524, 2009.

[7] S. L. Tomar, D. M. Winn, P. A. Swango, G. A. Giovino, and D. V. Kleinman, "Oral mucosal smokeless tobacco lesions among adolescents in the United States," *Journal of Dental Research*, vol. 76, no. 6, pp. 1277–1286, 1997.

[8] J. E. Henningfield, R. V. Fant, and S. L. Tomar, "Smokeless tobacco: an addicting drug," *Advances in dental research*, vol. 11, no. 3, pp. 330–335, 1997.

[9] D. M. Winn, "Tobacco use and oral disease," *Journal of Dental Education*, vol. 65, no. 4, pp. 306–312, 2001.

[10] A. K. Armitage and D. M. Turner, "Absorption of nicotine in cigarette and cigar smoke through the oral mucosa," *Nature*, vol. 226, no. 5252, pp. 1231–1232, 1970.

[11] H. Schievelbein, R. Eberhardt, and K. Loschenkohl, "Absorption of nicotine through the oral mucosa. I. Measurement of nicotine concentration in the blood after application of nicotine and total particulate matter," *Agents and Actions*, vol. 3, no. 4, pp. 254–258, 1973.

[12] J. Stamler and R. B. Shekelle, "Lower dietary cholesterol and saturated fat intake, lower serum cholesterol, and expected effects on coronary risk and on longevity," *Lipid Review*, vol. 3, pp. 89–96, 1989.

[13] P. C. Gupta and C. S. Ray, "Epidemic in India," in *Tobacco: Science, Policy and Public Health*, P. Boyle, N. Gray, J. Henningfield, J. Seffrin, and W. Zatonski, Eds., pp. 253–266, Oxford University Press, Oxford, UK, 2004.

[14] R. Shimkhada and J. W. Peabody, "Tobacco control in India," *Bulletin of the World Health Organization*, vol. 81, no. 1, pp. 48–52, 2003.

[15] D. Simpson, "India: tobacco toothpaste squeezed out," *Tobacco control*, vol. 6, no. 3, p. 171, 1997.

[16] D. N. Sinha, P. C. Gupta, and M. S. Pednekar, "Tobacco use in a rural area of Bihar, India," *Indian Journal of Community Medicine*, vol. 28, pp. 167–170, 2003.

[17] D. N. Sinha, P. C. Gupta, and M. S. Pednekar, "Tobacco use among students in the eight North-eastern states of India," *Indian Journal of Cancer*, vol. 40, no. 2, pp. 43–59, 2003.

[18] D. N. Sinha, P. C. Gupta, and M. S. Pednekar, "Use of tobacco products as dentifrice among adolescents in India: questionnaire study," *British Medical Journal*, vol. 328, no. 7435, pp. 323–324, 2004.

[19] J. M. Garrigues, A. Pérez-Ponce, S. Garrigues, and M. D. L. Guardia, "Fourier-transform infrared determination of nicotine in tobacco samples by transmittance measurements after leaching with CHCl3," *Analytica Chimica Acta*, vol. 373, no. 1, pp. 63–71, 1998.

[20] S. M. Rafferty, "Identification of nicotine by gas chromatography/mass spectroscopy analysis of smoking pipe residue," *Journal of Archaeological Science*, vol. 29, no. 8, pp. 897–907, 2002.

[21] S. Reddy and H. A. Shaik, "Estimation of nicotine content in popular Indian brands of smoking and chewing tobacco products," *Indian Journal of Dental Research*, vol. 19, no. 2, pp. 88–91, 2008.

[22] R. B. Bhonsle, P. R. Murti, and P. C. Gupta, "Tobacco habits in India," in *Proceedings of an International Symposium on Control of Tobacco-Related Cancers and Others Diseases (1990)*, P. C. Gupta, J. E. Hamner, and P. R. Murti, Eds., pp. 268–290, Oxford University Press, Bombay, India, 1992.

[23] R. Mythilli, "Efficacy of herbal-based toothpastes and conventional dentifrices on the control of plaque and gingivitis," *Bulletin of the Indian Society of Periodontology*, vol. 21, article 86, 1997.

[24] I. R. D'Silva, "The effect of neem gel on plaque and gingivitis," *Journal of Indian Society of Periodontology*, vol. 2, article 63, 1999.

[25] K. R. Seshan, "Efficacy of mineral product in the control of bleeding and spongy gums as an astringent, anti-inflammatory and dentifrice," *Journal of Indian Society of Periodontology*, vol. 2, article 66, 1999.

[26] K. S. Reddy and P. C. Gupta, Eds., *Report on Tobacco Control in India Ministry of Health and Family Welfare*, Government of India, New Delhi, India, 2004.

[27] R. V. Fant, J. E. Henningfield, R. A. Nelson, and W. B. Pickworth, "Pharmacokinetics and pharmacodynamics of moist snuff in humans," *Tobacco Control*, vol. 8, no. 4, pp. 387–392, 1999.

[28] N. Shah and P. P. Sharma, "Role of chewing and smoking habits in the etiology of oral submucous fibrosis (OSF): a case-control study," *Journal of Oral Pathology and Medicine*, vol. 27, no. 10, pp. 475–479, 1998.

[29] D. R. Sawyer and N. K. Wood, "Oral cancer. Etiology, recognition, and management," *Dental Clinics of North America*, vol. 36, no. 4, pp. 919–944, 1992.

[30] I. M. Shapiro, G. H. Cohen, H. L. Needleman, and O. C. Tuncay, "The presence of lead in toothpaste," *The Journal of the American Dental Association*, vol. 86, no. 2, pp. 394–395, 1973.

[31] C. P. Boghani, *Periodontal problems*, Dissertation, University of Dundee, Scotland, UK, 1971.

[32] R. Peto, A. D. Lopez, J. Boreham, M. Thun, and C. Heath, "Mortality from tobacco in developed countries: indirect estimation from national vital statistics," *Lancet*, vol. 339, no. 8804, pp. 1268–1278, 1992.

Measurement of Redox Potential in Nanoecotoxicological Investigations

Ratna Tantra,[1] Alex Cackett,[1] Roger Peck,[1] Dipak Gohil,[2] and Jacqueline Snowden[1]

[1] *Nanoanalysis Group, National Physical Laboratory, Hampton Road, Teddington, Middlesex TW11 0LW, UK*
[2] *Advanced Engineered Materials Group, National Physical Laboratory, Hampton Road, Teddington, Middlesex TW11 0LW, UK*

Correspondence should be addressed to Ratna Tantra, ratna.tantra@npl.co.uk

Academic Editor: Christian Gagnon

Redox potential has been identified by the Organisation for Economic Co-operation and Development (OECD) as one of the parameters that should be investigated for the testing of manufactured nanomaterials. There is still some ambiguity concerning this parameter, i.e., as to what and how to measure, particularly when in a nanoecotoxicological context. In this study the redox potentials of six nanomaterials (either zinc oxide (ZnO) or cerium oxide (CeO_2)) dispersions were measured using an oxidation-reduction potential (ORP) electrode probe. The particles under testing differed in terms of their particle size and dispersion stability in deionised water and in various ecotox media. The ORP values of the various dispersions and how they fluctuate relative to each other are discussed. Results show that the ORP values are mainly governed by the type of liquid media employed, with little contributions from the nanoparticles. Seawater was shown to have reduced the ORP value, which was attributed to an increase in the concentration of reducing agents such as sulphites or the reduction of dissolved oxygen concentration. The lack of redox potential value contribution from the particles themselves is thought to be due to insufficient interaction of the particles at the Pt electrode of the ORP probe.

1. Introduction

The size of engineered nanomaterials makes many novel and innovative products, as evident by the increasing number of commercially available nanotechnology products. Thus, there is a huge concern surrounding the potential toxicity of these nanomaterials and there is a need to sufficiently test such materials. The goal here is to understand and control risk, and both toxicity testing and physicochemical characterisation should be conducted. Although our current understanding of risk associated with nanomaterials is limited, attempts have been made in order to assess this systematically. Recently, Aschberger et al. [1] have carried out a risk assessment based on several case studies. They have indicated the risk expected from metal and metal oxide nanomaterials, which was particularly relevant in the case of algae and Daphnia. They have attributed the risk from such materials their exposure to both the particles and corresponding dissolved ions.

There is a general consensus within the nanoecotoxicological community that physicochemical characterisation of nanomaterials in complex media is not a trivial matter, and so the reliability of such measurements is vital if we are to understand and control the risk imposed by nanomaterials [2, 3]. In recent years, the OECD initiative has adopted a holistic approach to this problem and that physicochemical characterisation should be carried out with as many parameters as possible, to include redox potential. The PROSPEcT (Ecotoxicology Test Protocols for Representative Nanomaterials in Support of the OECD Sponsorship Programme) project is the UK's contribution to this OECD initiative, and the UK is responsible for two types of nanomaterials: cerium oxide (CeO_2) and zinc oxide (ZnO) [4]. Out of all seventeen OECD parameters identified, redox potential is the most ambiguous in its definition, what this parameter means and how it is measured, in a nanoecotoxicological context.

Integral to any ecotoxicological investigation is the ability to measure the redox conditions of a given system as indicated by the redox potential. In nature, redox reactions are an important part of phenomena such as mineral weathering, bacterial respiration, and degradation of pollutants [5]. In soil chemistry, for example, the redox potential value can estimate whether the soil is aerobic or anaerobic, and whether chemical compounds such as Fe oxides or nitrate have been chemically reduced or are present in their oxidised form. In natural waters, redox reactions include the oxidation of organic matter and various reduction reactions such as the reduction of oxygen to water, nitrate to elementary nitrogen dioxide, iron (III) to Fe (II), sulphate to sulphide, and carbon dioxide to methane [6]. In terms of nanomaterial toxicity, redox potential is a parameter that has been associated with inducing oxidative stress. Recently, Burello and Worth [7], in their prediction of a given nanomaterial to induce oxidative stress, have developed a theoretical framework that combines measurements of nanoparticle particle size and redox potential. The need to accurately measure redox potential is evident, in particular we need to understand the extent that nanomaterials can influence the natural redox phenomena should these materials be released into the environment.

Redox potential is a measure of a system's affinity for electrons, and the measurement of redox potential will only have meaning when there are reduced and oxidised species, called the redox couple, in the liquid media. The redox couple undergoes a redox reaction, in which the reduction (gain of electrons) of one redox species is accompanied by the oxidation (loss of electrons) of another [6]. The movement of electrons, governed by kinetics (e.g., transport limitations of the redox species to the electrode), creates an electric potential. The potential measured is determined by the ratio of activities of oxidised and reduced species, as defined by the Nernst equation; this is a thermodynamic property [8]. The redox potential can be directly measured using a potentiometer (high impedance voltmeter) with an oxidation-reduction potential (ORP) electrode [9]. This is the recommended technique under the current OECD guidelines for the testing of nanomaterials (NMs) [10]; essentially it is a measurement of potential difference (in mV) across a two-electrode system, that is, an inert platinum (Pt) electrode and silver-silver chloride (Ag/AgCl) reference electrode. Rogers et al. have recently adopted this approach to measure the redox potential of nanomaterial dispersions, that is, cerium oxide dispersed in synthetic freshwater algal medium [11].

There are theoretical and practical difficulties associated with the measurement of redox potential and these, although not well recognised, have already been discussed for many years [6]. Firstly, redox potential is based on the concepts of equilibrium thermodynamics, and as such it can only be adequately measured at equilibrium. A reliable redox potential measurement requires that equilibrium be established not only at the electrode, but also among the various redox couples in solution. Many redox reactions are slow and often are at nonequilibrium conditions. Secondly, most redox potential measurements represent mixed potentials, and certain redox species may not contribute significantly towards the redox potential value; that is, not all will react sufficiently fast enough at the electrode and therefore will not contribute towards stable and reliable redox potential measurements [12]. If the particles themselves act as a redox species, then there are various factors that may prevent them contributing towards the final ORP value, including sedimentation events, diffusion limitations, and the barrier of electron exchange at the Pt electrode. If this is true, then redox potentials of nanomaterial dispersions are likely to be solely dominated by dissolved redox species in the media, rather than contributions arising from the particles themselves. In this study, we aim to investigate if this is the case. Although the ORP probe has been conveniently used in the past by scientists to directly measure redox potential, it is essential that the reliability of such data should be questioned when measuring nanomaterial dispersions. There is the risk that researchers may treat such a tool as a *black box* and thus may not be fully aware of the inherent limitations in the use of such a tool in these measurements.

In this study, the ORP values of six nanomaterial (either ZnO or CeO_2 dispersed in one of the four liquid media) dispersions will be measured using an ORP probe. Dispersions will be carried out according to the dispersion protocol as recommended under PROSPEcT. The ORP values of the nanomaterial dispersions will be compared relative to each other and to the corresponding media blank, to identify if there is any evidence of redox contributions as a result of the particles themselves. If there are redox contributions from the particles themselves, then this is likely to happen when dispersions are stable, as this would allow sufficient time for the particles to interact with the Pt electrode. Consequently as part of the investigation, the properties associated with the different nanomaterials will be characterised, parameters of interest to include particle size, zetapotential, and dispersion stability (as reported by the so-called *half life* values). Zetapotential is a well-known parameter that characterizes the electric properties of solid surface in contact with liquid and is a way to probe surface charge. The magnitude of this value is related to dispersion stability, that is, the higher the value, the better the dispersion stability [13]. The concept of "half-life" has been put forward in the OECD guidelines as the measurand to indicate dispersion stability through time that is, the larger the half-life value; the longer it takes for the concentration to reduce by half and thus the more stable the dispersion. Lastly, the corresponding scanning electron microscopy (SEM) data, that is, the primary particle size (mean Feret diameter) and the corresponding standard deviation, will also be reported.

2. Experimental Section

All experiments were performed in a temperature-controlled laboratory, and for the redox potential measurements the temperature of the dispersions were monitored using a temperature probe (reported value of ~20°C) to ensure that any change in the readings was not attributed to temperature changes in the dispersions.

2.1. Materials. The NMs supplied from the PROSPEcT programme were of two types, either CeO_2 or ZnO, and are as follows:

(a) Nanograin CeO_2 (from Umicore Belgium),

(b) Nanosun ZnO (from Micronisers, Australia),

(c) Micron ZnO (from Sigma Aldrich, UK),

(d) Z-COTE ZnO (from BASF, Germany),

(e) Micron CeO_2 (from Sigma Aldrich, UK),

(f) Ceria dry CeO_2 (from Antaria, Australia).

The particles were used as received and did not contain any added surface stabilisers.

DI water (resistivity of 18 Mohm) from a Millipore, MilliQ system was used to prepare all aqueous solutions and suspensions.

For the purpose of zetapotential measurements, DI water with 5 mM sodium chloride (Sigma Aldrich, UK) was employed in addition to deionised water; the NaCl here served as background electrolyte for the measurement of zetapotential. The "recipes" (chemical compositions) used for making up the ecotox media were obtained from the University of Exeter, one of our collaborators in the PROSPEcT project.

Three types of ecotox relevant media were prepared accordingly and for long-term storage, the ecotox solutions were autoclaved and kept refrigerated until needed.

(a) Seawater, in which 25 g per L of Tropic Marine Sea Salt (Tropical and Marine Limited) was made up, resulting in pH ~8.8.

(b) Daphnia freshwater media. This was prepared by firstly dissolving appropriate salts (196 mg $CaCl_2 \cdot 2H_2O$, 82 mg $MgSO_4 \cdot 7H_2O$, 65 mg $NaHCO_3$, 0.002 mg Na_2SeO_3, as obtained by appropriate dilutions of a 2 mg/mL stock solution) in 1 L of DI water. Upon continued stirring, further DI water was added so that conductivity of the solution was between ~360 and 480 μS/cm. End volume ~1–1.5 L. Final pH ~7.9.

(c) Fish freshwater media. This was prepared in three separate steps. First, salts (11.76 g $CaCl_2 \cdot 2H2O$, 4.93 g $MgSO_4 \cdot 7H_2O$, 2.59 g $NaHCO_3$, 0.23 g KCl) were dissolved separately in 1 L of DI water to make four separate stock solutions. Second, 25 mL of each salt stock solution was aliquot into a clean bottle and diluted in DI water (made up to 1 L volume). Third, 200 mL of the stock solution from step 2 was aliquoted and further diluted with DI water (made up to 1 L volume). Final pH ~7.3.

Nanomaterials were dispersed using the protocol as previously reported (Tantra, Jing, Gohil 2010) (http://www.nanotechia-prospect.org/publications/basic). Briefly, this involved weighing the nanoparticle powder into small, clean vials using an analytical mass balance. Dispersion was carried out by adding the appropriate liquid media (fish, daphnia, seawater, or DI water) dropwise (5 drops from a Pasteur pipette) and mixing using a spatula so as to produce a thick paste before adding 15 mL of liquid media and stirring gently, using the same spatula. The formation of a thick paste as a first step was necessary to allow the efficient displacement of powder-air interface with the powder-liquid interface. The subsequent deagglomeration step was carried out using an ultrasonic probe (130 Watt Ultrasonic Processors); this was done by inserting the ultrasonic probe tip (6 mm Ti) half way down the 15 mL volume of dispersed nanoparticles, and sonication was carried out with 90% amplitude for 20 s. After sonication, the nanoparticle suspension was diluted using the appropriate liquid media, in order to make up to 1 L total volume. A glass rod was used to gently mix the final dispersion, to ensure homogeneity. The dispersions (in the four different media) were stored in separate precleaned 1 L media bottles and left undisturbed. Dispersion concentrations were 50 mg/L. Analyses of redox potentials, half-lives, and zetapotentials were conducted on the day immediately after the dispersions were made.

2.2. High-Resolution SEM. SEM images were obtained using a Supra 40 field emission scanning electron microscope from Carl Zeiss (Welwyn Garden City, Hertfordshire, UK), in which the optimal spatial resolution of the microscope is a few nanometres. In-lens detector images were acquired at an accelerating voltage of 15 kV, a working distance of $\approx$3 mm, and a tilt angle 0°. The SEM was calibrated using a SIRA grid calibration set (SIRA, Chislehurst, Kent, UK). These are metal replicas of cross-ruled gratings of area 60 mm^2 with 19.7 lines/mm for low magnification and 2160 lines/mm for high magnification calibrations, accurate to 0.2%. For analysis of the "as received" nanoparticle powders, a sample of each powder was sprinkled over a SEM carbon adhesive disc; one side of the carbon disc was placed securely on a metal stub, whilst the other side was exposed to the nanoparticle powder. Excess powder was removed by gently tapping the stub on its side until a light coating of powder on the surface became apparent. An adequate magnification was chosen for image acquisition for example, for the estimation of primary particle mean diameter, the shape and limits of the primary particles should become apparent. SEM micrographs were analysed by manually tracing contours of primary particles onto a transparency sheet. The transparency sheet was scanned for further image analysis using Image J software, which automatically calculated particle diameter dimensions.

2.3. Redox Potential Measurements. Redox potentials were measured using an ORP Oakton Waterproof ORP Testr, purchased from Cole-Parmer, UK. This, in effect, measures the potential difference across two electrodes (a Pt electrode against a double junction Ag/AgCl reference electrode). The ORP instrument manufacturer has specified a resolution of $\pm$1 mV, with an accuracy of $\pm$2 mV.

The electrode was used in accordance with the manufacturer's instructions. Prior to use, the electrode was preconditioned in clean tap water for 30 minutes before a final rinse with distilled water. When making measurements, the electrode was carefully placed in a vial containing the nanomaterial dispersion sample; there must be sufficient liquid sample to cover the sensing element. The electrode was carefully stirred a little and then placed in a fixed position, slightly above the bottom of the container. The signal output was allowed to settle for 5 minutes before a reading, the "field potential," was noted. At this point, the signal was stable and there was no further change observed within the next few minutes. After measurement, the electrode was cleaned with tap water and rinsed with distilled water, after which further measurements could be made. When not in use, the electrode was stored in Oakton electrode storage solution.

The redox potential ORP electrode was calibrated against YSI Zobell ORP Calibration Solution (purchased from Cole-Palmer). This reagent was made available in dry form and was reconstituted with 125 mL of DI water prior to use, after which the solution has ~6-month expiry date. This standard solution was used to verify the performance of the electrode at the beginning and end of the study. For Ag/AgCl reference, the redox potential value for Zobell solution was quoted to be 231 ± 10 mV (depending on temperature); at ~20°C, this value was ~237 mV.

Redox potential measurements were carried out on freshly dispersed nanomaterial in the four chosen media, as detailed above. All field potential values recorded were subjected to an additive correction factor of +206 mV. This was necessary so that the final value was reported as if the reference electrode was a standard hydrogen reference electrode (SHE) instead of the Ag/AgCl, as previously documented [9]. The conversion from Ag/AgCl′ to SHE is typically on the order of 200 to 220 mV, and voltage correction is temperature dependent and also varies slightly with the concentration of KCl (~3.5 M) in the electrode filling solution.

2.4. Measurement of Half-Lives through Turbidity Measurements. Turbidity was measured using an HF Scientific-Micro100 RI turbidity meter (Cole-Palmer, UK); this meter has an infrared light source that meets the international standard ISO 7027 for turbidity measurements. The meter was calibrated on standards, which are based on AMCO-AEPA-1 microspheres; these standards are traceable to standard formazin suspension. Standard values of 1000, 10 and 0.02 NTU were used to calibrate the meter. Prior to use, the meter was allowed to warm up for 30 minutes. Sample cuvettes (HF Scientific (USA)) were used to hold the samples. Note that glass thickness may vary from cuvette to cuvette and within the same cuvette. Hence, individual vials were indexed; indexing of the cuvette entails finding the point of the cuvette that light passes through that gives the lowest reading and, once indexed, the holder can be marked accordingly. Prior to their use, cuvettes were cleaned, in accordance with manufacturer's instructions. This involved washing the interior and exterior of the cuvette with a detergent (2% Hellmanex in DI water); it was then rinsed several times in distilled water before finally rinsing in DI water. The cuvette was further rinsed with the sample two times before filling (30 mL) and analysed. The cuvette was placed into the meter and signal allowed to settle before taking readings. Turbidity readings were taken at regular time intervals. When not in use, the vials (containing the dispersions) were stored in the dark.

2.5. Zetapotential Measurements. Electrophoretic measurements were obtained using a Zetasizer Nano ZS (Malvern Instruments, UK) equipped with a 633 nm laser. The reference standard (DTS1230, zetapotential standard from Malvern) was used to qualify the performance of the instrument. Sample preparation involved filling a disposable capillary cell (DTS1060, Malvern). Prior to their use, these cells were thoroughly cleaned with ethanol and deionised water, as recommended by the instrument vendor. For analysis, the individual cell was filled with the appropriate sample and flushed before refilling; measurement was carried out on the second filling. Malvern Instrument's Dispersion Technology software (Version 4.0) was used for data analysis, and zetapotential values were estimated from the measured electrophoretic mobility data using the Smoluchowski equation, as documented in a previous publication [13].

3. Results and Discussion

Table 1 shows the redox potential results associated with dispersions of the PROSPEcT nanomaterials in four different media. The table also contains the redox potential values of the corresponding blank media, that is, liquid media with no nanomaterial. The values in brackets show the difference of ORP readings upon addition of the nanomaterials with respect to the corresponding blank media.

Results show that ORP values are dominated by the type of liquid media used for dispersions. Nanomaterial dispersions in seawater resulted in a much smaller ORP values in comparison with dispersions made in other media. In addition, this is also the case with the ORP values of the corresponding blank media, that is, blank seawater having the smallest ORP value, of 384 mV, compared to the rest of the blank liquid media (redox potential values all above 400 mV). The ORP values reported here is not specific to a single chemical species and thus represent an aggregate oxidization-reduction of all species that can react at the Pt working electrode [14]. The fact that the type of liquid media itself seems to have some contribution to the final ORP values is not surprising, as dissolved redox species in the liquid can easily interact with the Pt electrode of the ORP probe. In fact, such ORP measurements are often employed as an accurate gauge of water quality and for the monitoring of dissolved species in the water [14]. Seawater in particular is shown to be more reducing in nature, that is, due to higher concentration of reducing agents (such as NO_2^-) in such media, if compared to the other liquid media. The presence of reducing agent has the effect of lowering the ORP value [15]. Furthermore, we expect a much-reduced level of oxidising agent such as dissolved oxygen in such a high saline solution, as the more saline the water can be the less oxygen the water can hold. If there is a reduction in oxidising agents, then this also has an effect of lowering the ORP value [16].

The ORP readings reported here were taken three times with very little variation among the replicates, that is, not more than ±2 mV. However, the second and third replicates were acquired soon after acquiring the 1st replicate, by taking the ORP probe out of the dispersion and reimmersing it back into the dispersion. The variations in the replicates here thus represent variations of the instrument's accuracy; they will not represent any variations that might be due

Table 1: Redox potential of nanomaterial dispersion in various liquid media; the value quoted (in mV) is relative to the standard hydrogen reference electrode. The values in bracket show the difference in value with respect to the corresponding blank liquid media.

Sample name	Redox potential (mV) of nanomaterial dispersions			
	DI water	Fish medium	Seawater	Daphnia medium
Liquid media with no nanomaterials	405	418	384	425
Nanograin CeO_2 (Umicore Belgium)	416 (11 mV)	439 (21 mV)	384 (0 mV)	415 (−10 mV)
Nanosun ZnO (Micronisers, Australia)	398 (−7 mV)	424 (6 mV)	380 (−4 mV)	415 (−10 mV)
Micron ZnO (Sigma Aldrich, UK)	398 (−7 mV)	430 (12 mV)	374 (−10 mV)	415 (−10 mV)
Z-COTE ZnO (BASF, Germany)	396 (−9 mV)	427 (9 mV)	379 (−5 mV)	422 (−3 mV)
Micron CeO_2 (Sigma Aldrich, UK)	422 (17 mV)	430 (12 mV)	382 (−2 mV)	429 (4 mV)
Ceria dry CeO_2 (Antaria, Australia)	414 (9 mV)	436 (18 mV)	387 (3 mV)	426 (1 mV)

Table 2: Mean values of zetapotential (of six replicates) for different nanomaterials dispersed in various media. DI water + 5 mM NaCl—this medium was employed to compare with the DI results when in the presence of inert background electrolyte. Values are the mean and ±1 SD of six replicates.

Sample name	DI water (mV)	DI water + 5 mM NaCl (mV)	Fish medium (mV)	Seawater (mV)	Daphnia medium (mV)
Nanograin CeO_2	33.0 ± 2.0	33.9 ± 1.7	−11.1 ± 1.0	N/A	1.2 ± 0.2
Nanosun ZnO	24.6 ± 0.4	25.2 ± 0.6	12.4 ± 0.3	N/A	4.9 ± 0.2
Micron ZnO	20.2 ± 0.4	13.9 ± 0.6	4.4 ± 0.4	N/A	−4.6 ± 0.4
Z-COTE ZnO	24.3 ± 0.4	20.8 ± 0.8	10.8 ± 0.1	N/A	1.3 ± 0.2
Micron CeO_2	−7.0 ± 6.0	−2.0 ± 2.0	−22.3 ± 0.5	N/A	−15.0 ± 0.3
Ceria Dry CeO_2	28.0 ± 2.0	23.0 ± 1.3	−15.3 ± 0.6	N/A	−17.4 ± 0.3

to other factors such as differences in dispersion quality. Table 1 also shows the change in ORP values (values reported in brackets) upon addition of the nanomaterials relative to the corresponding blank media. Results show that, in most cases, there is a change of less than ~10 mV associated upon addition of the nanomaterials. There are only three cases in which the ORP value change is greater than 15 mV: Nanograin CeO_2 in fish medium, Micron CeO_2 in DI water, and Ceria dry CeO_2 in fish media. Currently, we offer no explanation as to why there is a much larger change in ORP values in these three cases, apart from potential variations in dispersion quality, for example, due to potential redox contaminants associated with the different samples received. In addition, no real differentiation can be made between ZnO and CeO_2 particles, with Z-COTE ZnO (BASF, Germany) having the same 9 mV change as the Ceria dry CeO_2 (Antaria, Australia), when both are dispersed in DI water.

The other physicochemical characterization associated with the nanomaterials are shown in Tables 2, 3, and 4 below, which correspond to zetapotential, turbidity, and SEM particle size measurements, respectively.

Results show that zetapotential values of nanomaterials when dispersed in seawater cannot be successfully measured (due to high conductivity) and thus displayed as N/A in Table 2. Such unsuccessful measurements were reported in the corresponding "quality report" at the end of the measurement. In general, results indicate high zetapotential values for nanomaterials that are dispersed either in DI water or DI water + 5 mM NaCl. Results of the DI water are similar to the corresponding DI water + NaCl case; the addition of NaCl into the DI water was carried out so as to have greater confidence in the DI water results, as the measurement of zetapotential usually involves the presence of inert background electrolyte. Overall, results show that nanomaterials are most stable when dispersed in DI water (or DI water + NaCl) and least stable when in an ecotox media. This is true apart for the case of Micron CeO_2 showing that it is least stable in DI water, that is, −7 mV when compared to other ecotox media such as fish medium, that is, −22 mV. Currently, no explanation is available for this behaviour, and dispersion stability was further measured by using the concept of half-life values (as previously discussed in the introduction, the larger the half-life, the more stable the dispersion). Results in Table 3 show that, as with zetapotential measurements, results in DI water are generally more stable (with the largest associated with Z-COTE ZnO of 4038 minutes) than when in ecotox media. However, unlike the zetapotential values, Micron CeO_2 also shows the same trend, that is, most stable in DI water than when in an ecotox media. The reason for this discrepancy lies in the fact that dispersion stability was measured in two different ways: through the measurement of interparticle force (zetapotential) or through analyzing the stability via sedimentation measurements (turbidity with time). The former measurement is solely governed by the electric properties of the solid surface in contact with liquid, which will subsequently contribute towards sedimentation rate; the latter measurement is not only determined by the zetapotential value but also by other factors, for example, particle size (in which the larger particles are expected to sediment at a much faster rate) [17]. The SEM results (Table 4) show the mean (Feret) primary particle sizes and

Table 3: Dispersion stabilities, as measured by their corresponding "half-lives" (the time it takes for particle concentration to be reduced by half) of the different nanomaterials when dispersed in various media.

Sample name	DI water (min)	Fish media (min)	Seawater (min)	Daphnia media (min)
Nanograin CeO_2	2676	282	288	252
Nanosun ZnO	2526	498	402	444
Micron ZnO	966	216	228	324
Z-COTE ZnO	4038	816	738	768
Micron CeO_2	432	348	294	294
Ceria Dry CeO_2	780	438	534	600

Table 4: The size of primary particles (of the "as-received" powders), as defined by their corresponding Feret's diameter. Mean diameter (±1 SD) of a minimum of 50–100 particles measured in the SEM images; the SD here represents the broadness of the size distribution.

Sample name	Supplier	Mean Feret diameter (±1 SD) from SEM images
Nanograin CeO_2	Umicore Belgium	28.4 ± 10.4
Nanosun ZnO	Micronisers, Australia	42.5 ± 3.6
Micron ZnO	Sigma Aldrich, UK	891.8 ± 800.0
Z-COTE ZnO	BASF, Germany	151.0 ± 55.6
Micron CeO_2	Sigma Aldrich, UK	615.3 ± 430.5
Ceria dry CeO_2	Antaria, Australia	44.9 ± 14.6

the corresponding standard deviations (to reflect on the polydispersity of the primary particle size). Results presented in Table 4 show that the mean primary particle sizes of the samples range from ~30 nm to ~890 nm, the largest being the Micron ZnO and Micron CeO_2 from Sigma Aldrich. The SD values show the large degree of polydispersity associated with samples received: high polydispersity associated with Sigma Aldrich samples, less so with Nanosun ZnO, Microniser. The SEM micrographs indicated that all particles tested here were highly aggregated together into agglomerates of irregular shape.

If there is any particle contribution towards the final ORP values, then, out of the two types of nanomaterials tested, we expected CeO_2 to have a bigger contribution compared to ZnO. This is on the basis that CeO_2 particle can act as a redox couple of Ce(IV)/Ce(III), which is not the case for ZnO. If CeO_2 particles had contributed to the final ORP value, then we expect this to occur with Nanograin CeO_2 (having the smallest particle size of ~30 nm, as shown in Table 4) and when dispersed in DI water, as this resulted in a highly stable dispersion (noted by its high dispersion stability value of 2676 min and high zeta potential value of 33 mV, as shown in Tables 3 and 2, resp.). A highly stable dispersion will mean sufficient time to allow particles to diffuse to the Pt electrode, thus interacting with the Pt electrode in order to contribute towards the final ORP reading. Hence, we expected the redox potential to be affected most by the Nanograin CeO_2 in DI water and clearly this was not the case. As shown in Table 2, Nanograin CeO_2 in DI water only resulted in an ORP value change of 11 mV compared to a change of 21 mV when the same particles were dispersed in fish medium. Overall, results suggest that the particles have minor effects on the final ORP readings.

4. Conclusion

The study investigated the redox potential measurements, using ORP probe electrode, of different ZnO and CeO_2 dispersions, in various liquid media. The variations in the ORP readings for the different dispersions could not be regarded as being highly significant and were mainly governed by the type of liquid media that the nanomaterials were dispersed in. This is not surprising, as ORP values are dominated by the amount of dissolved chemical species in the liquid media. Dispersions in seawater resulted in the lowest ORP values, suggesting that the media is *reducing* in nature. This was attributed to a much higher concentration of reducing agents such as sulphites or a reduction in the concentration of dissolved oxygen under a high salinity environment. The study shows that there was little contribution from the particles themselves towards the final ORP reading, with no significant differentiation between CeO_2 and ZnO. As it is clear that redox potential measurements using an ORP electrode will not indicate a particle's contribution towards the final redox potential value, the work has highlighted the need to have better tools for such measurements. There are several alternatives to using the ORP probe, including X-ray photoelectron spectroscopy (XPS) and electron paramagnetic resonance (EPR) and electron energy loss spectroscopy (EELS) [18]. However, these technologies rely on the indirect measurement of redox potential and the accuracy of the values reported may come into question.

Acknowledgments

This work was conducted as part of PROSPEcT, which is a public-private partnership between DEFRA, EPSRC, and

TSB and the Nanotechnology Industries Association (NIA Ltd.) and its members, and was administered by the DEFRA LINK Programme. The authors would like to thank Dr. Alex Shard for continuing support and Mr. Jordan Tompkins for the initial handling and distribution of the nanomaterials. R. Tantra gratefully acknowledges Professor Philip N. Bartlett from the University of Southampton and Dr. Andy Wain, whose expertise in electrochemistry has immensely helped in our understanding of the study.

References

[1] K. Aschberger, C. Micheletti, B. Sokull-Klüttgen, and F. M. Christensen, "Analysis of currently available data for characterising the risk of engineered nanomaterials to the environment and human health—lessons learned from four case studies," *Environment International*, vol. 37, no. 6, pp. 1143–1156, 2011.

[2] K. W. Powers, S. C. Brown, V. B. Krishna, S. C. Wasdo, B. M. Moudgil, and S. M. Roberts, "Research strategies for safety evaluation of nanomaterials. Part VI. Characterization of nanoscale particles for toxicological evaluation," *Toxicological Sciences*, vol. 90, no. 2, pp. 296–303, 2006.

[3] R. Tantra, S. Jing, S. K. Pichaimuthu, N. Walker, J. Noble, and V. A. Hackley, "Dispersion stability of nanoparticles in ecotoxicological investigations: the need for adequate measurement tools," *Journal of Nanoparticle Research*, vol. 13, no. 9, pp. 3765–3780, 2011.

[4] R. Tantra, D. Gohil, S. Kaliyappan, and S. Jing, "Nanoparticle characterisation for ecotoxicological studies using imaging versus non-imaging based tools," *The International Journal of Sustainable Development and Planning*, vol. 6, no. 2, pp. 1–14, 2010.

[5] J. R. Lead and E. Smith, *Environmental and Human Health Impacts of Nanotechnology*, Wiley-Blackwell, 2009.

[6] J Schüring, H. D. Schulz, W. R. Fischer, J. Böttcher, and D. Schüring, *Redox: Fundamentals, Processes and Applications*, Springer, Berlin, Germany, 2010.

[7] E. Burello and A. P. Worth, "A theoretical framework for predicting the oxidative stress potential of oxide nanoparticles," *Nanotoxicology*, vol. 5, no. 2, pp. 228–235, 2011.

[8] S. S. Judd and T. Stephenson, *Process Science and Engineering for Water and Wastewater Treatment*, IWA Publishing, 2002.

[9] W. D. Weight, *Hydrogeology Field Manual*, Mcgraw-Hill Professional Publishing, 2008.

[10] ENV/JM/MONO, "Ref: no. 27–46 list of manufactured nanomaterials and list of endpoints for phase one of the sponsorship programme for the testing of manufactured nanomaterials: revision," 2010, http://www.oecd.org/document/53/0,3746,en_2649_37015404_37760309_1_1_1_1,00.html.

[11] N. J. Rogers, N. M. Franklin, S. C. Apte et al., "Physicochemical behaviour and algal toxicity of nanoparticulate CeO_2 in freshwater," *Environmental Chemistry*, vol. 7, no. 1, pp. 50–60, 2010.

[12] C. M. Bethke, *Geochemical and Biogeochemical Reaction Modeling*, Cambridge University Press, 2010.

[13] R. Tantra, P. Schulze, and P. Quincey, "Effect of nanoparticle concentration on zeta-potential measurement results and reproducibility," *Particuology*, vol. 8, no. 3, pp. 279–285, 2010.

[14] W. J. Sutherland, *Ecological Census Techniques: A Handbook*, Cambridge University Press, 2nd edition, 2006.

[15] V. Shah, *Emerging Environmental Technologies*, Springer, 2008.

[16] H. J. G. Baretta-Bekker, E. K. Duursma, and B. R. Kuipers, *Encyclopedia of Marine Sciences*, Springer, 2nd edition, 2002.

[17] E. E. Kissa, *Dispersions: Characterization, Testing, and Measurement*, CRC Press, 1999.

[18] G. Yang, S. Cook, R. J. Hand, and G. Möbus, "CeO_2 nanoprecipitation in borosilicate glasses: a redox study using EELS," *Journal of the European Ceramic Society*, vol. 30, no. 4, pp. 831–838, 2010.

Quantitative Property-Property Relationship for Screening-Level Prediction of Intrinsic Clearance of Volatile Organic Chemicals in Rats and Its Integration within PBPK Models to Predict Inhalation Pharmacokinetics in Humans

Thomas Peyret and Kannan Krishnan

Département de Santé Environnementale et Santé au Travail, Université de Montréal, C.P. 6128, Succursale Centre-Ville, Montréal, QC, Canada H3C 3J7

Correspondence should be addressed to Kannan Krishnan, kannan.krishnan@umontreal.ca

Academic Editor: Jane C. Caldwell

The objectives of this study were (i) to develop a screening-level Quantitative property-property relationship (QPPR) for intrinsic clearance (CL_{int}) obtained from *in vivo* animal studies and (ii) to incorporate it with human physiology in a PBPK model for predicting the inhalation pharmacokinetics of VOCs. CL_{int}, calculated as the ratio of the *in vivo* V_{max} (μmol/h/kg bw rat) to the K_m (μM), was obtained for 26 VOCs from the literature. The QPPR model resulting from stepwise linear regression analysis passed the validation step ($R^2 = 0.8$; leave-one-out cross-validation $Q^2 = 0.75$) for CL_{int} normalized to the phospholipid (PL) affinity of the VOCs. The QPPR facilitated the calculation of CL_{int} (L PL/h/kg bw rat) from the input data on log P_{ow}, log blood: water PC and ionization potential. The predictions of the QPPR as lower and upper bounds of the 95% mean confidence intervals (LMCI and UMCI, resp.) were then integrated within a human PBPK model. The ratio of the maximum (using LMCI for CL_{int}) to minimum (using UMCI for CL_{int}) AUC predicted by the QPPR-PBPK model was 1.36 ± 0.4 and ranged from 1.06 (1,1-dichloroethylene) to 2.8 (isoprene). Overall, the integrated QPPR-PBPK modeling method developed in this study is a pragmatic way of characterizing the impact of the lack of knowledge of CL_{int} in predicting human pharmacokinetics of VOCs, as well as the impact of prediction uncertainty of CL_{int} on human pharmacokinetics of VOCs.

1. Introduction

The evolving scientific and regulatory activities in Europe and North America emphasize the need for the development of tools that refine, replace, or reduce the use of animals and human volunteers in pharmacokinetic and toxicity tests [1–3]. The ability to base the toxic responses on the target tissue dose or internal concentration of the toxic moiety of the chemicals is key to the predictive tools reflective of the current state of science. Therefore, physiologically based pharmacokinetic (PBPK) models that are capable of providing *a priori* prediction of the time course of chemicals in blood and tissues is of tremendous interest [4]. PBPK models are mechanistically based mathematical descriptions of the absorption, distribution, metabolism, and excretion of chemicals or pharmaceutical compounds. In PBPK models, the organism is represented as a set of several tissue compartments interconnected by blood flows. In these models, the internal dose measures (e.g., blood or tissue concentrations, amount metabolized) of a chemical are described on the basis of mass-balance differential equations requiring species-specific properties (e.g., alveolar ventilation rate, cardiac output, regional blood flows, and tissue volumes) and chemical-specific input parameters (e.g., partition coefficients and metabolic constants). Although the species-specific values of several physiological parameters are available in the literature [4–6], the partition coefficients (PCs) and metabolic constants need to be determined experimentally or calculated by using animal-replacement methods for each chemical individually [7]. The values of tissue : blood or tissue : plasma partition coefficients essential for developing PBPK models have been estimated for a wide range of chemicals and chemical classes, including drugs, with the use of tissue composition-based algorithms or QSAR methods (e.g., [8–19]).

Regarding the metabolism parameters (i.e., hepatic clearance, intrinsic clearance, V_{max}, K_m, K_{cat}, free energy of binding, energy of activation, or activation enthalpy), some studies have developed 2-D and 3-D QSARs but with a specific focus on either a single isozyme, a single reaction or a single class of substances [8, 20–38]. None of these past efforts succeeded in predicting both V_{max} and K_m (or CL_{int}) of environmental chemicals for direct incorporation within animal or human PBPK models. Alternatively, few studies utilized the group contribution method of Gao [39–43], to predict metabolic rates for PBPK models. In this method, the chemical is decomposed into different structural fragments or groups, the contributions of which are obtained by regression analysis [39]. Accordingly, these publications demonstrated the feasibility of developing structure-property relationships for the metabolism rates. The group contribution method was successfully used to develop quantitative structure-property relationships (QSPRs) for the tissue : air partition coefficients as well as intrinsic (CL_{int}) and hepatic clearance (CL_h for a group of low-molecular-weight volatile organic chemicals (VOCs) in rats [41, 42]. These QSPR models, in turn, were incorporated within PBPK models to predict reasonably well the blood kinetics of inhaled VOCs in rats. As these QSPRs are species specific, they could not be used to conduct interspecies extrapolations. To overcome this limitation, Béliveau et al. [40] developed biologically based algorithms for PCs and CL_h to conduct rat to human extrapolations of the inhalation toxicokinetics of VOCs. In this study, QSPRs based on the group contribution method were developed for the chemical-specific input parameters of the biological algorithms for PCs (i.e., oil : air, water : air,and blood protein : air) and CL_{int} (intrinsic clearance normalized for cytochrome P450 2E1 content). More recently, QSPRs were developed for the metabolic constants V_{max} (maximum velocity of reaction) and K_m (Michaelis constant) [43] and were further incorporated within a rat PBPK model to predict the toxicokinetics of mixtures of VOCs. Despite the successful use of the group contribution method in QSPR modeling of metabolism rates, their principal limitation relates to the fact that the chemical space they cover is extremely limited (low-molecular-weight VOCs containing one or more of the following fragments: CH_3, CH_2, CH, C, C=C, H, Br, Cl, F, benzene ring, and H on benzene ring). More experimental data on diverse chemicals would be needed to determine the contributions of other molecular fragments, as has been done with P_{ow} (e.g., estimation of the contribution of 130 fragments (i.e., groups) required 1200 measurements of P_{ow}) [44]. To extend the currently available QSPR for CL_{int} to cover more diverse fragments and at the same time respect a reasonable ratio of the number of parameters to the number of observations, extensive experimental data would be required.

Since the critical limitation in the construction of PBPK models for new substances continues to be the metabolism rate, a pragmatic approach—particularly for inhaled VOCs—is to evaluate the maximum and minimum possible blood concentration profiles in exposed individuals. Thus, using a hepatic extraction ratio (E) of 0 and 1 in the PBPK models, Poulin and Krishnan [45] obtained simulations of the physiological limits (i.e., maximal and minimal blood concentration profiles) for inhaled VOCs in humans. Assuming the conceptual PBPK model and the values of its physiological parameters are reliable, the real answer, that is, the actual concentrations and kinetic curve, would be somewhere in between the theoretical limits simulated with these PBPK models [45]. The uncertainty associated with these theoretical bounds can be reduced by developing better estimates of the metabolism constants. This could be done, at a practical level, by developing *in silico* tools that provide a range of plausible values, in lieu of a single accurate point estimate. Such a tool might be of use for the toxicokinetic screening of substances, until the time when the chemical-specific measurements are obtained *in vivo*, *in vitro*, or with a highly precise mechanistic *in silico* method.

Since human exposures to environmental contaminants in most cases do not attain levels that approach or exceed saturation, it is not crucial to predict V_{max} and K_m separately, particularly for simulating kinetics in humans exposed to low atmospheric concentrations of VOCs. Therefore, the availability of *in silico* approaches based on easily available parameters to predict plausible range of CL_{int} would be desirable as a screening-level tool. The objective of this study was therefore to develop a quantitative property-property relationship (QPPR) model of animal data to generate initial estimates (or bounds) of intrinsic clearance of VOCs, for eventual incorporation within a human PBPK model to simulate blood concentration profiles associated with inhalation exposures. In this regard, we focused on evaluating the impact of the uncertainty associated with QPPR predictions of CL_{int} on the blood kinetics of VOCs in humans, relative to that of the uncertainty associated with the total lack of knowledge of the metabolic rate in humans. Furthermore, the reliability of applying the QPPR to predict the area under the blood concentration versus time curve (AUC) of parent chemicals was evaluated, as a function of the sensitivity of the metabolism parameter in the PBPK model and the prediction uncertainty of QPPR model.

2. Methods

A QPPR model for CL_{int} was developed using a calibration set of 26 VOCs. The QPPR predictions were then compared with experimental data for several VOCs and the pharmacokinetics in humans were simulated using integrated QPPR-PBPK models for these 26 VOCs. The predictions of QPPR were evaluated further with an external data set of CL_{int} for 11 VOCs.

2.1. QPPR Modeling for Intrinsic Clearance

2.1.1. Chemicals and Data Sources. The development of a global QPPR model for metabolism was initially undertaken using experimental data on the *in vivo* intrinsic clearance of 26 VOCs in rats, collated and evaluated in previous studies by Béliveau et al. [40, 41] (1,1,1,2-tetrachloroethane; 1,1,2,2-tetrachloroethane; 1,1,2-trichloroethane; 1,1-dichloroethane; 1,1-dichloroethylene; 1,2-dichloroethane; benzene; bromochloromethane; bromodichloromethane; carbon tetrachloride; chloroethane; chloroform; *cis*-1,2-dichloroethylene; dibromomethane; dichloromethane; ethylbenzene; hexachloroethane; isoprene; methyl chloride; *m*-xylene; *n*-hexane; pentachloroethane; styrene; toluene; trichloroethylene; vinyl chloride) [24, 46–53].

Subsequently, the resulting QPPR model was evaluated with experimental *in vivo* data on CL_{int} for 11 additional VOCs in rats (1,1,1-trichloroethane; 1,2,4-trimethylbenzene; bromoform; dibromochloromethane; furan; halothane; *o*-xylene; *trans*-1,2-dichloroethylene; tetrachloroethylene; propylene; ethylene) [46, 48, 54–61]. These 11 chemicals outside the calibration set were also lipophilic, low-molecular-weight VOCs and likely substrates of cytochrome P450 2E1 [32, 62]. Moreover except for halothane and 1,2,4-trimethylbenzene, the chemicals of the evaluation dataset possess values of P_{ow}, ionization potential, and blood : water PC within the range of values for the chemicals in the QPPR calibration set.

2.1.2. Modeling Endpoint. For QPPR modeling, CL_{int} (expressed in units of L blood, CL_{intblood}, or L phospholipids, CL_{intPL}) was used as the endpoint. Initially, CL_{intblood} (L blood/h/kg$^{0.75}$) for all the studied chemicals was computed as allometrically scaled $V_{\max}$ (μmol/h/kg$^{0.75}$)/K_m (μmol/L blood). Since CYPs are located in the endoplasmic reticulum embedded in the phospholipidic bilayer [63], the CL_{intPL} values reflecting chemical affinity for the phospholipids (PL) were subsequently computed. The values of CL_{intPL} (L phospholipid/h/kg$^{0.75}$) were obtained by dividing $V_{\max}$ (μmol/h/kg$^{0.75}$) with K_m expressed as μmol/L PL. The K_m values in μM of PL were obtained by multiplying the values of K_m expressed as μmol/L blood with the chemical-specific phospholipid : blood partition coefficients (P_{plb}) calculated as follows:

$$P_{\text{plb}} = \frac{0.3 \cdot P_{\text{oa}} + 0.7 \cdot P_{\text{wa}}}{P_{\text{ba}}}, \quad (1)$$

where P_{oa} is the *n*-octanol : air PC, P_{wa} the water : air PC, and P_{ba} the blood : air PC.

The above equation computes P_{plb} as the ratio of phospholipid : air to blood : air PCs of the VOCs, based on Poulin and Krishnan [10, 12].

2.1.3. Input Parameters for Transforming the Endpoint. The input parameters required for converting the CL_{int} obtained from the literature were P_{oa}, P_{wa}, and P_{ba}.

(1) P_{oa} and P_{wa}. The *n*-octanol : air PC (P_{oa}), was calculated as the product of the *n*-octanol : water PC (P_{ow}) and P_{wa} (inverse of Henry's law constant at 37.5°C). The values of P_{ow} and P_{wa} were predicted using U.S. EPA's freeware EPISUITE (http://www.epa.gov/opptintr/exposure/pubs/episuite.htm).

(2) P_{ba}. Experimental values were used for rat blood : air [54, 56, 59, 64–68]. The calculated values of P_{plb} for the chemicals used for the development and for the evaluation of the QPPR are reported in Table 1.

2.1.4. Variable Selection. A priori list of variables was developed on the basis on mechanistic considerations. The rate and affinity for P450-mediated metabolism would appear to be related to the size, shape, charge, and energy of the substrate; therefore variables that reflect these properties were chosen for the QPPR analysis [21, 23, 27, 28, 32, 69–71]. The descriptors of the size and shape of the molecule were the molecular length, width, depth, volume, surface, and the Kappa 2 index [72], as well as two descriptors used in the work of Lewis et al. [23], namely, the ratio of the molecular length to the molecular width (L/W) and the ratio of the area of the molecule (i.e., length times width) to the square of the depth (a/d^2). The dipole moment and ionization potential (IP) were used as measure of the charge disposition and the energy in the molecule, respectively. The values of all the previously cited descriptors were calculated using commercially available software (Molecular Modeling Pro, Chem SW, Fairfield, CA). Before calculating the molecular descriptors with Molecular Modeling Pro, the 3D molecules were drawn and minimized using the full MM2 (molecular mechanics program) method provided in the software. The dipole moment and the ionization potential were calculated using MOPAC/PM3 program, included in Molecular Modeling Pro.

Hydrophobic descriptors such as $\log P_{\text{ow}}$ (log of the *n*-octanol : water PC) that reflect hydrogen bonding and π-π stacking have already been correlated to the values of metabolic constants [69–71]. In this study, the following physicochemical parameters were chosen to describe the relative solubility and partitioning into diverse biological media: $\log P_{\text{ow}}$, log phospholipid : water PC ($\log P_{\text{plw}}$); log blood : water PC ($\log P_{\text{bw}}$), and log water : air PC ($\log P_{\text{wa}}$). The blood : water and phospholipid : water PCs were obtained by dividing the blood : air and phospholipid : air PCs values by the water : air PC values. The values of P_{ow}, P_{wa}, blood : air, and phospholipid : air PCs were obtained as described for the calculation of P_{plb} (1).

2.1.5. Statistical Analysis. Multilinear regression analysis approach was chosen for the QPPR analysis of CL_{int} because linear regression models are simple, transparent, and easy to reproduce [73]. The regression analysis was performed using SPSS v16 for Windows (SPSS Inc., Chicago, IL). Stepwise regression analysis was performed to select the QPPRs based on the most statistically significant independent variable(s) from an *a priori* list (see Section 2.1.4). The coefficient of determination R^2, the adjusted R^2 (R^2_{adj}; adjusted for number of variables) [73], the standard error of the estimate *s*, and the value and significance of the *F* statistic were calculated. The

Table 1: Partition coefficients used in the human PBPK models.

Chemicals[a]	Partition coefficient (PC)[b]						Reference
	P_{ba}	P_{lb}	P_{rb}	P_{pb}	P_{fb}	P_{plb}	
Benzene	8.19	2.08	2.08	1.26	60.93	4.55	[66]
Bromochloromethane	10.4	2.81	2.81	1.07	31.5	2	[66, 77]
Bromodichloromethane	26.6	1.15	1.15	0.47	19.77	2.48	[78, 79]
Carbon tetrachloride	2.73	5.2	5.2	1.67	131.5	8.57	[66]
Chloroethane	2.69	1.34	1.34	1.2	14.3	4.42	[66]
Chloroform	6.85	3.08	3.08	2.03	29.6	1.93	[66]
Dibromomethane	19.9	3.42	3.42	2.03	39.8	1.78	[66, 77]
Dichloroethane (1,1-)	4.94	2.19	2.19	1.04	33.2	4.27	[66]
Dichloroethane (1,2-)	19.5	1.83	1.83	1.2	17.64	9.25	[66]
Dichloroethylene (1,1-)	0.81	5.46	5.46	2.53	84.69	4.82	[66, 77]
Dichloroethylene (*cis*-1,2)	9.85	1.55	1.55	0.62	23	5.2	[66]
Dichloromethane	9.7	1.46	1.46	0.82	12.4	1.79	[80]
Ethylbenzene	28	2.99	2.15	0.93	55.6	13.2	[67]
Hexachloroethane	52.4	7.04	7.04	1.43	63.4	156	[66]
Hexane (*n*-)	2.13	5.2	5.2	2.9	159	1.89	[47]
Isoprene	0.75	2.57	2.45	1.97	82	11.84	[52]
Methyl chloride	2.48	1.4	1.4	0.39	5.44	3.04	[66]
Pentachloroethane	50.3	5.17	5.17	1.44	81.9	21.7	[66, 77]
Styrene	52	2.7	5.7	1	50	30.2	[50]
Tetrachloroethane (1,1,1,2-)	30.2	2.92	2.92	1.31	71.1	37.3	[66]
Tetrachloroethane (1,1,2,2-)	116	1.69	1.69	0.87	32.47	14.3	[66]
Toluene	15.6	5.36	5.36	1.77	65.4	13.8	[67]
Trichloroethane (1,1,2-)	35.7	2.05	2.05	0.64	40.3	10.1	[66]
Trichloroethylene	8.11	3.35	3.35	1.24	68.3	5.73	[66]
Vinyl chloride	1.16	1.38	1.38	1.81	17.2	4.87	[66]
Xylene (*m*-)	26.4	3.44	3.44	1.59	70.4	15.1	[67]
Bromoform	102.3	2.06	2.06	1.12	40.4	2.44	[78, 79]
Dibromochloromethane	49.2	2.56	2.56	1.13	38.96	1.48	[78, 79]
Dichloroethylene (trans-1,2-)	6.04	1.48	1.48	0.58	24.5	11.7	[66]
Ethylene	0.22	2.05	2.18	2.95	8.73	1.05	[59]
Furan	6.59	0.9	0.9	0.64	9.72	2.75	[56]
Halothane	3.3	2.42	2.42	2.91	44.2	5.82	[58]
Propylene	0.44	1.09	1.2	1.25	11.7	1.52	[54]
Tetrachloroethylene	10.3	5.88	5.88	3.1	119.1	11.1	[57]
Trichloroethane (1,1,1-)	2.53	1.24	3.4	3.4	103.9	21.7	[48]
Trimethylbenzene (1,2,4-)	85	4.4	4.4	2.11	109	19	[61]
Xylene (o-)	34.9	3.09	3.09	1.47	53.8	22.6	[66]

[a] Chemicals in italics were not included in the dataset for the calibration of the model.
[b] P_{ba}: blood : air PC; P_{lb}: liver blood PC; P_{rb} : richly perfused tissues : blood PC; P_{pb}: poorly perfused tissues : blood PC; P_{fb}: fat : blood PC; P_{plb}: phospholipids : blood PC.

normality of the residuals was checked visually on normal probability plots of the standardized residuals (i.e., expected normal cumulative probability versus observed cumulative probability). Leave-one-out cross-validation was conducted and the results were expressed in terms of Q^2, a measure of precision error of the model. The Q^2 was computed as follows [74]:

$$Q^2 = 1 - \frac{\text{PRESS}}{\text{SSY}}, \tag{2}$$

where PRESS is that predicted residual sum of squares and SSY the sum of squares of the response values. The statistical significance ($p < 0.05$) of the regression coefficients was estimated by a t statistic test. Multicollinearity refers to the occurrence of correlation between two independent variables in the multiple linear regression model. Multicollinearity of the variables in the model was assessed by calculating the variance inflation factor (VIF) for all independent variables [75]. The value of VIF was calculated as follows [75]:

$$\mathrm{VIF}_i = \frac{1}{1 - R_i^2}, \tag{3}$$

where VIF_i is the variance inflation factor of the independent variable i in the multilinear regression model and R_i^2 the coefficient of determination of the regression between the independent variable i and the other independent variables in the multilinear regression model.

For each model, the application domain was documented by reporting the ranges of values of the descriptors, the modeled response, and the endpoint.

A QPPR model was considered adequate when: the values of R^2 and R^2_{adj} were ≥ 0.6 [73], the value of Q^2 was ≥ 0.6 [76], and the independent variables were not highly correlated (i.e., VIF < 4) [75].

The predictions of the QPPR model were obtained in terms of lower and upper bounds of the 95% mean confidence intervals (LMCI and UMCI, resp.) in order to represent the uncertainty associated with the mean predicted value. The LMCI and UMCI for the 11 VOCs, not in the QSPR calibration dataset, were obtained by adding them in the SPSS file containing the data used for the QPPR, along with the values of their independent variables only.

2.2. Translation of QPPR Predicted Intrinsic Clearance Values to In Vivo Metabolism Rate and Integration within Human PBPK Models. In the PBPK model, the value of intrinsic clearance was calculated as the product of the QPPR value of CL_{intPL} (L of PL/h/kg$^{0.75}$) and the phospholipid : blood PC (values of P_{plb} in Table 1). The intrinsic clearance (L blood/h/kg$^{0.75}$) was used within the human PBPK models to compute the hepatic clearance.

The rate of metabolism was calculated on the basis of hepatic clearance (i.e., hepatic clearance times the arterial concentration) [4, 40, 41, 45]. For chloroethane, dichloromethane, vinyl chloride, and dibromomethane a first-order constant (1, 2, 1, and 0.7 h^{-1}, resp.) was included in the calculation of the hepatic clearance, CL_h (L/h) [41]:

$$CL_h = Q_L \cdot E, \tag{4}$$

where $E = (CL_{\mathrm{int}} + K_f \cdot V_L)/((CL_{\mathrm{int}} + K_f \cdot V_L) + Q_L)$, Q_L is the blood flow through the liver (L/h), CL_{int} the intrinsic clearance (L blood/h), K_f the first order metabolic constant (h^{-1}), and V_L the liver volume (L).

2.3. PBPK Modeling. The QPPR values of CL_{int} were included in a human PBPK model for inhaled VOCs [50]. Briefly, the PBPK model consisted in four tissue compartments (i.e., liver, fat, richly, and poorly perfused tissues) and a gas exchange lung, which were interconnected by blood flows. The distribution of VOCs into tissue compartments was described as perfusion limited, and the metabolism was limited to liver.

To evaluate the impact of uncertainty on the metabolic rate, for all the chemicals, PBPK simulations were also conducted by setting the value of E to 0.999 ($E_{\max}$) and then to 0.001 ($E_{\min}$), respectively.

The human physiological parameters of the PBPK model (i.e., body weight = 70 kg; cardiac output = 18 L/h/kg$^{0.74}$; alveolar ventilation = 18 L/h/kg$^{0.74}$; tissue compartment volumes, fraction of body weight:liver = 0.026; richly perfused tissues = 0.05; poorly perfused tissues = 0.62; fat = 0.19; perfusion of the tissue compartments, fraction of cardiac output:liver = 0.26; richly perfused tissues = 0.44; poorly perfused tissues = 0.25; fat = 0.05) were obtained from Tardif et al. [67]. Table 1 presents the value of the partition coefficients used in the PBPK model (i.e., blood : air, tissue : blood, and phospholipid : blood PCs). The phospholipid : blood PC was calculated using (1), whereas the blood : air PC and tissue : blood PCs were gathered from the literature [48, 50, 52, 54, 56–59, 61, 66, 67, 77–80].

The PBPK model (differential and algebraic mass-balance equations, physiological parameters, QSPR equations for metabolic constants, and PCs) was written in ACSL (acslX, version 2.5, Aegis Technologies Group, Inc, Huntsville, AL). The model code is included in the supplementary data available online at doi:10.1155/2012/286079. To compare the impact of different (uncertain) scenarios of rate of metabolism on the pharmacokinetics in human, simulations were carried out by setting (i) the value of CL_{int} equal to the lower and upper bound of the QPPR predicted mean 95% confidence interval, or (ii) the liver extraction ratio to 0.001 (no metabolism) and 0.999 (maximum extraction). The 24 h venous blood kinetics corresponding to the four scenarios of metabolism were simulated for an 8 h exposure to 1 ppm of each VOC. The 24 h area under the curve (AUC_{24}) of the venous blood kinetics was also calculated to compare the four scenarios of metabolism simulated with PBPK models. Additionally, the venous blood kinetics of *m*-xylene, toluene, ethylbenzene, dichloromethane, styrene, 1,2,4-trimethylbenzene, and 1,1,1-trichloroethane were compared to experimental data [61, 67, 81–83].

2.4. Analysis of Applicability of the CL_{int} QPPR to PBPK Modeling. The applicability of the QPPR model was evaluated on the basis of the level of uncertainty in the QPPR estimate and the impact (sensitivity) of metabolism on the AUC_{24}. Figure 1 illustrates the role of uncertainty and sensitivity in the reliability of the QPPR-PBPK modeling framework, based on reference [84]. The sensitivity of the metabolism to the AUC was estimated by the ratio of the AUC_{24} obtained with no metabolism ($E_{\min}$) to that obtained with the maximum theoretical metabolism ($E_{\max}$). The sensitivity of AUC_{24} to metabolism was considered to be low, medium, or high if the ratio ($AUC_{E_{\min}}/AUC_{E_{\max}}$) was within a factor of 2, within an order of magnitude, or greater. The uncertainty in the QPPR prediction was evaluated by comparing it

Confidence in the QPPR-PBPK model		Impact of metabolism on AUC ($AUC_{E_{min}}/AUC_{E_{max}}$): Low (<2)	Medium (2–10)	High (>10)
QPPR prediction uncertainty ($Pred. CL_{inPL}/exp. CL_{inPL}$)	Low (<2)	High	High	High
	Medium (2–10)	High	Medium	Medium
	High (>10)	High	Medium	Low

FIGURE 1: Evaluation of the confidence in applying the QPPR for CL_{intPL} in a PBPK model using a sensitivity/uncertainty approach.

to the experimental data. The prediction uncertainty was considered to be low, medium or high if the prediction was within a factor of two, within an order of magnitude and above 10-fold of the experimental data, respectively.

This approach was applied to evaluate the reliability of applying the QPPR within the PBPK model for two situations: (i) for the calibration set of chemicals, for which the uncertainty of the QPPR was evaluated by comparing the predictions of CL_{intPL} with the experimentally derived CL_{intPL} values and (ii) for chemicals in the evaluation dataset, for which the uncertainty in the QPPR prediction was considered to be "high", to replicate the "data poor" situations with new or tested chemicals with unknown experimental CL_{int} values.

3. Results

3.1. QPPR Development. The initial effort to develop a QPPR model for metabolism rate (expressed as $CL_{intblood}$, in units of L blood/hr), based on a stepwise analysis of its relationship to various molecular descriptors and physicochemical properties, was not successful (not shown). Same analysis, repeated for CL_{int} expressed in units of L PL/h (CL_{intPL}), yielded a QPPR that consisted of $\log P_{plw}$, $\log P_{bw}$, and IP (ionization potential, eV) as input parameters. This model satisfied the criteria for an acceptable model in terms of coefficient of determination ($R^2 = 0.802$; $R^2_{adj} = 0.775$), leave-one-out cross validation ($Q^2 = 0.755$), and multicollinearity (VIFs: $\log P_{plw} = 2.42$; $\log P_{bw} = 2.38$; IP $= 1.04$). The values of the regression coefficients were significant (P value < 0.001 for the constant, $\log P_{plw}$ and $\log P_{bw}$, and 0.007 for IP).

However, as the value of $\log P_{ow}$ can be obtained more readily than $\log P_{plw}$, the regression analysis was repeated by using $\log P_{ow}$, $\log P_{bw}$, and calculated IP, and it yielded the following QPPR:

$$\log CL_{intPL} = 5.63(\pm 1.187) - 1.287(\pm 0.149) \cdot \log P_{ow} + 1.08(\pm 0.233) \cdot \log P_{bw} - 0.328(\pm 0.111) \cdot \text{IP}. \quad (5)$$

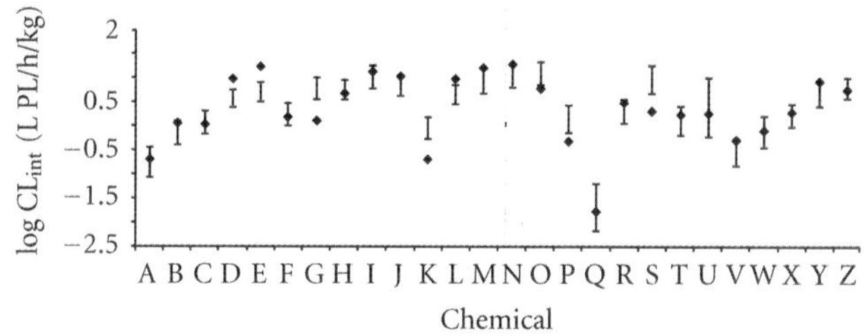

FIGURE 2: Experimental and predicted values of $\log CL_{int}$ for 26 VOCs. The horizontal bars represent the QPPR predicted LMCI and UMCI, the symbols represent the experimental data. A: 1,1,1,2-tetrachloroethane; B: 1,1,2,2-tetrachloroethane; C: 1,1,2-trichloroethane; D: 1,1-dichloroethane; E: 1,1-dichloroethylene; F: 1,2-dichloroethane; G: 1,2-dichloroethylene (*cis*-); H: benzene; I: bromochloromethane; J: bromodichloromethane; K: carbon tetrachloride; L: chloroethane; M: chloroform; N: dibromomethane; O: dichloromethane; P: ethylbenzene; Q: hexachloroethane; R: isoprene; S: methyl chloride; T: *m*-xylene; U: *n*-hexane; V: pentachloroethane; W: styrene; X: toluene; Y: trichloroethylene; Z: vinyl chloride.

This QPPR model satisfied the criteria for an acceptable model in terms of coefficient of determination ($R^2 = 0.796$; $R^2_{adj} = 0.768$), leave-one-out cross validation ($Q^2 = 0.748$), and multicollinearity (VIFs: $\log P_{ow} = 2.42$; $\log P_{bw} = 2.38$; IP $= 1.04$). The application domain of the model can be described with [min; max] as follows: $\log P_{ow} = [1.09; 4.03]$; $\log P_{bw}$ [0.16; 2.49]; calculated ionization potential [9.13; 11.28].

The QPPR (5) was subsequently applied to calculate the CL_{intPL} of the VOCs in the calibration set. Table 2 presents the values of the input parameters, along with the experimental data for the 26 VOCs used in QPPR development. Figure 2 illustrates the comparison of the predicted values of CL_{intPL} (LMCI and UMCI) and the experimental data. The uncertainty in the predicted log CL_{intPL} can be characterized by the difference between the UMCI and the LMCI; this value ranged from 0.37 (1,1-dichloroethane) to 1.23 (*n*-hexane) with a mean of 0.54 and a standard deviation of 0.18. The nearest confidence bounds of the predicted log CL_{intPL} were higher than 5-fold of the experimental value (exp.) for three substances (*cis*-1,2-dichloroethylene, LMCI $= 0.55$ versus exp. $= 0.09$; styrene, LMCI $= -0.45$ versus exp. $= -0.09$; and 1,1,2-trichloroethane, UMCI $= 0.46$ versus exp. $= 0.02$). The impact of the imprecision of these QPPR predictions of the metabolic constants on the pharmacokinetics in humans was then evaluated by PBPK modeling.

Figure 3 presents the predictions of the 24 h blood pharmacokinetics following 8 h exposure to 1 ppm of each of the 26 VOCs used in the QPPR analysis. The bold lines represent the simulations obtained using 0 and 1 as the hepatic extraction ratio, whereas the grey area encompassed by thin lines represents the simulation obtained using LMCI and UMCI of predicted CL_{int} in PBPK models. Overall, the envelope of the concentrations predicted using the QPPR predictions reduced the region of uncertainty associated with

Table 2: Input parameters and experimental data of log CL_{intPL}.

Chemical	Input parameters			Log Cl_{intPL} [a] (L_{PL}/h/kg)	Ref V_{max}, K_m
	Log P_{ow}	Log P_{bw}	Ionization potential (eV)		
Benzene	1.99	0.820	9.743	0.667	[53]
Bromochloromethane	1.43	0.642	10.562	1.118	[49]
Bromodichloromethane	1.61	0.717	10.676	1.029	[46]
Carbon tetrachloride	2.44	0.988	10.985	−0.700	[24]
Chloroethane	1.58	0.438	10.410	0.987	[24]
Chloroform	1.52	0.741	10.839	1.192	[24]
Dibromomethane	1.52	0.777	10.587	1.275	[51]
Dichloroethane (1,1-)	1.76	0.624	10.577	0.974	[24]
Dichloroethane (1,2-)	1.83	0.356	10.446	0.163	[24]
Dichloroethylene (1,1-)	2.12	0.922	9.748	1.223	[24]
Dichloroethylene (*cis*-1,2)	1.98	0.752	9.493	0.092	[24]
Dichloromethane	1.34	0.608	10.582	0.777	[24]
Ethylbenzene	3.03	1.386	9.406	−0.334	[49]
Hexachloroethane	4.03	1.315	10.843	−1.767	[24]
Hexane (*n*-)	3.29	2.492	11.276	0.252	[47]
Isoprene	2.58	0.987	9.349	0.472	[52]
Methyl chloride	1.09	0.160	10.473	0.299	[24]
Pentachloroethane	3.11	1.251	10.763	−0.297	[24]
Styrene	2.89	0.889	9.130	−0.088	[50]
Tetrachloroethane (1,1,1,2-)	2.93	0.836	10.728	−0.693	[24]
Tetrachloroethane (1,1,2,2-)	2.19	0.519	10.736	0.051	[24]
Toluene	2.54	0.879	9.442	0.282	[49]
Trichloroethane (1,1,2-)	2.01	0.491	10.689	0.018	[24]
Trichloroethylene	2.47	1.192	9.368	0.916	[24]
Vinyl chloride	1.62	0.433	9.833	0.741	[24]
Xylene (*m*-)	3.09	1.388	9.308	0.218	[48]

[a]: EXP. experimental data (references in Section 2); LMCI and UMCI: lower and upper bound of the 95% mean confidence interval, respectively.

the complete lack of knowledge of hepatic extraction ratio in humans (i.e., ranging from 0 to 1).

The average ratio (± standard deviation) of the PBPK model simulated values of the end-of-exposure blood concentrations (i.e., C_{max}) obtained with E_{min} and E_{max} was 4.19 ± 1.81. The lowest and highest ratios, based on the theoretical bounds of hepatic extraction (i.e., E_{min} and E_{max}), were observed for isoprene (1.63) and 1,1,2,2-tetrachloroethane (8.05), respectively. However, the average ratio (± standard deviation) of the PBPK model simulated values of the end-of-exposure blood concentrations, based on QPPR-generated bounds (LMCI, UMCI), was 1.29 ± 0.27. This ratio was the highest for hexachloroethane (2.39) and the lowest for 1,1-dichloroethylene (1.06).

For the 26 VOCs used in the development of the QPPR, the values of AUC_{24}s for a 1 ppm continuous exposure are reported in Table 3. The ratio of the highest to the lowest AUC predicted with E_{min} and E_{max} was 4.3 ± 1.94 ranging from 1.63 (isoprene) to 8.7 (1,1,2,2-tetrachloroethane). The ratio of the maximum to minimum concentrations predicted using the QPPR metabolism rate was 1.36 ± 0.4 ranging from 1.06 (1,1-dichloroethylene) to 2.8 (isoprene).

Figure 4 illustrates the range of predictions of venous blood pharmacokinetics compared to experimental data [67, 81, 82]. Overall, the predicted envelope of concentrations approximated reasonably the experimental data for dichloromethane, ethylbenzene, styrene, toluene, and *m*-xylene.

3.2. Analysis of Applicability of the CL_{int} QPPR to PBPK Modeling. The reliability of applying the QPPR within the PBPK model was assessed for the 26 VOCs in the calibration dataset (Table 4). The uncertainty of the QPPR prediction was estimated as the ratio of predicted CL_{intPL} to experimental CL_{intPL}. For 3 VOCs (isoprene, 1,1-dichloroethylene, and vinyl chloride) the sensitivity of AUC to CL_{int} was low (ratio of AUCs < 2) whereas uncertainty of the CL_{int} QPPR was low for isoprene and vinyl chloride and medium for 1,1-dichloroethylene. For the other 23 VOCs, the ratio of AUCs was between 2 and 5. For 16 of the later 23 VOCs (benzene; bromochloromethane; bromodichloromethane; chloroform; dibromomethane; 1,2-dichloroethane; hexachloroethane; *n*-hexane; pentachloroethane; styrene;

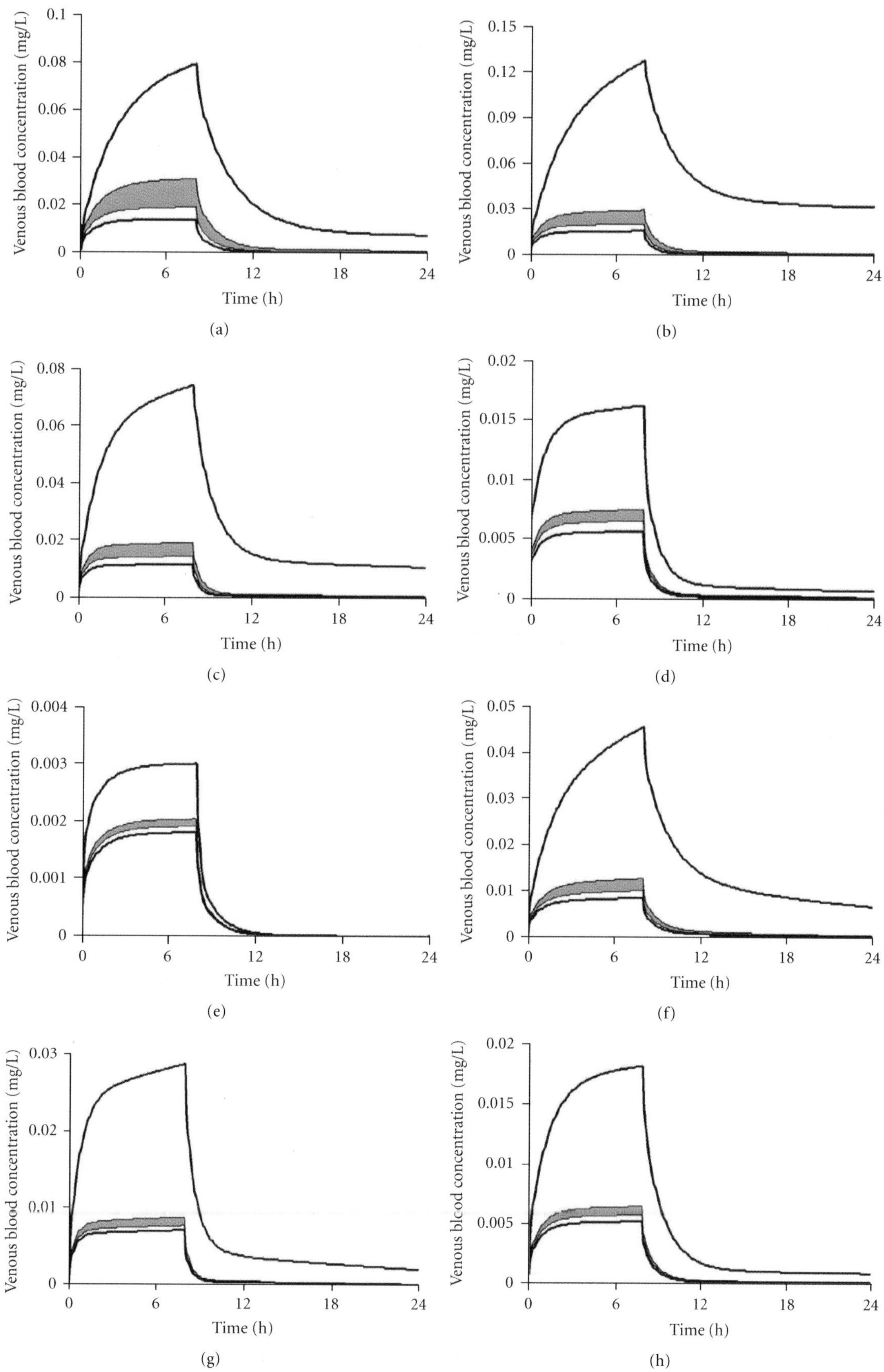

FIGURE 3: Continued.

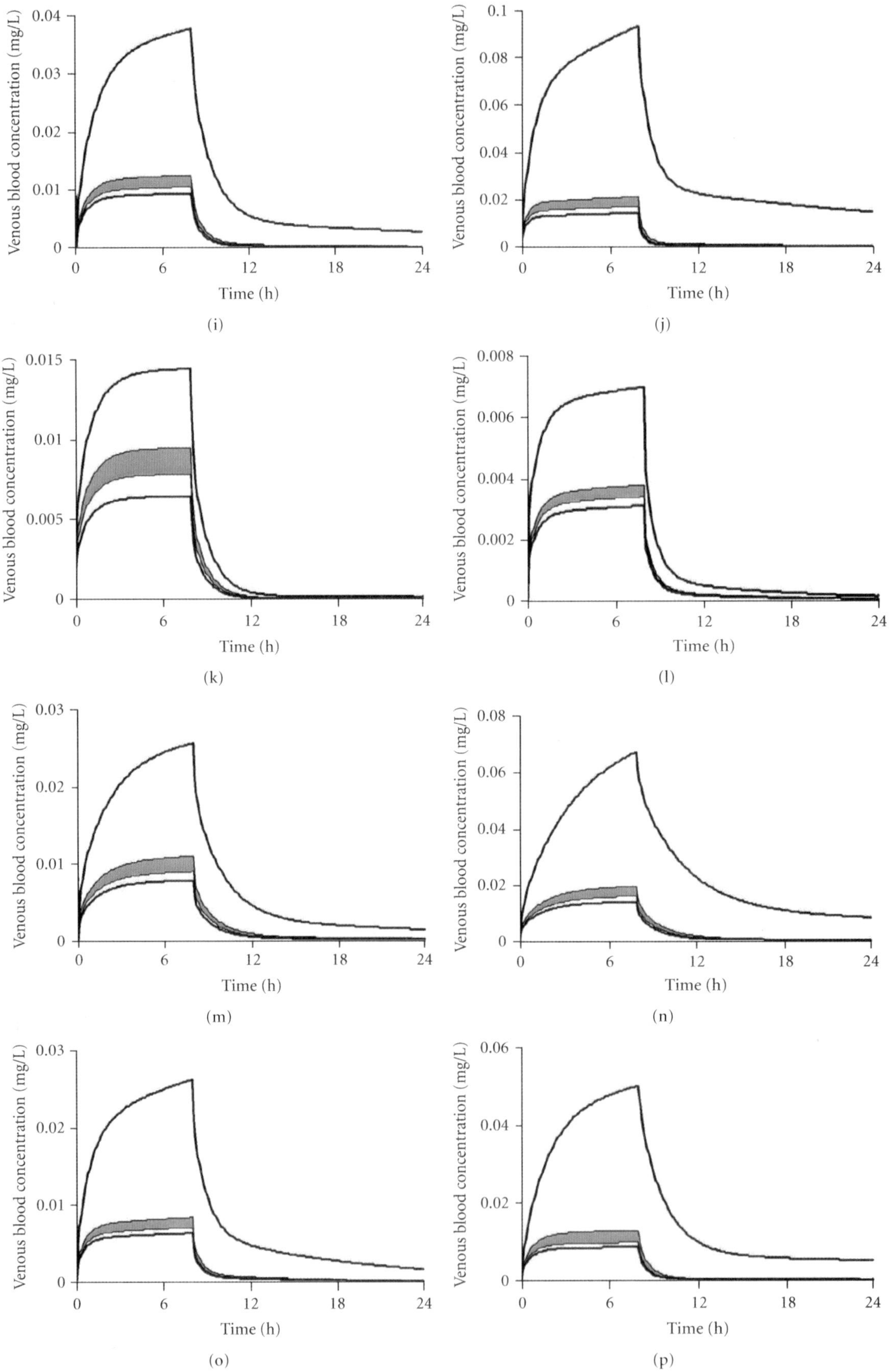

Figure 3: Continued.

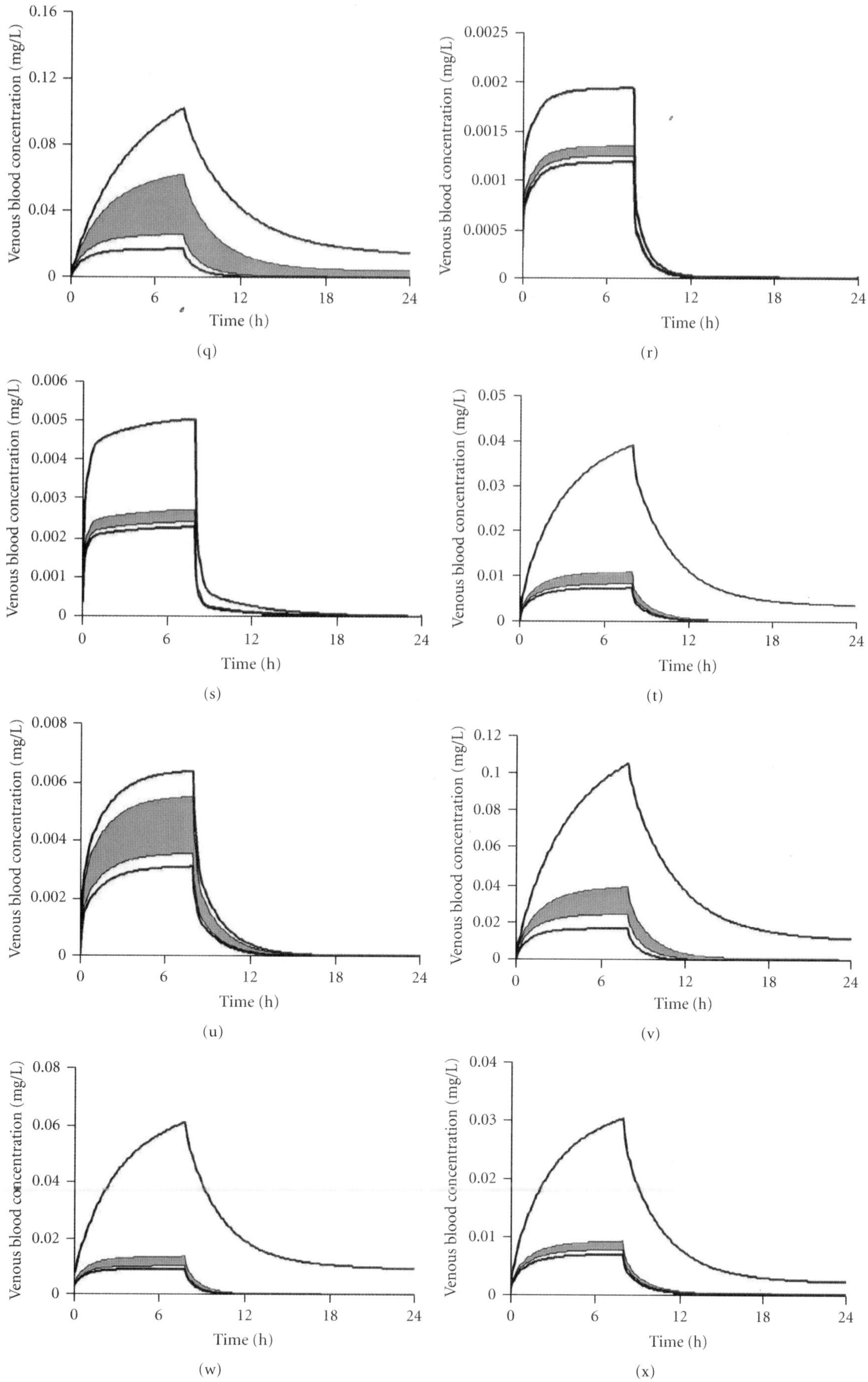

FIGURE 3: Continued.

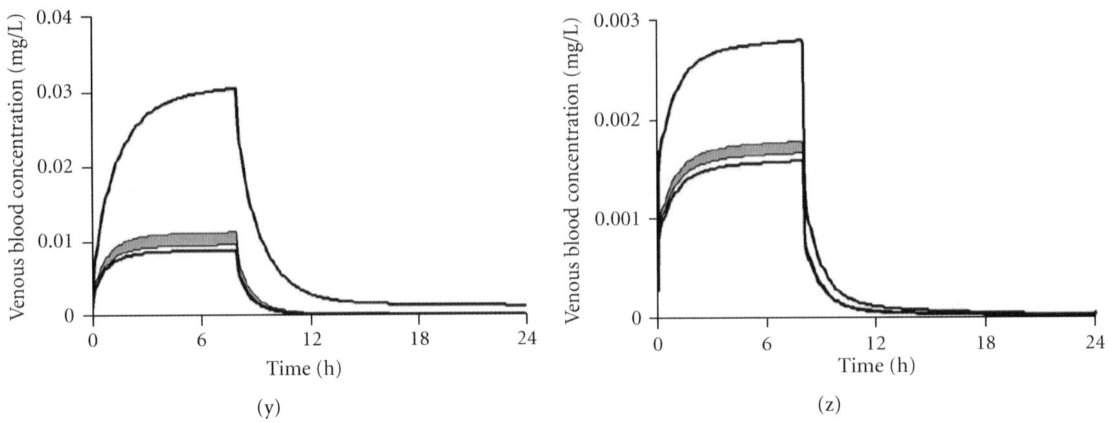

Figure 3: 24 h simulation of the venous blood concentration following inhalation exposure to 1 ppm, 8 h for 26 volatile organic compounds considering maximum and minimum (bold lines) and QPPR-based hepatic extraction (grey area). (a) 1,1,1,2-Tetrachloroethane; (b) 1,1,2,2-tetrachloroethane; (c) 1,1,2-trichloroethane; (d) 1,1-dichloroethane; (e) 1,1-dichloroethylene; (f) 1,2-dichloroethane; (g) 1,2-dichloroethylene (*cis*-); (h) benzene; (i) bromochloromethane; (j) bromodichloromethane; (k) carbon tetrachloride; (l) chloroethane; (m) chloroform; (n) dibromomethane; (o) dichloromethane; (p) ethylbenzene; (q) hexachloroethane; (r) isoprene; (s) methyl chloride; (t) *m*-xylene; (u) *n*-hexane; (v) pentachloroethane; (w) styrene; (x) toluene; (y) trichloroethylene; (z) vinyl chloride.

Table 3: Area under the curve for four metabolic scenarios for the VOCs used in the QPPR development.

Chemicals	24 h Area under the curve (mg/L-h) Metabolic scenario[a]			
	E_{min}	E_{max}	LMCI	UMCI
Benzene	0.437	0.125	0.155	0.138
Bromochloromethane	0.913	0.229	0.305	0.257
Bromodichloromethane	2.380	0.356	0.523	0.422
Carbon tetrachloride	0.34	0.153	0.224	0.186
Chloroethane	0.156	0.069	0.084	0.076
Chloroform	0.599	0.185	0.257	0.211
Dibromomethane	1.659	0.336	0.466	0.384
Dichloroethane (1,1-)	0.391	0.138	0.181	0.158
Dichloroethane (1,2-)	1.142	0.205	0.305	0.241
Dichloroethylene (1,1-)	6.98×10^{-2}	4.22×10^{-2}	4.76×10^{-2}	4.47×10^{-2}
Dichloroethylene (*cis*-1,2)	0.702	0.174	0.214	0.188
Dichloromethane	0.65	0.157	0.206	0.174
Ethylbenzene	1.247	0.216	0.32	0.246
Hexachloroethane	3.071	0.494	1.774	0.738
Hexane (*n*-)	0.15	0.073	0.129	0.084
Isoprene	4.59×10^{-2}	2.81×10^{-2}	0.084	2.95×10^{-2}
Methyl chloride	0.119	0.054	0.064	0.057
Pentachloroethane	2.584	0.418	0.929	0.595
Styrene	1.497	0.222	0.322	0.246
Tetrachloroethane (1,1,1,2-)	1.911	0.337	0.739	0.457
Tetrachloroethane (1,1,2,2-)	3.337	0.384	0.717	0.495
Toluene	0.74	0.168	0.223	0.188
Trichloroethane (1,1,2-)	1.876	0.284	0.474	0.355
Trichloroethylene	0.721	0.209	0.267	0.227
Vinyl chloride	6.68×10^{-2}	3.79×10^{-2}	4.25×10^{-2}	3.98×10^{-2}
Xylene (*m*-)	1.117	0.209	0.308	0.236

[a]: E_{min}: no metabolism; E_{max}: maximum hepatic extraction; LMCI and UMCI: lower and upper bound of the 95% mean confidence interval, respectively.

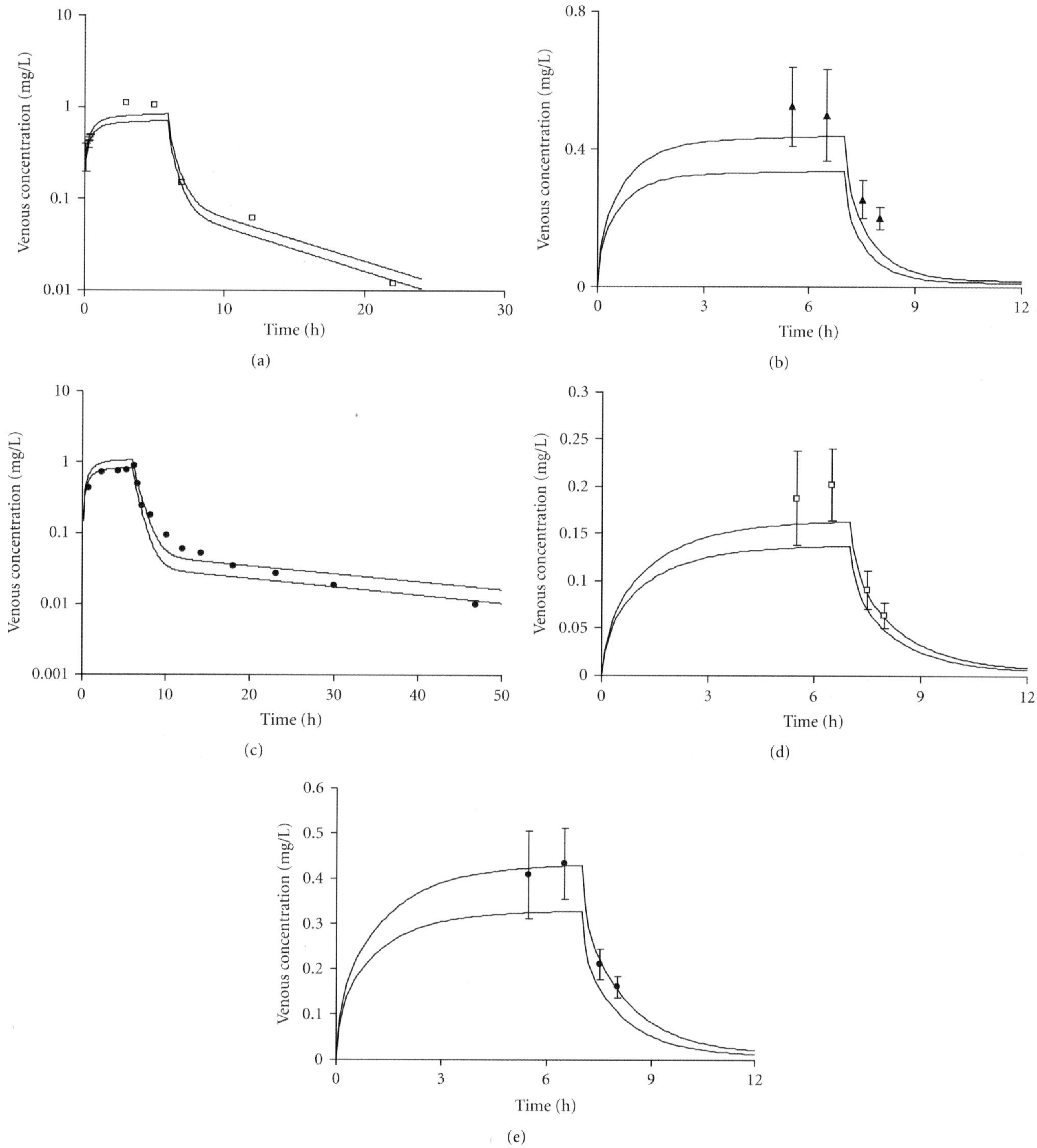

FIGURE 4: Comparison of PBPK model simulation with experimental data of venous blood concentration following inhalation exposure to (a) 100 ppm, 6 h dichloromethane [77]; (b) 33 ppm, 7 h ethylbenzene [67]; (c) 80 ppm, 6 h styrene [78]; (d) 17 ppm, 7 h toluene [67]; (e) 33 ppm, 7 h *m*-xylene [67]. Bold lines: predicted LMCI and UMCI for CL_{int}.

1,1,1,2-tetrachloroethane; 1,1,2,2-tetrachloroethane; toluene; 1,1,2-trichloroethane; trichloroethylene; *m*-xylene) the prediction uncertainty was low, thus the confidence in using the QPPR in the PBPK model is high for these compounds. The uncertainty was medium for the prediction of CL_{intPL} for 7 VOCs (carbon tetrachloride; chloroethane; 1,1-dichloroethane; *cis*-1,2-dichloroethylene; dichloromethane; ethylbenzene; methyl chloride). Therefore, for these chemicals, the confidence in using the QPPR in an inhalation PBPK model to evaluate the AUC is medium.

TABLE 4: Reliability analysis of the QPPR for CL_{int} on the PBPK predicted AUC.

		Impact of metabolism on AUC ($AUC_{E_{min}}/AUC_{E_{max}}$)[a]		
		Low (<2)	Medium (2–5)	High (>5)
QPPR prediction uncertainty (Pred./Exp. CL_{intPL})[b]	Low (<2)	Isoprene, vinyl chloride	Benzene; bromochloromethane; bromodichloromethane; chloroform; dibromomethane; 1,2-dichloroethane; hexachloroethane; *n*-hexane; pentachloroethane; styrene; 1,1,1,2-tetrachloroethane; 1,1,2,2-tetrachloroethane; toluene; 1,1,2-trichloroethane; trichloroethylene; *m*-xylene	
	Medium (2–5)	1,1,-Dichloroethylene	Carbon tetrachloride; chloroethane; 1,1-dichloroethane; *cis*-1,2-dichloroethylene; dichloromethane; ethylbenzene; methyl chloride	
	High (>5)			

[a] Calculated as the ratio of the PBPK simulations of 24 h AUC (of venous blood concentration, 1 ppm VOC, 24 h exposure) obtained by setting $E = 0$ (i.e., $CL_{int} = 0$) to that setting $E = 1$ (i.e., $CL_{int} = 1000$).
[b] Calculated as the ratio of the predicted to the experimental values of CL_{intPL}.

TABLE 5: Input parameters and experimental data on log CL_{int} for VOCs of QPPR evaluation.

Chemical	Input parameters log P_{ow}	log P_{bw}	IP (eV)	Log Cl_{intPL}[a] (L_{PL}/h/kg)	Ref V_{max}, K_m
Bromoform	1.79	0.896	10.837	1.006	[46]
Dibromochloromethane	1.70	1.025	10.702	1.108	[46]
Dichloroethylene (*trans*-1,2-)	1.98	0.484	9.512	0.438	[55]
Ethylene	1.27	0.776	10.638	1.208	[59]
Furan	1.36	0.441	9.375	1.773	[56]
Halothane	2.26	0.977	11.039	1.104	[58]
Propylene	1.68	0.995	10.103	1.118	[54]
Tetrachloroethylene	2.97	1.404	9.217	−1.804	[57]
Trichloroethane (1,1,1-)	2.68	0.823	10.751	−2.467	[48]
Trimethylbenzene (1,2,4-)	3.63	1.829	9.084	−0.132	[61]
Xylene (*o*-)	3.09	1.213	9.304	0.163	[60]

[a] Experimental data (references in Section 2).

3.3. QPPR Evaluation. The QPPR model was applied to predict the CL_{intPL} of 11 VOCs that were not in the calibration dataset. Table 5 presents the values of the input parameters along with the experimental data for the 11 VOCs used in QPPR evaluation. Figure 5 illustrates the comparison of the predicted values of CL_{intPL} (LMCI and UMCI) and the experimental data. The average difference ($\pm$ standard deviation) between the UMCI and the LMCI was 0.57 ± 0.11 ranging from 0.46 (bromoform) to 0.84 (1,2,4-trimethylbenzene). The highest UMCI-LMCI ranges were obtained for furan (0.62), tetrachloroethylene (0.63), and 1,2,4-trimethylbenzene (0.84). The nearest predicted values of UMCI and LMCI on log CL_{intPL} were greater than 5-fold of the experimental data for tetrachloroethylene (LMCI = 0.02 versus exp = −1.8). As in the QPPR development section, the impact of the imprecision on these log CL_{int} predictions on the pharmacokinetics in humans was evaluated by PBPK modeling.

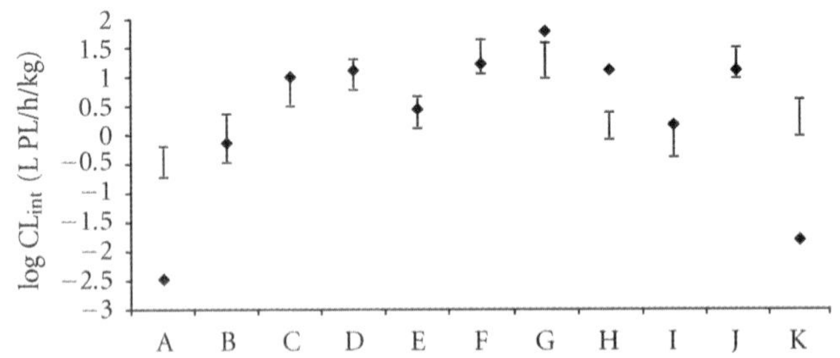

FIGURE 5: Comparison of the predicted log CL_{int} (LMCI and UMCI) with the experimental data on 11 VOCs. The bars represent the QPPR predictions and the symbols the experimental values. A: 1,1,1-trichloroethane; B: 1,2,4-trimethylbenzene; C: 1,2-dichloroethylene (*trans*-); D: bromoform; E: dibromochloromethane; F: ethylene; G: furan; H: halothane; I: *o*-xylene; J: propylene; K: tetrachloroethylene.

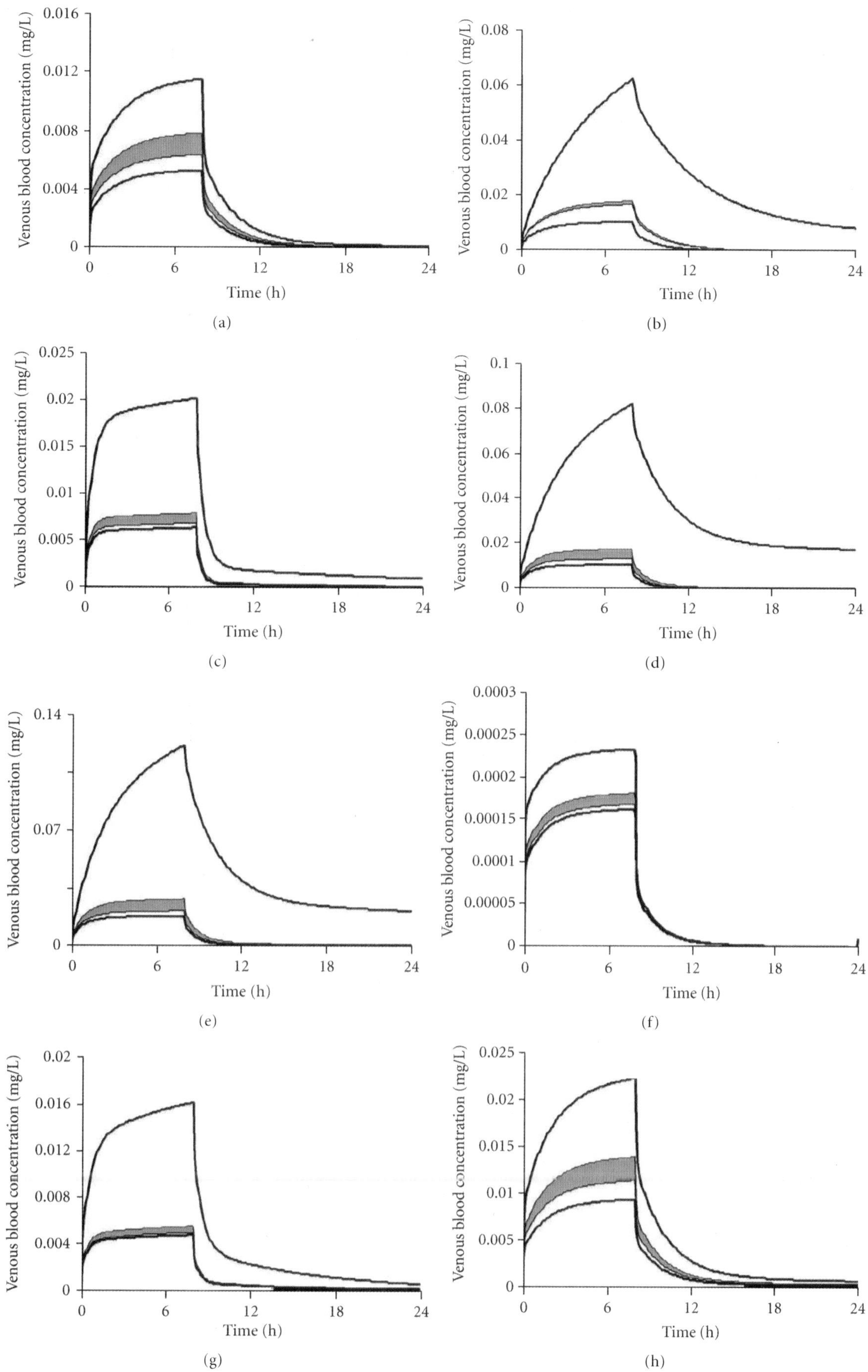

FIGURE 6: Continued.

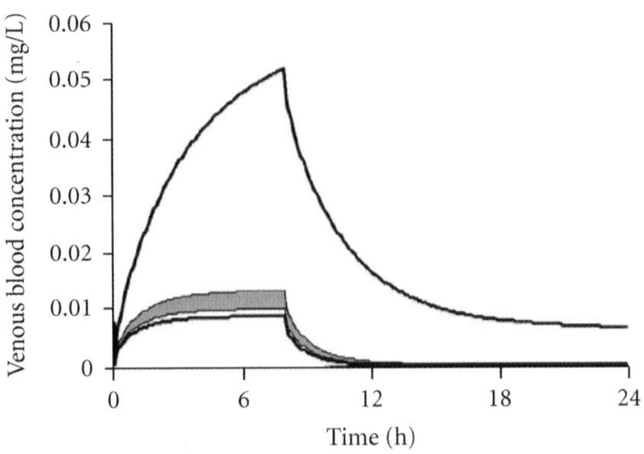

(i)

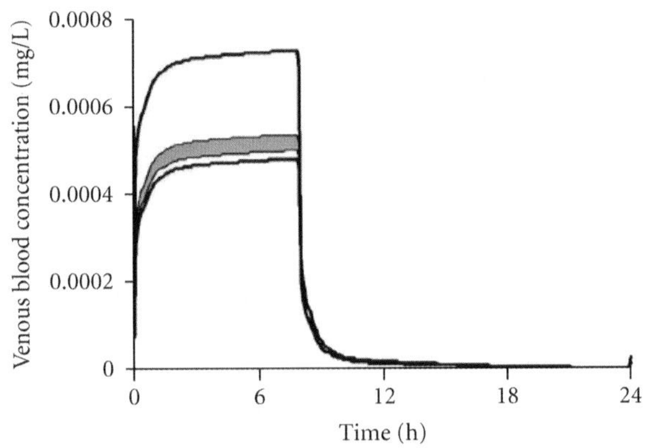

(j)

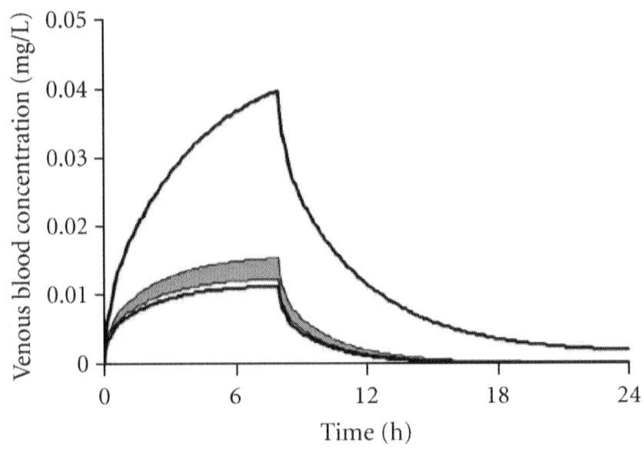

(k)

FIGURE 6: 24 h simulation of the venous blood concentration following inhalation exposure to 1 ppm, 8 h for 11 volatile organic compounds considering maximum and minimum (bold lines) and QPPR-based hepatic extraction (grey area). (a) 1,1,1-Trichloroethane; (b) 1,2,4-trimethylbenzene; (c) 1,2-dichloroethylene (*trans*-); (d) bromoform; (e) dibromochloromethane; (f) ethylene; (g) furan; (h) halothane; (i) *o*-xylene; (j) propylene; (k) tetrachloroethylene.

Figure 6 presents the predictions of the 24 h blood pharmacokinetics following 8 h exposure to 1 ppm of each of the 11 VOCs used in the QPPR evaluation. The bold lines represent the simulations obtained using 0 and 1 as the hepatic extraction ratio, whereas the grey area encompassed by thin lines represents the simulation obtained using LMCI and UMCI of predicted CL_{int} in PBPK models. The reduction of the region of uncertainty associated with the complete lack of knowledge of hepatic extraction ratio in humans (i.e., ranging from 0 to 1) by the envelope of the concentrations predicted using the QPPR predictions was observed for the 11 VOCs.

The mean ratio ($\pm$ standard deviation) of the PBPK model simulated values of the end-of-exposure blood concentrations obtained with E_{min} and E_{max} was 3.92 $\pm$ 2.13 ranging from 1.42 (ethylene) to 7.45 (bromoform). However, the same average ratio ($\pm$ standard deviation) of PBPK simulated blood concentrations, based on QPPR-generated bounds (LMCI and UMCI) was 1.2 $\pm$0.1, ranging from 1.07 (ethylene) to 1.33 (bromoform).

Table 6 presents the values of the AUC_{24}s (mg/L-h) for the 11 VOCs used in the evaluation of the QPPR. The average ratio of the highest to lowest AUC predicted using E_{min} and E_{max} was 4.08 $\pm$ 2.31 (mean $\pm$ SD). The lowest and highest ratios, based on the theoretical bounds of hepatic extraction (i.e., $E = 0.001$ or 0.999), were observed for ethylene (1.44) and bromoform (7.96), respectively.

The ratio of the maximum to minimum concentrations predicted using the QPPR metabolism rate was 1.2 $\pm$ 0.1, ranging from 1.07 (propylene) to 1.33 (dibromochloromethane).

Figure 7 illustrates the range of predictions for two of the chemicals in the external dataset (1,2,4-trimethylbenzene and 1,1,1-trichloroethane) venous blood pharmacokinetics compared to experimental data [61, 85]. The QPPR-PBPK model-generated "envelope" of concentrations simulated reasonably the experimental data for 1,2,4-trimethylbenzene whereas the blood concentrations of 1,1,1-trichloroethane were underestimated by about 30%.

3.4. Analysis of Applicability of the CL_{int} QPPR to PBPK Modeling. The reliability of applying the QPPR within the PBPK model was assessed for the 11 VOCs in the evaluation dataset, using the framework shown in Figure 1. Considering that the experimental data of CL_{intPL} for new or untested chemicals will be essentially unknown, it is realistic to consider the uncertainty of the QPPR prediction of CL_{intPL} to be high for all chemicals in the evaluation dataset.

TABLE 6: Area under the curve for four metabolic scenarios, for VOCs in the evaluation dataset.

Chemicals	24 h Area under the curve (mg/L-h) Metabolic scenario[a]			
	E_{min}	E_{max}	LMCI	UMCI
Bromoform	2.122	0.267	0.434	0.328
Dibromochloromethane	3.114	0.45	0.7	0.527
Dichloroethylene (*trans*-1,2-)	0.472	0.149	0.185	0.16
Ethylene	5.87×10^{-3}	4.08×10^{-3}	4.55×10^{-3}	4.23×10^{-3}
Furan	0.388	0.113	0.131	0.118
Halothane	0.523	0.22	0.325	0.266
Propylene	1.76×10^{-2}	1.16×10^{-2}	1.3×10^{-2}	1.21×10^{-2}
Tetrachloroethylene	0.953	0.266	0.363	0.291
Trichloroethane (1,1,1-)	0.271	0.125	0.184	0.15
Trimethylbenzene (1,2,4-)	1.577	0.249	0.425	0.395
Xylene (*o*-)	1.297	0.218	0.325	0.248

[a]: E_{min}: no metabolism; E_{max}: maximum hepatic extraction; LMCI and UMCI: lower and upper bound of the 95% mean confidence interval, respectively.

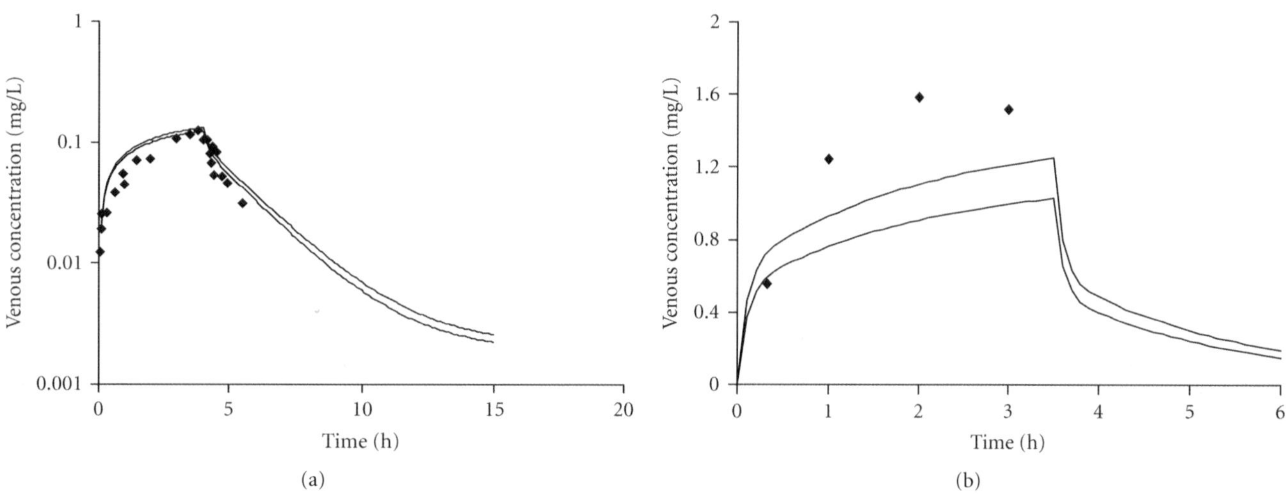

FIGURE 7: Comparison of PBPK model simulations (bold lines: predicted LMCI and UMCI for CL_{int}) with experimental data of venous blood concentration following inhalation exposure to (a) 8 ppm, 4 h 1,2,4-trimethylbenzene [59] and (b) 175 ppm, 3.5 h 1,1,1-trichloro ethane [85].

The results of the analysis of applicability for the chemicals in the evaluation dataset are reported in Table 7. For 3 VOCs (ethylene; propylene; 1,1,1-trichloroethane) the sensitivity was low (ratio of AUCs < 2) thus the reliability of using their CL_{int} QPPR in the PBPK was considered high. For the other 8 VOCs (bromoform; dibromochloromethane; *trans*-1,2-dichloroethylene; furan; halothane; tetrachloroethylene; 1,2,4-trimethylbenzene; *o*-xylene), the ratio of the maximum to the minimum possible AUCs was between 2 and 5, such that the confidence in using the QPPR in an inhalation PBPK model to evaluate the AUCs is medium for these chemicals.

4. Discussion

SARs, QSAR, QSPRs, and QPPRs have been developed for various toxicological and chemical properties but only very few studies have focused on developing such models to parameterize PBPK models [8, 86]. A limitation in developing PBPK models relates to the availability of the metabolic constants (CL_{int}, V_{max}, and K_m) [8]. Quantitative relationships between structure and metabolism rates have been investigated for a limited number of closely related compounds, even though their applicability to PBPK modeling has not been demonstrated (e.g., QSPR models for K_{cat} and $1/K_m$ [87]). Other works in this area relate to the development of quantum chemical or quantum dynamic methods for prediction of activation energy or enthalpy of activation of P450 mediated reactions [20, 25, 26, 31, 36, 38, 88–91], which have not been used to derive metabolism constants for direct incorporation within rodent or human PBPK models.

The use of the group contribution method to develop QSPRs for integration within PBPK models has been successfully demonstrated, particularly for the inhalation toxicokinetics of VOCs [40–43]. This approach however is limited to VOCs containing one or more of the molecular groups

TABLE 7: Reliability analysis for the chemicals in the QPPR evaluation dataset.

		Impact of metabolism on AUC ($AUC_{E_{min}}/AUC_{E_{max}}$)[a]		
		Low (<2)	Medium (2–5)	High (>5)
QPPR prediction uncertainty (Pred./Exp. CL_{intPL})[b]	Low (<2)			
	Medium (2–5)			
	High (>5)	Ethylene; propylene; 1,1,1-trichloroethane	Bromoform; dibromochloromethane; *trans*-1,2-dichloroethylene; furan; halothane; tetrachloroethylene; 1,2,4-trimethylbenzene; *o*-xylene	

[a] Calculated as the ratio of the PBPK simulations of 24 h AUC (of venous blood concentration, 1 ppm VOC, 24 h exposure) obtained by setting $E = 0$ (i.e., $CL_{int} = 0$) to that setting $E = 1$ (i.e., $CL_{int} = 1000$).
[b] Calculated as the ratio of the predicted to the experimental values of CL_{intPL}.

or fragments for which the contribution has been evaluated (i.e., CH_3, CH_2, CH, C, C=C, benzene ring, H on benzene ring, and halogens). In order to extend the applicability domain then, it is important to investigate the feasibility of developing QSPRs based on more global, physicochemical properties. In this regard, the present study investigated the development of a QPPR, that used chemical properties rather than chemical structure as input, and it was calibrated to predict CL_{int} expressed in terms of chemical affinity to phospholipids in the endoplasmic reticulum in which CYP enzymes are embedded [63]. This logical transformation of CL_{int} data, reported here for the first time in literature, facilitated the development of more adequate QPPR than the conventional CL_{int} based on blood concentrations. All efforts to develop QPPRs for predicting CL_{int} based on blood concentrations were unsuccessful. The QPPR based chemical affinity to phospholipids–obtained in this study should be regarded as a screening level tool to provide plausible range of metabolism rates in order to facilitate a first-cut evaluation of the blood concentration of inhaled VOCs in humans. The uncertainty associated with this QPPR tool should be evaluated along with the sensitivity of CL_{int} on the dose metrics of the chemical of interest, in the perspective of intended precision. Accordingly, if the dose metric is highly sensitive to CL_{int} and the QPPR predictions of CL_{int} are highly uncertain, then the present tool is of limited use even for screening purposes. In such cases, then *in vivo* or *in vitro* studies can be undertaken to get chemical-specific estimates of CL_{int}.

The QPPR predictions were reasonably in accordance with experimental values for most but not all chemicals in the calibration and evaluation datasets. For some chemicals, the predicted values of log CL_{int} for 1,1,1-trichloroethane (Figure 5(A)) and tetrachloroethylene (Figure 5(K)) exceeded the experimental values by two orders of magnitude. The QSPR for rat hepatic clearance developed by Béliveau and colleagues [41] also overestimated the metabolic rate of these two VOCs. However the PBPK model for 1,1,1-trichlorethane indicated that the AUC of parent chemical in venous blood is not sensitive to V_{max} and K_m [92, 93]. This was demonstrated in Figure 6(a), showing that QPPR-overestimation of CL_{intPL} of 1,1,1-trichloroethane led only to a minimal impact, in terms of the underestimation of the venous blood concentration. In the case of tetrachloroethylene, a poorly metabolized halogenated VOC, the overestimation of the CL_{intPL} led to a 3-fold underestimation of the C_{max} (Figure 6(k)) or a 4-5-fold underestimation of the AUC_{24} (Table 7). If this magnitude of error is not acceptable for screening-level evaluation, then the metabolic rate should be experimentally determined. The combined assessment of the uncertainty/sensitivity of metabolic constants in PBPK models would facilitate the determination of the applicability of the QPPR model, given the level of precision need for an application (Figure 1)

The QPPR developed in this study is a generic tool to provide initial estimates of CL_{int} of VOCs metabolized by hepatic CYP. It does not take into account stereochemistry or other pathway-specific rates and processes, which may be important for some chemicals (e.g., predicted values of CL_{int} are almost identical for 1,1-dichloroethylene and *cis*-1,2-dichloroethylene but experimental values vary by log units of 1.06). Therefore, predictions of CL_{int} based on generic considerations are likely to be inaccurate for specific chemicals but are of limited use in that the estimates (along with the bounds, representing the level of uncertainty) can be integrated with human physiology to provide a first-cut view of the plausible kinetic profiles.

The utility of the QPPR models depends, in part, on the ability to reproducibly calculate the descriptors [74]. Hence, in this study, the descriptors that could be easily calculated and interpreted were chosen and obtained using EPISUITE (for log P_{ow} and P_{wa}) and MMPro (for the ionization potential). However, the blood solubility parameter (i.e., blood : air PC) is additionally required and this can either be obtained experimentally *in vitro* or using other QSARs that account for protein (i.e., haemoglobin and plasma protein) binding in addition to solubility considerations. There are some algorithms and QSARs available in this regard, but further development is necessary to adequately account for the protein binding phenomena in human blood for various classes of chemicals [8].

The QPPR developed in this study computes CL_{intPL}, which can then be converted to CL_{intblood} for use in PBPK modeling. In an effort to evaluate whether the same input parameters can be used to relate to CL_{intblood}, additional analyses were performed. These yielded the following equation (significant terms only):

$$\log CL_{\text{intblood}} = 5.117 - 0.305 \cdot \log P_{\text{ow}} - 0.324 \cdot \text{IP}. \quad (6)$$

Even though (5) and (6) give almost identical results (one for CL_{intPL} and the other for CL_{intblood}) despite the differing R^2 values (0.796 versus 0.402), it should be noted that (5) was obtained based on statistical analysis of calibration dataset (i.e., modeling) whereas (6) was derived simply by fitting CL_{intblood} to the specific input parameters. Further rearrangements and simplifications of the QPPR, as well as the loss of accuracy associated with such attempts, were not performed in the current study.

The output of the QPPR developed in the present study is $\log CL_{\text{int}}$, which is useful for simulating pharmacokinetics in humans of chemicals at low levels of exposure. CL_{int} is applicable to first-order situations (i.e., when blood levels in humans are much lower than the K_m for metabolizing enzyme) and is derived by dividing the $V_{\max}$ (i.e., the enzyme turn-over) with K_m (representing the affinity of the substrate for the enzyme). The input parameters of the QPPR, namely, $\log P_{\text{ow}}$ and $\log P_{\text{bw}}$, are estimates of the relative solubility in octanol, water, and blood. Then, an interpretation of the model for CL_{int} could be that the binding to the P450 enzyme is a result of hydrophobic interactions [94] which, in turn, can be estimated with parameters reflective of the solubility in *n*-octanol and blood. The solubility in blood is the sum of the solubility in its components (water, phospholipids, neutral lipids, and proteins). Most of the studied VOCs are likely to bind to hemoglobin because of their lipophilicity ($\log P_{\text{ow}}$ value above 1) and low molecular volume [40]. The P_{bw}, thus, is likely an indicator of the binding to proteins, whereas the $\log P_{\text{ow}}$ reflects more the affinity for biotic lipids in the metabolism microenvironment. Similar to $\log P_{\text{ow}}$, the ionization potential has already been correlated with metabolic rates, namely, the $V_{\max}$ and $V_{\max}/k_m$ [23], as this latter parameter could be correlated with the energy needed to break a covalent bond for the oxidation of the substrate.

The QSPR model for CL_{int} developed in this study has a defined theoretical endpoint, is nonambiguous, has a defined domain of application, was analyzed using appropriate goodness-of-fit (R^2) and robustness (Q^2), and has an attempt of mechanistic interpretation. The *in vivo* dataset on 26 VOCs used for the QPPR calibration was chosen because it was previously collated and used in QSPR analyses [40, 41]. These values were taken mainly from the work of Gargas et al. [24]. The QSPR analysis was also attempted with the entire dataset of 37 VOCs (calibration + external dataset) but it did not improve the goodness-of-fit statistics (not shown).

The predicted bounds of the 95% confidence interval of intrinsic clearance were incorporated within a PBPK model to predict the blood toxicokinetics of VOCs. The simulations of blood kinetics were comparable to experimental data for 6 VOCs (toluene, *m*-xylene, ethylbenzene, styrene, dichloromethane,1,2,4-trimethylbenzene, and 1,1,1-trichloroethane, Figures 4 and 7). The simulations obtained in the present study, using lower and upper confidence intervals on the mean predicted CL_{int}, reduced clearly the uncertainty bounds associated with the total lack of knowledge (i.e., E ranging anywhere between 0 and 1). Furthermore, the present study incorporated the QPPR predictions of CL_{int} along with physiological parameters, such that impact on *in vivo* kinetics could be simulated. In effect, in some cases where the uncertainty on CL_{int} predictions was high, it did not translate into a proportionate error on the predictions of kinetics, due to the additional consideration of physiological constraints, and such observations are critical in data-poor situations for designing focused studies to generate chemical-specific data *in vitro* or *in vivo*.

The QPPR developed in this study approximated the experimental rat metabolic constants for the various low-molecular-weight VOCs; and it was used along with the human physiology to generate initial or screening level values of CL_{int} to construct human PBPK models that could be of potential use to interpret data such as measured biomarker levels or for designing kinetic studies to reduce database uncertainty. As shown with some VOCs (e.g., Figure 3: 1,1,1,2-tetrachloroethane, hexachloroethane, and *n*-hexane), the blood concentration profile is extremely influenced by CL_{int}, such that metabolism cannot be neglected in simulating or interpreting human exposure data. And in such cases, the ability to generate at least a range of plausible values of CL_{int}, as done in the present study, would facilitate first in-human simulations of pharmacokinetics of parent chemicals. Integrating information on the impact of metabolism on dose metrics (i.e., AUC) along with prediction uncertainty of the QPPR facilitates the determination of the level of confidence in using this screening level tool. Depending upon the overall confidence in the QPPR application for predicting dose metrics (low, medium, and high) relative to the use purposes, decisions can be made as to the specific studies needed.

Overall, the QPPR developed in the present study allows to predict the CL_{int} of VOCs on the basis of generic molecular descriptors rather than with fragment constants as done previously. The chemical concentration in phospholipids, for the first time, was found to be a dose metric amenable to QPPR analysis. The QPPR was then used to generate range of values of CL_{int}; the level of confidence in these estimates was assessed by considering the impact of CL_{int} on the simulated dose metrics (i.e., AUC of parent chemical in venous blood). For other dose metrics and situations, a more robust QPPR needs to be developed, and such efforts can be based on the methodological developments accomplished in this study. The QPPR-based simulation of pharmacokinetics reduced the range of uncertainty for few substances relative to complete lack of knowledge of the CL_{int}, but it needs to be evaluated/refined with much larger dataset should this screening-level approach be adopted for providing more precise estimates of metabolism rates. Overall, the integrated

QPPR-PBPK model developed in this study is a potentially useful tool for characterizing and reducing the uncertainty associated with the complete lack of knowledge of CL_{int} in predicting human pharmacokinetics of inhaled VOCs.

Acknowledgments

Financial support by Agence Française de Sécurité Sanitaire de l'Environnement et du Travail (AFSSET; EST-2007-85) and Natural Sciences and Engineering Research Council of Canada (NSERC; Discovery grant 138195-2007 RGPIN) is acknowledged.

References

[1] Commission des communautés européennes, *LIVRE BLANC Stratégie pour la future politique dans le domaine des substances chimiques*, 2001.

[2] CEPA, "Loi canadienne sur la protection de l'environnement (1999), Règlement sur les renseignements concernant les substances nouvelles (substances chimiques et polymères)," in *Gazette du Canada partie II*, pp. 1850–2221, Queen's Printer for Canada, Ottawa, Canada, 2005.

[3] United States Environmental Protection Agency, "The U.S. Environmental Protection Agency's strategic plan for evaluating the toxicity of chemicals," Tech. Rep. EPA/100/K-09/001, Office of the Science Advisor, Science Policy Council, Washington, DC, USA, 2009.

[4] K. Krishnan and M. E. Andersen, "Physiologically based pharmacokinetic modeling in toxicology," in *Principles and Methods of Toxicology*, A. W. Hayes, Ed., pp. 231–292, Taylor & Francis, Boca Raton, Fla, USA, 2007.

[5] A. D. Arms and C. C. Travis, "Reference physiological parameters in pharmacokinetic modeling," Tech. Rep. EPA/600/6-88/004, United States Environmental Protection Agency, Washington, DC, USA, 1988.

[6] R. P. Brown, M. D. Delp, S. L. Lindstedt, L. R. Rhomberg, and R. P. Beliles, "Physiological parameter values for physiologically based pharmacokinetic models," *Toxicology and Industrial Health*, vol. 13, no. 4, pp. 407–484, 1997.

[7] M. Béliveau and K. Krishnan, "In Silico approaches for developing physiologically based pharmacokinetic (PBPK) models," in *Alternative Toxicological Methods*, H. Salem and S. A. Katz, Eds., pp. 479–532, CRC Press, Boca Raton, Fla, USA, 2003.

[8] T. Peyret and K. Krishnan, "QSARs for PBPK modelling of environmental contaminants," *SAR and QSAR in Environmental Research*, vol. 22, no. 1-2, pp. 129–169, 2011.

[9] J. DeJongh, H. J. M. Verhaar, and J. L. M. Hermens, "A quantitative property-property relationship (QPPR) approach to estimate in vitro tissue blood partition coefficients of organic chemicals in rats and humans," *Archives of Toxicology*, vol. 72, no. 1, pp. 17–25, 1997.

[10] P. Poulin and K. Krishnan, "An algorithm for predicting tissue: blood partition coefficients of organic chemicals from n-octanol: water partition coefficient data," *Journal of Toxicology and Environmental Health*, vol. 46, no. 1, pp. 117–129, 1995.

[11] P. Poulin and K. Krishnan, "A biologically-based algorithm for predicting human tissue: blood partition coefficients of organic chemicals," *Human and Experimental Toxicology*, vol. 14, no. 3, pp. 273–280, 1995.

[12] P. Poulin and K. Krishnan, "A tissue composition-based algorithm for predicting tissue: air partition coefficients of organic chemicals," *Toxicology and Applied Pharmacology*, vol. 136, no. 1, pp. 126–130, 1996.

[13] P. Poulin and K. Krishnan, "A mechanistic algorithm for predicting blood: air partition coefficients of organic chemicals with the consideration of reversible binding in hemoglobin," *Toxicology and Applied Pharmacology*, vol. 136, no. 1, pp. 131–137, 1996.

[14] P. Poulin and F. P. Theil, "A priori prediction of tissue:plasma partition coefficients of drugs to facilitate the use of physiologically-based pharmacokinetic models in drug discovery," *Journal of Pharmaceutical Sciences*, vol. 89, no. 1, pp. 16–35, 2000.

[15] P. Poulin and F. P. Theil, "Prediction of pharmacokinetics prior to in vivo studies. 1. Mechanism-based prediction of volume of distribution," *Journal of Pharmaceutical Sciences*, vol. 91, no. 1, pp. 129–156, 2002.

[16] T. Rodgers, D. Leahy, and M. Rowland, "Physiologically based pharmacokinetic modeling 1: predicting the tissue distribution of moderate-to-strong bases," *Journal of Pharmaceutical Sciences*, vol. 94, no. 6, pp. 1259–1276, 2005.

[17] T. Rodgers and M. Rowland, "Physiologically based pharmacokinetic modelling 2: predicting the tissue distribution of acids, very weak bases, neutrals and zwitterions," *Journal of Pharmaceutical Sciences*, vol. 95, no. 6, pp. 1238–1257, 2006.

[18] W. Schmitt, "General approach for the calculation of tissue to plasma partition coefficients," *Toxicology in Vitro*, vol. 22, no. 2, pp. 457–467, 2008.

[19] T. Peyret, P. Poulin, and K. Krishnan, "A unified algorithm for predicting partition coefficients for PBPK modeling of drugs and environmental chemicals," *Toxicology and Applied Pharmacology*, vol. 249, no. 3, pp. 197–207, 2010.

[20] P. Rydberg, U. Ryde, and L. Olsen, "Prediction of activation energies for aromatic oxidation by cytochrome P450," *Journal of Physical Chemistry A*, vol. 112, no. 50, pp. 13058–13065, 2008.

[21] D. Zhou, L. Afzelius, S. W. Grimm, T. B. Andersson, R. J. Zauhar, and I. Zamora, "Comparison of methods for the prediction of the metabolic sites for CYP3A4-mediated metabolic reactions," *Drug Metabolism and Disposition*, vol. 34, no. 6, pp. 976–983, 2006.

[22] C. Hansch, S. B. Mekapati, A. Kurup, and R. P. Verma, "QSAR of Cytochrome P450," *Drug Metabolism Reviews*, vol. 36, no. 1, pp. 105–156, 2004.

[23] D. F. V. Lewis, C. Sams, and G. D. Loizou, "A quantitative structure-activity relationship analysis on a series of alkyl benzenes metabolized by human cytochrome P450 2E1," *Journal of Biochemical and Molecular Toxicology*, vol. 17, no. 1, pp. 47–52, 2003.

[24] M. L. Gargas, P. G. Seybold, and M. E. Andersen, "Modeling the tissue solubilities and metabolic rate constant V_{max} of halogenated methanes, ethanes, and ethylenes," *Toxicology Letters*, vol. 43, no. 1–3, pp. 235–256, 1988.

[25] K. R. Korzekwa, J. P. Jones, and J. R. Gillette, "Theoretical studies on cytochrome P-450 mediated hydroxylation: a predictive model for hydrogen atom abstractions," *Journal of the American Chemical Society*, vol. 112, no. 19, pp. 7042–7046, 1990.

[26] H. Yin, M. W. Anders, K. R. Korzekwa et al., "Designing safer chemicals: predicting the rates of metabolism of halogenated alkanes," *Proceedings of the National Academy of Sciences of the*

United States of America, vol. 92, no. 24, pp. 11076–11080, 1995.

[27] C. L. Waller, M. V. Evans, and J. D. Mckinney, "Modeling the cytochrome P450-mediated metabolism of chlorinated volatile organic compounds," *Drug Metabolism and Disposition*, vol. 24, no. 2, pp. 203–210, 1996.

[28] J. Ishizaki, K. Yokogawa, E. Nakashima, and F. Ichimura, "Relationships between the hepatic intrinsic clearance or blood cell-plasma partition coefficient in the rabbit and the lipophilicity of basic drugs," *Journal of Pharmacy and Pharmacology*, vol. 49, no. 8, pp. 768–772, 1997.

[29] D. F. V. Lewis, "Modelling human cytochromes P450 for evaluating drug metabolism: an update," *Drug Metabolism and Drug Interactions*, vol. 16, no. 4, pp. 307–324, 2000.

[30] D. F. V. Lewis, "Quantitative structure-activity relationships (QSARs) within the cytochrome P450 system: QSARs describing substrate binding, inhibition and induction of P450s," *Inflammopharmacology*, vol. 11, no. 1, pp. 43–73, 2003.

[31] J. P. Jones, M. Mysinger, and K. R. Korzekwa, "Computational models for cytochrome P450: a predictive electronic model for aromatic oxidation and hydrogen atom abstraction," *Drug Metabolism and Disposition*, vol. 30, no. 1, pp. 7–12, 2002.

[32] D. F. V. Lewis, "On the recognition of mammalian microsomal cytochrome P450 substrates and their characteristics: towards the prediction of human P450 substrate specificity and metabolism," *Biochemical Pharmacology*, vol. 60, no. 3, pp. 293–306, 2000.

[33] D. F. V. Lewis, S. Modi, and M. Dickins, "Structure-activity relationship for human cytochrome P450 substrates and inhibitors," *Drug Metabolism Reviews*, vol. 34, no. 1-2, pp. 69–82, 2002.

[34] K. V. Balakin, S. Ekins, A. Bugrim et al., "Quantitative structure-metabolism relationship modeling of metabolic N-dealkylation reaction rates," *Drug Metabolism and Disposition*, vol. 32, no. 10, pp. 1111–1120, 2004.

[35] S. Ekins, S. Andreyev, A. Ryabov et al., "Computational prediction of human drug metabolism," *Expert Opinion on Drug Metabolism and Toxicology*, vol. 1, no. 2, pp. 303–324, 2005.

[36] P. N. D'Yachkov, N. V. Kharchevnikova, A. V. Dmitriev, A. V. Kuznetsov, and V. V. Poroikov, "Quantum chemical simulation of cytochrome P450 catalyzed aromatic oxidation: metabolism, toxicity, and biodegradation of benzene derivatives," *International Journal of Quantum Chemistry*, vol. 107, no. 13, pp. 2454–2478, 2007.

[37] G. P. Miller, "Advances in the interpretation and prediction of CYP2E1 metabolism from a biochemical perspective," *Expert Opinion on Drug Metabolism and Toxicology*, vol. 4, no. 8, pp. 1053–1064, 2008.

[38] A. N. Mayeno, J. L. Robinson, R. S. H. Yang, and B. Reisfeld, "Predicting activation enthalpies of cytochrome-P450-mediated hydrogen abstractions. 2. Comparison of semiempirical PM3, SAM1, and AM1 with a density functional theory method," *Journal of Chemical Information and Modeling*, vol. 49, no. 7, pp. 1692–1703, 2009.

[39] C. Gao, R. Goind, and H. H. Tabak, "Application of the group contribution method for predicting the toxicity of organic chemicals," *Environmental Toxicology and Chemistry*, vol. 11, no. 5, pp. 631–636, 1992.

[40] M. Béliveau, J. Lipscomb, R. Tardif, and K. Krishnan, "Quantitative structure-property relationships for interspecies extrapolation of the inhalation pharmacokinetics of organic chemicals," *Chemical Research in Toxicology*, vol. 18, no. 3, pp. 475–485, 2005.

[41] M. Béliveau, R. Tardif, and K. Krishnan, "Quantitative structure-property relationships for physiologically based pharmacokinetic modeling of volatile organic chemicals in rats," *Toxicology and Applied Pharmacology*, vol. 189, no. 3, pp. 221–232, 2003.

[42] E. Kamgang, T. Peyret, and K. Krishnan, "An integrated QSPR-PBPK modelling approach for in vitro-in vivo extrapolation of pharmacokinetics in rats," *SAR and QSAR in Environmental Research*, vol. 19, no. 7-8, pp. 669–680, 2008.

[43] K. Price and K. Krishnan, "An integrated QSAR-PBPK modelling approach for predicting the inhalation toxicokinetics of mixtures of volatile organic chemicals in the rat," *SAR and QSAR in Environmental Research*, vol. 22, no. 1-2, pp. 107–128, 2011.

[44] W. M. Meylan and P. H. Howard, "Atom/fragment contribution method for estimating octanol-water partition coefficients," *Journal of Pharmaceutical Sciences*, vol. 84, no. 1, pp. 83–92, 1995.

[45] P. Poulin and K. Krishnan, "Molecular structure-based prediction of the toxicokinetics of inhaled vapors in humans," *International Journal of Toxicology*, vol. 18, no. 1, pp. 7–18, 1998.

[46] S. Haddad, G. C. Tardif, and R. Tardif, "Development of physiologically based toxicokinetic models for improving the human indoor exposure assessment to water contaminants: trichloroethylene and trihalomethanes," *Journal of Toxicology and Environmental Health A*, vol. 69, no. 23, pp. 2095–2136, 2006.

[47] N. Ali and R. Tardif, "Toxicokinetic modeling of the combined exposure to toluene and n-hexane in rats and humans," *Journal of Occupational Health*, vol. 41, no. 2, pp. 95–103, 1999.

[48] R. Tardif and G. Charest-Tardif, "The importance of measured end-points in demonstrating the occurrence of interactions: a case study with methylchloroform and m-xylene," *Toxicological Sciences*, vol. 49, no. 2, pp. 312–317, 1999.

[49] M. L. Gargas, M. E. Andersen, and H. J. Clewell III, "A physiologically based simulation approach for determining metabolic constants from gas uptake data," *Toxicology and Applied Pharmacology*, vol. 86, no. 3, pp. 341–352, 1986.

[50] J. C. Ramsey and M. E. Andersen, "A physiologically based description of the inhalation pharmacokinetics of styrene in rats and humans," *Toxicology and Applied Pharmacology*, vol. 73, no. 1, pp. 159–175, 1984.

[51] M. L. Gargas, H. J. Clewell III, and M. E. Andersen, "Metabolism of inhaled dihalomethanes in vivo: differentiation of kinetic constants for two independent pathways," *Toxicology and Applied Pharmacology*, vol. 82, no. 2, pp. 211–223, 1986.

[52] J. G. Filser, G. A. Csanády, B. Denk et al., "Toxicokinetics of isoprene in rodents and humans," *Toxicology*, vol. 113, no. 1–3, pp. 278–287, 1996.

[53] S. Haddad, R. Tardif, G. Charest-Tardif, and K. Krishnan, "Physiological modeling of the toxicokinetic interactions in a quaternary mixture of aromatic hydrocarbons," *Toxicology and Applied Pharmacology*, vol. 161, no. 3, pp. 249–257, 1999.

[54] J. G. Filser, R. Schmidbauer, F. Rampf, C. M. Baur, C. Putz, and G. A. Csanady, "Toxicokinetics of inhaled propylene in mouse, rat, and human," *Toxicology and Applied Pharmacology*, vol. 169, no. 1, pp. 40–51, 2000.

[55] M. L. Gargas, H. J. Clewell, and M. E. Andersen, "Gas uptake inhalation techniques and the rates of metabolism of chloromethanes, chloroethanes and chloroethylenes in the rat," *Inhalation Toxicology*, vol. 2, no. 3, pp. 295–319, 1990.

[56] G. L. Kedderis and S. D. Held, "Prediction of furan pharmacokinetics from hepatocyte studies: comparison of bioactivation and hepatic dosimetry in rats, mice, and humans"," *Toxicology and Applied Pharmacology*, vol. 140, no. 1, pp. 124–130, 1996.

[57] R. H. Reitz, M. L. Gargas, A. L. Mendrala, and A. M. Schumann, "In vivo and in vitro studies of perchloroethylene metabolism for physiologically based pharmacokinetic modeling in rats, mice, and humans," *Toxicology and Applied Pharmacology*, vol. 136, no. 2, pp. 289–306, 1996.

[58] R. J. Williams, A. Vinegar, J. N. Mcdougal, A. M. Jarabek, and J. W. Fisher, "Rat to human extrapolation of HCFC-123 kinetics deduced from halothane kinetics: a corollary approach to physiologically based pharmacokinetic modeling," *Fundamental and Applied Toxicology*, vol. 30, no. 1, pp. 55–66, 1996.

[59] G. A. Csanády, B. Denk, C. Pütz et al., "A physiological toxicokinetic model for exogenous and endogenous ethylene and ethylene oxide in rat, mouse, and human: formation of 2-hydroxyethyl adducts with hemoglobin and DNA," *Toxicology and Applied Pharmacology*, vol. 165, no. 1, pp. 1–26, 2000.

[60] J. E. Dennison, M. E. Andersen, and R. S. H. Yang, "Characterization of the pharmacokinetics of gasoline using PBPK modeling with a complex mixtures chemical lumping approach," *Inhalation Toxicology*, vol. 15, no. 10, pp. 961–986, 2003.

[61] A. M. Hissink, J. Krüse, B. M. Kulig et al., "Model studies for evaluating the neurobehavioral effects of complex hydrocarbon solvents. III. PBPK modeling of white spirit constituents as a tool for integrating animal and human test data," *NeuroToxicology*, vol. 28, no. 4, pp. 751–760, 2007.

[62] D. F. V. Lewis, *Guide to Cytochromes P450: Structure and Function*, Taylor & Francis, London, UK, 2001.

[63] A. I. Archakov and G. I. Bachmanova, Eds., *Cytochrome P-450 and Active Oxygen*, Taylor & Francis, London, UK, 1990.

[64] Z. Fang, J. Sonner, M. J. Laster et al., "Anesthetic and convulsant properties of aromatic compounds and cycloalkanes: implications for mechanisms of narcosis," *Anesthesia and Analgesia*, vol. 83, no. 5, pp. 1097–1104, 1996.

[65] P. D. Lilly, M. E. Andersen, T. M. Ross, and R. A. Pegram, "Physiologically based estimation of in vivo rates of bromodichloromethane metabolism," *Toxicology*, vol. 124, no. 2, pp. 141–152, 1997.

[66] M. L. Gargas, R. J. Burgess, D. E. Voisard, G. H. Cason, and M. E. Andersen, "Partition coefficients of low-molecular-weight volatile chemicals in various liquids and tissues," *Toxicology and Applied Pharmacology*, vol. 98, no. 1, pp. 87–99, 1989.

[67] R. Tardif, G. Charest-Tardif, J. Brodeur, and K. Krishnan, "Physiologically based pharmacokinetic modeling of a ternary mixture of alkyl benzenes in rats and humans," *Toxicology and Applied Pharmacology*, vol. 144, no. 1, pp. 120–134, 1997.

[68] M. Béliveau and K. Krishnan, "Estimation of rat blood: air partition coefficients of volatile organic chemicals using reconstituted mixtures of blood components," *Toxicology Letters*, vol. 116, no. 3, pp. 183–188, 2000.

[69] C. Hansch and L. Zhang, "Quantitative structure-activity relationships of cytochrome P-450," *Drug Metabolism Reviews*, vol. 25, no. 1-2, pp. 1–48, 1993.

[70] D. F. V. Lewis and M. Dickins, "Baseline lipophilicity relationships in human cytochromes P450 associated with drug metabolism," *Drug Metabolism Reviews*, vol. 35, no. 1, pp. 1–18, 2003.

[71] D. F. V. Lewis and Y. Ito, "Human P450s involved in drug metabolism and the use of structural modelling for understanding substrate selectivity and binding affinity," *Xenobiotica*, vol. 39, no. 8, pp. 625–635, 2009.

[72] L. B. Kier, "A shape index from molecular graphs," *Quantitative Structure-Activity Relationships*, vol. 4, no. 3, pp. 109–116, 1985.

[73] Organisation for Economic Co-operation and Development, "Guidance document on the validation of (quantitative) structure-activity relationship [(Q)SAR] models," Tech. Rep., OECD-OCDE, Paris, France, 2007, OECD Environment Health and Safety Publications, Editor.

[74] P. Gramatica, "Principles of QSAR models validation: Internal and external," *QSAR and Combinatorial Science*, vol. 26, no. 5, pp. 694–701, 2007.

[75] S. A. Glantz and B. K. Slinker, *Primer of Applied Regression and Analysis of Variance*, McGraw-Hill, New York, NY, USA, 2nd edition, 2001.

[76] S. Wold, "Validation of QSARs," *Quantitative Structure Activity Relashionship*, vol. 10, pp. 191–193, 1991.

[77] C. J. W. Meulenberg and H. P. M. Vijverberg, "Empirical relations predicting human and rat tissue: air partition coefficients of volatile organic compounds," *Toxicology and Applied Pharmacology*, vol. 165, no. 3, pp. 206–216, 2000.

[78] S. Batterman, L. Zhang, S. Wang, and A. Franzblau, "Partition coefficients for the trihalomethanes among blood, urine, water, milk and air," *Science of the Total Environment*, vol. 284, no. 1–3, pp. 237–247, 2002.

[79] L. M. da Silva, G. Charest-Tardif, K. Krishnan, and R. Tardif, "Influence of oral administration of a quaternary mixture of trihalomethanes on their blood kinetics in the rat," *Toxicology Letters*, vol. 106, no. 1, pp. 49–57, 1999.

[80] M. E. Andersen, H. J. Clewell, M. L. Gargas, F. A. Smith, and R. H. Reitz, "Physiologically based pharmacokinetics and the risk assessment process for methylene chloride," *Toxicology and Applied Pharmacology*, vol. 87, no. 2, pp. 185–205, 1987.

[81] J. C. Ramsey, J. D. Young, R. J. Karbowski, M. B. Chenoweth, L. P. McCarty, and W. H. Braun, "Pharmacokinetics of inhaled styrene in human volunteers," *Toxicology and Applied Pharmacology*, vol. 53, no. 1, pp. 54–63, 1980.

[82] M. E. Andersen, H. J. Clewell, M. L. Gargas et al., "Physiologically based pharmacokinetic modeling with dichloromethane, its metabolite, carbon monoxide, and blood carboxyhemoglobin in rats and humans," *Toxicology and Applied Pharmacology*, vol. 108, no. 1, pp. 14–27, 1991.

[83] T. M. Cahill, I. Cousins, and D. Mackay, "Development and application of a generalized physiologically based pharmacokinetic model for multiple environmental contaminants," *Environmental Toxicology and Chemistry*, vol. 22, no. 1, pp. 26–34, 2003.

[84] International Programme on Chemical Safety, *Characterization and Application of Physiologically Based Pharmacokinetic Models in Risk Assessment*, International Programme on Chemical Safety, 2010.

[85] C. J. MacKay, L. Campbell, A. M. Samuel et al., "Behavioral changes during exposure to 1,1,1-trichloroethane: time-course and relationship to blood solvent levels," *American Journal of Industrial Medicine*, vol. 11, no. 2, pp. 223–239, 1987.

[86] M. T. D. Cronin and D. Livingstone, *Predicting Chemical Toxicity and Fate*, CRC Press, Boca Raton, Fla, USA, 2004.

[87] H. Gao and C. Hansch, "QSAR of P450 oxidation: on the value of comparing kcat and km with kcat/km," *Drug Metabolism Reviews*, vol. 28, no. 4, pp. 513–526, 1996.

[88] J. P. Jones, K. R. Korzekwa, F. J. Eric, and R. W. Michael, "Predicting the rates and regioselectivity of reactions mediated by the P450 superfamily," in *Methods in Enzymology*, pp. 326–335, Academic Press, New York, NY, USA, 1996.

[89] D. L. Harris, J.-Y. Park, L. Gruenke, and L. Waskell, "Theoretical study of the ligand-CYP2B4 complexes: effect of structure on binding free energies and heme spin state," *Proteins*, vol. 55, no. 4, pp. 895–914, 2004.

[90] L. Olsen, P. Rydberg, T. H. Rod, and U. Ryde, "Prediction of activation energies for hydrogen abstraction by cytochrome P450," *Journal of Medicinal Chemistry*, vol. 49, no. 22, pp. 6489–6499, 2006.

[91] D. N. Kim, K. H. Cho, W. S. Oh et al., "EaMEAD: activation energy prediction of cytochrome p450 mediated metabolism with effective atomic descriptors," *Journal of Chemical Information and Modeling*, vol. 49, no. 7, pp. 1643–1654, 2009.

[92] Y. Lu, S. Rieth, M. Lohitnavy et al., "Application of PBPK modeling in support of the derivation of toxicity reference values for 1-trichloroethane," *Regulatory Toxicology and Pharmacology*, vol. 50, no. 2, pp. 249–260, 2008.

[93] R. H. Reitz, J. N. McDougal, M. W. Himmelstein, R. J. Nolan, and A. M. Schumann, "Physiologically based pharmacokinetic modeling with methylchloroform: implications for interspecies, high dose/low dose, and dose route extrapolations," *Toxicology and Applied Pharmacology*, vol. 95, no. 2, pp. 185–199, 1988.

[94] M. H. Wang, D. Wade, L. Chen, S. White, and C. S. Yang, "Probing the active sites of rat and human cytochrome P450 2E1 with alcohols and carboxylic acids," *Archives of Biochemistry and Biophysics*, vol. 317, no. 1, pp. 299–304, 1995.

14

In Vivo Toxicity of Silver Nanoparticles and Silver Ions in Zebrafish (*Danio rerio*)

Katrine Bilberg,[1,2] Mads Bruun Hovgaard,[1] Flemming Besenbacher,[1] and Erik Baatrup[2]

[1] *Interdisciplinary Nanoscience Center (iNANO) and Department of Physics and Astronomy, Aarhus University, 8000 Aarhus C, Denmark*

[2] *Section of Zoophysiology, Department of Biological Sciences, Aarhus University, C.F. Moellers Allé 3, Building 1131, 8000 Aarhus C, Denmark*

Correspondence should be addressed to Erik Baatrup, erik.baatrup@biology.au.dk

Academic Editor: Christian Gagnon

The influence of water chemistry on characterised polyvinyl pyrrolidone- (PVP-) coated silver nanoparticles (81 nm) was investigated. NaCl solution series of 100–800 mg L^{-1} lead to initial and temporal increase in nanoparticles size, but agglomeration was limited. pH variation (5–8) had only minor influence on the hydrodynamic particle size. Acute toxicity of nanosivler to zebrafish (*Danio rerio*) was investigated in a 48-hour static renewal study and compared with the toxicity of silver ions ($AgNO_3$). The nanosilver and silver ion 48-hour median lethal concentration (LC_{50}) values were 84 μg L^{-1} and 25 μg L^{-1}, respectively. To investigate exposure-related stress, the fish behaviour was observed visually after 0, 3, 6, 12, 24, 27, 30, and 48 hours of both nanosilver and ionic silver treatments. These observations revealed increased rate of operculum movement and surface respiration after nanosilver exposure, suggesting respiratory toxicity. The present study demonstrates that silver nanoparticles are lethal to zebrafish.

1. Introduction

Silver is a rarely occurring element in the earth's crust (0.05–0.1 ppm) but is deposited at much higher concentrations in ores in association with other elements [1]. In the aquatic environment, silver originates from leaching, mining, or anthropogenic sources [2]. It is traditionally incorporated in, for example, coins, jewellery, electronics, and photographic manufacturing [3]. In addition, the antibacterial capacity of both ionic silver and nanosilver has expanded its use significantly [3, 4], being incorporated in a variety of products, including clothing, paints, plastics, food containers packaging, wound dressings, bandages, and household appliances such as refrigerators and washing machines [3, 5].

The concentration of silver has been found to be less than 5 ng L^{-1} in three Connecticut undeveloped headwaters and between 25 and 100 ng L^{-1} in rivers from industrialised and urban areas [6]. In rivers in Texas, particulate silver concentrations range from <0.01 to 62 ng L^{-1} [7]. Generally, the concentration of silver ions is extremely low in surface waters, because ionic silver binds to a variety of negatively charged ligands [2, 8]. The concentration of silver nanoparticles from consumer products in the aquatic environment is predicted to be about 0.01 μg L^{-1} [9]. In 2010, the silver concentration in courses of the Rhine, receiving outlets of textiles and plastics containing nanosilver, was estimated to be between 4 and 40 ng silver L^{-1}, accounting for 15% of the total silver release [10]. Future discharge of nanosilver to the aquatic environment will undoubtedly increase seriously due to the expected extensive use of nanosilver.

The silver ion is toxic to fish [11–13], and therefore it is crucial also to establish the toxicity of nanosilver. Metal nanoparticles of cupper have been demonstrated to be acutely toxic to zebrafish with an LC_{50} value of 1–1.5 mg L^{-1} [14, 15]. In contrast, aluminium, cobalt, nickel, and titanium dioxide nanoparticles were found to be less toxic to adult zebrafish with a 48-hour median lethal concentration (LC_{50}) >10 mg L^{-1} [14].

Metal nanoparticles possess unique properties due to their size, shape, surface structure, aggregation characteristics, and chemical composition [16–18] that differ from their respective soluble metal. How water chemistry such as salinity and pH influence the toxicity of nanoparticle is sparsely investigated [19] but possibly affects the size and shape of the particles [20]. Consequently, it is important to characterize the nanoparticles in the actual environment in order to know how they chemically interact as this likely alters their toxicity.

The aim of this study was to establish the 48-hour lethal concentration (LC_{50}) of waterborne 81 nm mean size silver nanoparticles to zebrafish (*Danio rerio*) and to compare the toxicity of these silver nanoparticles with silver ions (administered as silver nitrate). In addition, the effects of water chemistry on nanosilver characteristics were investigated.

2. Methods

2.1. Experimental Animal. Zebrafish (*Danio rerio*) were purchased from Credo Fish (Aalborg, Denmark). The fish were acclimatised for at least two weeks in a 26°C stock aquarium containing aerated head tank water. Head tank water consists of demineralised water mixed with nonchlorinated tap water- (16 : 1) added NaCl to a conductivity of approximately 275 μS (132 mg L^{-1}), which is optimal for zebrafish according to Nüsselin-Volhard and Dahm [21], and also prevents fungi growth. The concentrations (in mg L^{-1}) of the predominant ions in the head tank water were: SO_4^{2-} 4.25, Na^+ 43.19, NO_3^- 0.09, Mg^{2+} 0.75, K^+ 0.21, Cl^- 63.93, Ca^{2+} 5.31, and HCO_3^- 19.31, in total ~137 mg L^{-1}. The photoperiod was 14 : 10 (light : dark) where the light period was initiated by an artificial sunrise. The sunrise was made by gradually increasing the voltage to a weak luminous lamp ten minutes before the luminous intensity rose in the room. The aquaria were illuminated with 95–105 LUX from an artificial light source.

2.2. Preparation of Silver Nanoparticle Suspension and Ionic Silver Solution. Silver nanoparticle powder (stated by the manufacturer to be spherical 30–40 nm particles), coated with 0.2% polyvinyl pyrrolidone (PVP) and a purity of 99.5%, was purchased from NanoAmor (Houston, USA). PVP-coated silver nanoparticles were chosen, as they are easily dispersed in water. A water dispersion of silver nanoparticles was prepared by suspending 0.5 g silver nanoparticle powder in 100 mL Milli-Q water, followed by immediate ultra sonication (Ultrasonic Homogenizer, BioLogics, Inc, Virgina, USA) in order to deaggregate the suspension. The sonicator was mounted with a solid titanium tip with a diameter of 9.5 mm. The suspension was placed on a magnetic stirrer and sonicated four times of 15 min over a 2-hour time span with pulses of half a second duration. The power output was 100 Watt and the output frequency was 20 kHz. Following sonication, the suspension was centrifuged at 1000 g for 2 hours (Sigma 3k 30, Struers KEBO lab., Demark), and finally the supernatant was filtrated through a 0.2 μm mixed cellulose ester filter (Frisenette ApS, Denmark). The stock nanosilver suspension had a clear yellow colour and was stored in darkness at 6°C until use.

To determine the concentration of silver in the stock nanosilver suspension, equal volumes of the suspension and 69% nitric acid (HNO_3) were mixed resulting in dissolution of the nanosilver. This solution was then diluted with Milli-Q water until the silver concentration was within the linear measuring range of the Atomic Absorption Spectrophotometer (AAS). The concentrations of silver were determined using a Perkin-Elmer Aanalyst 300 AAS (Perkin-Elmer, Hvidovre, Denmark) mounted with a silver lumina hollow cathode lamp (Perkin-Elmer, Hvidovre, Denmark). In all cases, double measurements were performed, and the instrument detection limit for silver was 36 μg L^{-1}.

Free silver ions in the silver nanoparticle stock suspension were measured by a silver ion-selective electrode (ISE) ISE225 (Hach Lange APS, 2700 Brønshøj, Denmark). The calibration curve was constructed from diluting $AgNO_3$ solutions in the silver ion range 0.1–1 mg L^{-1}. The ISE is sensitive to interferences from sulphides, which, however, are not likely to be present in the suspension. The amount of dissolved silver was also determined by ultracentrifugating the stock suspension 30 min at 100 000 g (Optima L80xp centrifuge, sw55 snE17986 rotor); whereafter the silver content in the supernatant was determined by AAS. The applied methods have previously been used to determine the content of dissolved metal nanoparticles [15, 22]. Double measurements estimated that in the nanosilver suspension, approximately 40% of the silver was in the form of silver ions.

To determine if the concentration of silver changed over time in the test tanks, water samples were obtained from a tank containing fish 0, 2, and 24 hours after the application of 80 μg L^{-1} silver nanoparticles. Using AAS, no decline in silver concentrations was found two hours after nanosilver application, whereas the concentration was reduced by 41% after 24 hours.

Silver nitrate ($AgNO_3$) pellets (SigmaAldrich, Steinheim, Germany) with a purity >99.5% were dissolved in Milli-Q water.

2.3. Silver Nanoparticle Characterisation

2.3.1. Powder X-Ray Diffraction. Crystallite size and crystalline phase were evaluated by powder X-ray diffraction (PXRD) using a STOE STAPI P (STOE & Cie GmbH, Darmstadt, Germany) powder diffractometer emitting $CuK\alpha_1$ (λ = 0.15405 nm) radiation, equipped with a curved 1D-PSD detector [23]. For analysis, the silver nanoparticle powder was mixed with diluted wood glue, allowing a fixation of the highly electrostatic sample between two Mylar discs, whilst providing a mounting transparent to the incident and diffracted X-ray radiation. Diffraction profiles were inspected to determine the presence of nanocrystallite domains (i.e., if the material was amorphous or not) and to identify the crystalline phase by direct comparison to reference libraries (International Centre for Diffraction Data, PDF-2). Further, an estimate of the crystallite domain size was obtained by fitting the 111 diffraction peak to a Voigt function (Origin7.5, OriginLab Corporation, USA), using the Scherrer formula [24, 25] on the full width half maximum (FWHM) peak value, after a linear background subtraction and instrumental profile correction of both the Gaussian and Lorentzian profile components [25]. The instrumental profile broadening was estimated from the fit of a Voigt function to the diffraction line profiles of a NIST LaB6 standard sample.

2.3.2. Transmission Electron Microscopy. The primary nanoparticle size and morphology were assessed using a Phillips CM20 transmission electron microscope (TEM) working at 200 keV. For TEM analysis, stock nanoparticle suspensions were diluted 1 : 100 and 10 μL were pipetted onto holey carbon grids (S147-4, Plano GmbH, Germany) and subsequently left to evaporate in a laminar flow hood. A series of images was selected to manually establish size distributions by tracing single particle contours using the scanning probe image software SPIP (Image Metrology ApS, Lyngby, Denmark).

2.3.3. Dynamic Light Scattering and Zeta Potential Measurements. The hydrodynamic diameter and zeta potential of the nanoparticles were characterised by dynamic light scattering (DLS) using a Malvern Zetasizer Nano (Malvern Instruments Ltd, Worcestershire, UK). Besides characterising the stock suspension (pH 3.9, Milli-Q water), a series of varying aqueous conditions were tested by mixing the stock silver nanoparticle suspension in a 1 : 1 ratio with preadjusted solutions of well-defined pH values, sodium chloride (NaCl) concentrations, or combinations thereof, 5 min prior to DLS measurements. The resulting pH and NaCl concentrations were pH 5–8 (steps of pH 1) and (100, 200, 400, 600, and 800) mg L^{-1} NaCl, respectively; with the latter NaCl series run both at pH 3.9 (stock suspension pH) and at pH 6.9 (head tank water pH). Also included in the series was head tank water. All measurements were performed at 26°C and repeated after initial (5 min), 30 min or 1 hour, 12 hours (data not shown), and 24 hours, with samples kept between measurements under conditions identical to the fish tanks used for nanosilver toxicity assessment. Each DLS measurement was run in triplicate using automated, optimal measurement time and laser attenuation settings. The recorded correlation functions and measured particle mobilities were converted into size distributions and zeta potentials, respectively, using the Malvern Dispersion Software (V5.10, http://www.zetasizer.com/).

2.4. Acute Toxicity Testing of Silver Nanoparticles and Silver Ions. A 48-hour acute toxicity (LC_{50}) test of silver nanoparticles on adult male zebrafish (standard length 28.1 ± 0.2 mm weighing 0.42 ± 0.04 g; $n = 110$) was conducted in a static water renewal experiment, according to the Organisation for Economic Cooperation and Development (OECD) guideline for testing of chemicals (OECD, 1992). The eight silver nanoparticle nominal exposure concentrations of 18, 36, 54, 72, 89, 107, 125, and 143 μg L^{-1} plus an unexposed control were determined from a preliminary exposure study. In addition, two PVP controls (Sigma-Aldrich, Steinheim, Germany) were included to assess the possible toxicity of the PVP coating. Zebrafish were exposed to PVP concentrations equalling half of the nanosilver LC_{50} value (42 μg L^{-1}) and hundred times the nanosilver LC_{50} value (8400 μg L^{-1}). Ten randomly selected male zebrafish were exposed to each concentration in 14 L aerated seamless glass tanks (29 cm × 21 cm × 23 cm) (length x width x height) containing five L of head tank water. After 24 h of treatment, the fish were transferred to new tanks containing their respective concentrations of nanosilver. The zebrafish were not fed 24 hours prior to or during the experiment in order to maintain constant exposure concentrations, given that nanoparticles might adhere to food and faeces particles [26].

A similar 48-hour acute toxicity (LC_{50}) test of silver ions was conducted with zebrafish of standard length 28.6 ± 0.3 mm and weighing 0.45 ± 0.03 g; $n = 80$, in order to compare the toxicity of silver nanoparticles with silver ions. The nominal exposure concentrations were 13, 21, 23, 25, 29, 37, and 47 μg silver ions L^{-1} administered as silver nitrate plus an unexposed control group.

As an indicator of exposure-related stress, the fish behaviour was assessed by a human observer after 0, 3, 6, 12, 24, 27, 30, and 48 hours of both silver nanoparticles and silver ion treatments. The behavioural components considered were operculum movements (ventilation rate), loss of equilibrium, surface respiration, body colour (pigmentation), circular swimming, jerk movement, bottom resting, and aggressive behaviour. Further, excess mucus production was recorded. Mortality was monitored continuously and fish were considered dead when operculum movement and response to mechanical stimuli could no longer be detected. After termination of the experiment, the remaining fish were killed in ice water and the gender was verified by means of the macroscopic appearance of the gonads.

Following exposure, all water quality values were satisfactory and there were no treatment differences. Oxygen saturation was 91.2 ± 2.5%, pH 6.9 ± 0.1, temperature 25–26°C, and conductivity 280.3 ± 8.4 μS. The load of ammonium, nitrate, and nitrite was measured with Tetra *test* (Tetra Werke, Melle; Germany) and phosphate with JBL test (JBL GmbH & Co. KG, Neuhofen, Germany); Ammonia <0.25 mg L^{-1}, nitrate <12.5 mg L^{-1}, nitrite <0.3 mg L^{-1}, and phosphate 0.25 mg L^{-1}.

2.5. Statistical Analysis. LC_{10} and LC_{50} values plus their 95% confidence intervals were calculated using the probit analysis in SPSS version 13.0 (SPSS Inc. Chicago, Il, USA).

3. Results

3.1. Silver Nanoparticle Characterisation. A representative TEM image of the primary silver nanoparticles is shown in Figure 1(a). The nanoparticles were found to predominantly have a slightly elliptical or multifaceted shape, although a few large or triangular particles present. The silver nanoparticle stock preparation had a mean primary size of 81 ± 2 nm and an aspect ratio of 1.2 ± 0.2. The reported size is defined as the maximum distance between two points on the particle circumference, equivalent to the diameter for spherical particles.

The PXRD analysis of the silver nanoparticle powder confirmed the presence of Ag nanocrystallites with a single Ag cubic crystalline orientation (Figure 1(b)) and showed no sign of oxidation or other crystalline phases present. The crystallite domain size estimated by the Sheerer formula was ~78.1 nm.

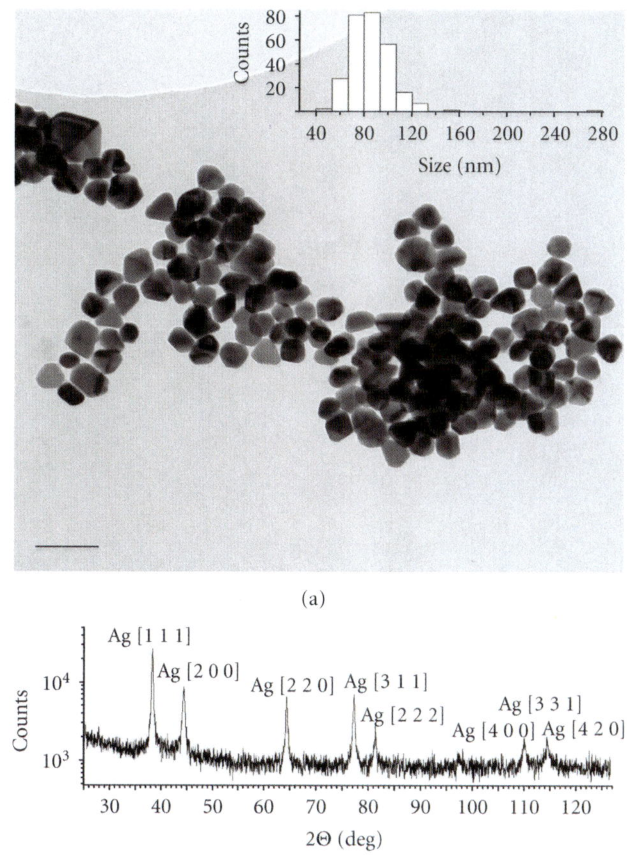

FIGURE 1: (a) Representative TEM image of stock nanosilver suspension along with size statistics (insert). (b) PXRD pattern for the nanosilver powder with the indexed diffraction lines of silver.

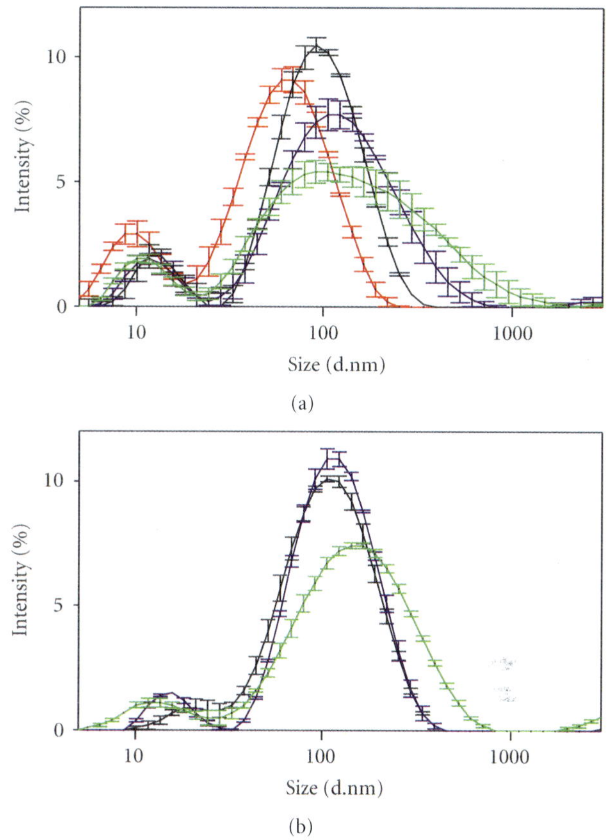

FIGURE 2: Dynamic Light Scattering (DLS) size distributions for (a) the nanosilver stock preparation (red line) along with the pH 6.9 200 mg L^{-1} NaCl solvent condition 5 min (black line), 1 hour (blue line), and 24 hours (green line). (b) The nanosilver mixed with head tank water directly (1 : 1) (black line), after 30 min (blue line), and 24 hours (green line). Data are presented as mean value ± SE.

As prepared for stock suspension, the silver nanoparticles were characterised using dynamic light scattering (DLS). In general, the DLS analysis presented bimodal distributions, for the stock preparation specifically (Figure 2(a), red curve); the distribution had a major peak at (73.55 ± 1.19) nm (~83% area intensity) and a minor peak around (10.8 ± 0.3) nm (~10% area intensity). In the following, the position of the major peak (73.55 ± 1.19) nm is referenced to as the measured hydrodynamic diameter or size of the nanoparticles under a given set of experimental conditions. Throughout the pH series pH (5–8), the measured silver nanoparticle diameter changed only slightly (~change of −0.1–17 nm), with the offset being evident from the initial mixing (5 min) and then approximately constant throughout the entire time series (5 min, 1 hour, 24 hours) for each pH. The stability of the nanoparticle suspensions under variations in salt concentrations (100–800 mg L^{-1}) was tested at two pH values, either as prepared for stock solution (pH 3.9) or equivalent to the head tank water (pH 6.9). For both pH values, the stability of the nanoparticle suspension had pronounced response to salt variations (see Supplementary results, Tables 1(a) and 1(b) available online at doi: 10.1155/2012/293784). At pH 6.9, an initial size increase of ~33–65 nm was observed for all NaCl concentrations, and after 1 h and 24 h, the size continued to increase significantly along with NaCl concentration and time, as exemplified by the pH 6.9 200 mg L^{-1} NaCl experiment in Figure 2(a) after 5 min (black), 1 h (blue) and 24 hours (green). Most pronounced was the increase in hydrodynamic radius of the 600 mg L^{-1} NaCl experiments after 24 hours, reaching (260 ± 29) nm. Besides the increase in size, a temporal development in the width of the DLS size distributions was also observed for all NaCl concentrations (Figure 2(a) and supplementary results, Tables 1(a) and 1(b)). For instance, for the pH 6.9 200 mg L^{-1} experiment (Figure 2(a)), the polidispersity index increased from 0.42 ± 0.02 to 0.507 ± 0.004 ending at 0.54 ± 0.04 for the 5 min, 1 hour, and 24 hours' time points, respectively. At stock preparation pH value 3.9, a likewise trend for the NaCl concentration series was observed concerning the development of the hydrodynamic size with NaCl concentration, reaching a maximum value of (311 ± 9) nm for 800 mg L^{-1} NaCl after 24-hour incubation (supplementary results, Table 1(a)).

Approaching the in vivo conditions, the head tank water preparation (1 : 1) revealed an initial hydrodynamic diameter of (121 ± 3) nm, increasing to (128 ± 3) nm after 30 min ending at (173 ± 3) nm at 24 hours as displayed in Figure 2(b).

In addition to hydrodynamic size measurements, the zeta potential was measured after 24 hours of incubation for the stock nanosilver preparation along with the tested pH and salt variations, including the in vivo relevant head tank water preparation. The stock nanosilver suspension was found to have a zeta potential of (−28.5 ± 0.75) mV, below the head tank water preparations with a zeta potential of (−38.4 ± 0.4) mV. For the variations in pH and salt concentrations, all potentials were measured to be between −27 mV and −48 mV, with no clear correlation between solution conditions and the exact zeta potential value.

3.2. Toxicity of Silver Nanoparticles. Silver nanoparticles are acutely toxic to male zebrafish (Figure 3(a)) with a semistatic 48-hour exposure LC_{50} of 84 $\mu g\ L^{-1}$ (95% CL = 74–93 $\mu g\ L^{-1}$) and LC_{10} of 57 $\mu g\ L^{-1}$ (95% CL = 36–68 $\mu g\ L^{-1}$). A narrow margin was found between the LC_{50} 24 h of 89 $\mu g\ L^{-1}$ (95% CL = 79–100 $\mu g\ L^{-1}$) and the LC_{50} 48 hour. There was no mortality in the control tank or at the three lowest silver nanoparticle concentrations. After 3 hours of exposure, the first fish started dying, and after 24 hours, all fish in the two highest test concentrations were dead. Extravasations of blood were observed in the anterior ventral surface of the body, just behind the head of the dead fish. This was not found in dead fish exposed to ionic silver.

The toxic action of silver nanoparticles was relatively rapid with signs of stress appearing within 30 min of exposure. At higher silver nanoparticle concentrations (>72 $\mu g\ L^{-1}$), toxicity stress signs emerged, starting with zebrafish lying on the tank bottom with increased respiratory rate. Hereafter surface respiration took place, and finally the fish stood still in the middle of the water column where they ultimately lost equilibrium and sank to the bottom. A few fish displayed jerky movements and circular swimming just before they lost equilibrium. No signs of aggressive behaviour or changes in body colour were observed in any of the tanks. After 24 hours of exposure, there were no longer visible differences in behaviour between the control and the lowest exposure groups. Fish mucus (thin white branched threads), likely secreted from the gills, was observed at the bottom of tanks exposed to at least 89 $\mu g\ L^{-1}$ silver nanoparticles. Mucus secretion was not observed in the control or the lower concentration exposure tanks.

As expected, no deaths or aberrant behaviour were observed in the groups of fish exposed to PVP alone.

3.3. Toxicity of Silver Ions. Mortality increased with increasing concentrations of ionic silver (Figure 3(b)). The 24-hour silver ion LC_{50} was estimated to 28 $\mu g\ L^{-1}$ (95% CL = 26–31 $\mu g\ L^{-1}$) and the estimated 48-hour LC_{50} was 25 $\mu g\ L^{-1}$ (95% CL = 23–26 $\mu g\ L^{-1}$). No mortality was recorded in the two lowest concentrations or in the control group. Signs of stress were revealed by the fish displaying increased swimming activity and attempts to escape from the tank. Behavioural stress signs were the same as described above for silver nanoparticles. In addition, elevated mucus secretion with strands of sloughed mucus appeared in the tank after exposure to higher concentrations of silver ions.

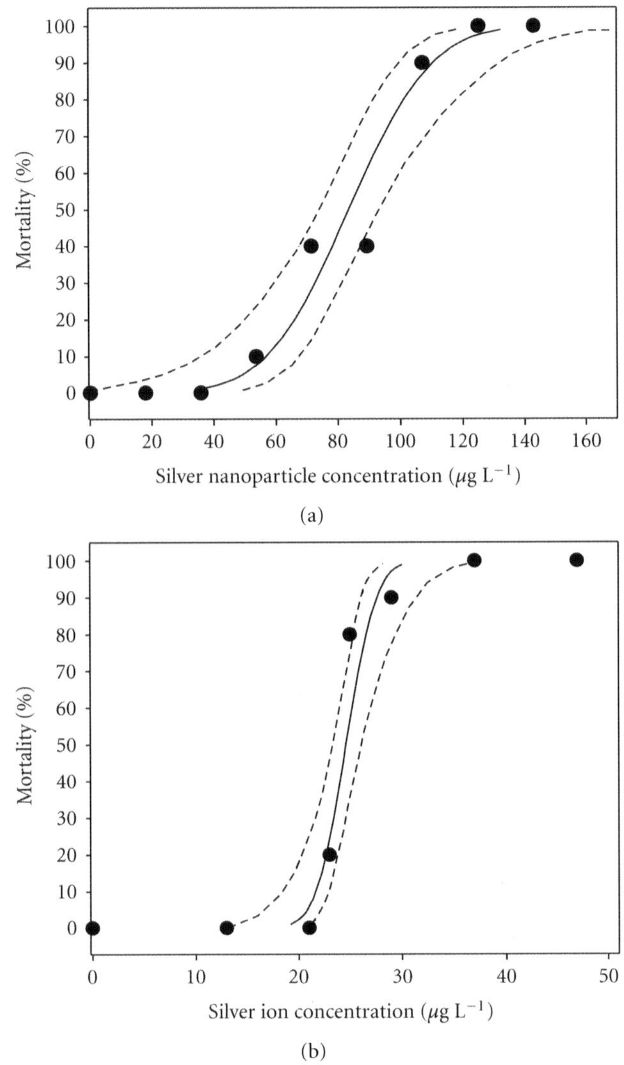

FIGURE 3: Toxicity of 81 nm silver nanoparticles (a) and silver ions (b) after 48 hours exposure to adult male zebrafish (*Danio rerio*) in a static renewal experiment. Black circles (•) represent the mean survival in percent after exposure to a given concentration ($n = 10$). Solid lines indicate the calculated lethality using probit analysis after exposure to silver nanoparticles and silver ions, respectively. Dashed lines indicate the 95% confidence intervals.

4. Discussion

4.1. Silver Nanoparticle Characterisation. The nanoparticle characterisation was conducted using a range of complementary techniques in order to characterise both the primary nanoparticle size distribution; and the in-suspension agglomeration under varying aqueous conditions.

The primary size was determined by image analysis on a representative selection of TEM images. Statistically, the TEM analysis demonstrated both a larger size and a particle morphology differing from the nominal spherical 30–40 nm particles. In line with previous work on a larger range of metal nanoparticles [27] this emphasises the importance of an in-house size characterisation for nanotoxicology studies.

The primary nanoparticle is not necessarily homogeneous in terms of chemical or crystalline properties. Metallic nanoparticles samples can contain both amorphous and various crystalline phases in elaborate geometrical configurations (e.g., core-shell), and nanoparticle materials can additionally be affected by postsynthesis oxidation. The PXRD analysis for the silver nanoparticles was consistent with a single Ag cubic crystalline phase present and showed no sign of oxidation or other crystalline phases. The estimate of crystallite size provided by the FWHM Scheerer formula is only accurate in the absence of additional contributions to the observed line broadening, like lattice strain caused by; for example, point defects or plastic deformations [28]. Additionally, it is important to emphasise that crystallite size is not generally the same as particle size, but only a measure of the size of a coherently diffracting domain; this is why we rely on TEM and DLS accurate particle sizing in the presented work. However, while a full analysis addressing microstrain is beyond the scope of this text, the agreement between the TEM primary partice size characterization and the Scheerer estimate of crystallite size suggests that the nanosilver particles have a good degree of crystallinity, with a limited amorphous component only.

Determining particle sizes via TEM or PXRD facilitates insight to the primary and crystalline sizes, but the techniques do not bring knowledge on how the nanoparticles agglomerate or behave in suspension under relevant aqueous conditions, which may affect aggregation significantly. A key element to investigating the biological response to nanoparticle exposure via liquid delivery is the ability to actually have free nanoparticles in suspension, as quantified by the difference between the primary nanoparticle size and in-suspension agglomeration and resulting size-distribution. The nanosilver utilised in the present study was synthesised with 0.2% PVP. PVP is a general metal-oxide chelating agent, allowing a strong binding to the silver nanoparticles while stabilising the particle suspension and redispersion by steric repulsion [29]. The stock preparation of silver nanoparticles had a bimodal size distribution; yet no clear evidence of a bimodal distribution was found by TEM. We thus attribute the minor peak at ~11 nm to scattering on free PVP in suspension in correspondence with DLS studies on PVP polymers [30]. The peak hydrodynamic size of the stock silver suspension was in good correspondence with the established TEM size statistics, signifying an only limited agglomeration of the silver nanoparticles when prepared following our specific redispersion protocol. This limited aggregation is in good agreement with the absolute value of the zeta potential measurements, as absolute zeta potentials in the range or above 30 mV indicate particle agglomeration stability.

During an in vivo experiment, both the ionic strength and the pH of the water will differ from those of the stock silver nanoparticle suspension and potentially change over time. The pH value of head tank water was measured to be pH 6.9; this is higher than the pH 3.9 observed for the stock preparation; this is why the nanoparticle suspension was subjected to a pH (5–8) variation test. The eight most abundant ionic species in the utilised head tank water preparation (SO_4^{2-}, Na^+, NO_3^-, Mg^{2+}, K^+, Cl^-, Ca^{2+}, HCO_3^-) have a total concentration of ~137 mg L^{-1}. The effective screening of these eight predominant ions can be quantified by the Debye length [31] with each ionic species, however, having a unique impact on the effective Debye length depending on both their specific molar concentration and charge. The combined Debye length was calculated as 6.3 nm, with clear dominating contributions from Na^+ and Cl^-. The silver nanoparticles were, therefore, subjected to a salt solution series of (100–800) mg L^{-1} NaCl, with 138 mg L^{-1} NaCl constituting a head tank water equivalent at a Debye length of 6.3 nm, situated reasonably between the 100 mg L^{-1} and 200 mg L^{-1} measurements. Throughout the pH series, only a minor change in the nanoparticle hydrodynamic size was observed, signifying that the PVP encapsulation and steric repulsion is stable against pH variations. For the variations in salt (100–800) mg L^{-1}, however, both an initial and temporal increase in size occurred. Synthesised silver nanoparticle suspensions without the addition of stabilisers, like PVP, are susceptible to agglomeration upon an increase in salt concentrations. The observed agglomeration, with a maximum at 600 mg L^{-1} pH 6.9, indicates defects and/or incomplete coverage of the PVP encapsulation. The fact that the peak-agglomerated size is only 3-4-fold the peak size of the stock suspension demonstrates, however, that the agglomeration is limited even in this worst case scenario.

For the in vivo relevant head tank water conditions, the peak-agglomerated size represented a 2-3-fold increase compared with stock conditions, thus performing better than the above described worst case scenario. The measured DLS size distribution agreed well with the corresponding pH value and ionic screening conditions (pH 6.9; 200 mg L^{-1}), both strengthening the DLS head tank water results and suggesting that the pH and salt solution series provide a valid insight to the behaviour of the silver nanoparticles under in vivo conditions.

Measured after 24 hours, the zeta potentials of the varying aqueous conditions (pH, salt variations, and head tank water) were all below −27 mV agreeing well with the observed limited agglomeration, but also indicating that some steady state or equilibrium size distribution was reached within the 24-hour observation time.

Concerning variations in pH, ionic concentrations, and dispersion in tank water, the nanoparticle characterisation shows the silver nanoparticles to have good stability against agglomeration, ensuring a population of free nanosized particles at the relevant time-scale of the in vivo experiments. For the initial exposure of silver nanoparticles, we thus argue that the current characterisation gives an adequate description of the silver nanoparticle particle distribution during the LC_{50} assessments.

4.2. Acute Toxicity of Silver Nanoparticles and Silver Ions. The present study demonstrates that the silver nanoparticles used are acutely lethal to adult zebrafish. Previously, the 48-hour nanosilver LC_{50} value has been found to be 7.07 mg L^{-1} in zebrafish exposed to metal oxide-coated silver nanoparticles with a size of 44.5 and 216 nm in suspension [14]. In another study on zebrafish, Choi et al. [32] reported the 24-hour LC_{50} to be 250 mg L^{-1} for 5–20 nm silver nanoparticles, which is far less toxic than the LC_{50} value found by Griffitt et al. [14] and in the present study. In Japanese medaka (*Oryzias latipes*), the 96-hour LC_{50} has been demonstrated to be 34.6 $\mu g\ L^{-1}$ for 50 nm uncoated silver particles [33]. Accordingly, it is clear that silver nanoparticles of different size and with or without different stabilisation agents process different degrees of toxicity in different organisms, under different exposure times and conditions.

Dynamic light scattering showed that the intensity of silver nanoparticles in the tank water decreased after 24 hours, indicating a concentration decline. Also, AAS measurements of water samples revealed a decline in silver concentration after 24 hours. This decline is likely due to particle adhesion to the sides of the tank. Accordingly, the actual silver nanoparticle exposure concentration available to the fish is presumably lower than the reported nominal concentration. This can explain that the reverted behaviour where the fish exposed to the lowest nanosilver concentrations after 24 hours resembled the behaviour of the control fish.

The demonstrated toxicity of the silver nanoparticles was attributed to the silver and not the PVP coating. Besides, PVP has successfully been applied as a nontoxic additive in a broad range of products, such as shampoo, toothpaste, contact lens solution, as a binder in pharmaceutical tablets, and as a food additive stabilizer.

As expected, the results of the present study confirmed that ionic silver is also acutely toxic to zebrafish at concentrations consistent with a prior estimation for zebrafish [14] and within the 96-hour LC_{50} range (5–70 $\mu g\ L^{-1}$) for other teleosts [8]. Given that tank water contained NaCl, it cannot be excluded that some of the silver existed as silver chloride. In rainbow trout (*Oncorhyncus mykiss*), Hogstrand et al. [34] found that dissolved silver chloride is at least ten times less toxic than silver ions to fish and particulate silver chloride is nontoxic. Similarly, Bury et al. [35] reported that increasing chloride concentrations decreased silver toxicity in rainbow trout whereas chloride ions did not significantly affect the 96-hour LC_{50} values for fathead minnows (*Pimephales promelas*).

The silver ions were approximately 3.4 times more toxic than the silver nanoparticles by mass of silver added to the tanks. In an in vitro study, PVP-coated nanosilver from the same supplier as the particles in the present study was found to be approximately four times less toxic than silver ions [36], indicating that nanoparticulate forms of silver are less toxic than their soluble forms by mass added. As with silver, this has also been shown to be the case for copper [14, 15] and aluminium nanoparticles [14]. In contrast, in a study on juvenile Japanese medaka (*Oryzias latipes*) Chae et al. [33] reported that nanosilver was more toxic than ionic silver after 24 hours of exposure and similar in toxicity after 96 hours.

The fraction of nanosilver that is chemically available is worth considering. If the nanosilver toxicity is caused by chemical interactions, the toxic portion of nanoparticles must originate either from silver ions dissolved from the particle or from the exposed silver atoms on the particle surface. For 80 nm particles using the bulk silver density and a hexagonal packing of 0.29 diameter silver atoms, the percentage of surface atoms is ~0.2%. Thus, the vast majority of the silver (>99.8%) is expected to be contained within the core of the nanoparticles. Silver ions can be released from the surface of silver nanoparticles [37] and the ISE and ultracentrifugation methods surprisingly estimated that up to 40% of the silver by mass existed as ionic silver in the nanosilver suspension. In contrast, Navarro et al. [22] estimated that 1% of the silver in a carbonate-coated nanosilver suspension was free silver ions. This underlines the importance of estimating the dissolution of metal nanoparticles. In fathead minnow embryo, the 96-hour LC_{50} of nanosilver was lower than the 15 $\mu g\ L^{-1}$ silver nitrate LC_{50} value, even though the amount of dissolved silver from nanosilver was 18–95 $\mu g\ L^{-1}$ [38]. Laban et al. [38] therefore presented the idea that silver ions dissociated from silver nitrate process a different toxicity than silver ions released from silver nanoparticles. In fact, this is in accordance with our results, because the silver ion LC_{50} value is below the amount of dissolved silver from the nanoparticles. Furthermore, only zebrafish exposed to silver ions as silver nitrate displayed an avoidance reaction, which was not observed in nanosilver exposed fish. Silver ions most likely contributed to the toxicity of the nanoparticle suspension. On the other hand, nanoparticles undoubtedly have an inherent toxicity. For example, extravasations of blood were only observed in fish exposed to silver nanoparticles. The precise mechanism whereby silver nanoparticles exert their toxicity to fish is to our knowledge unknown. The observed increased ventilation rate, surface respiration, and excessive gill mucus secretion during nanosilver exposure suggest the gills as target organs of nanosilver toxicity. Likewise, during ionic silver exposure, hyperventilation was observed in rainbow trout (*Oncorhynchus mykiss*) and attributed to counteracting metabolic acidosis [39]. Increased mucus secretion after ionic silver application has previously been noticed [40]. When a toxicant irritates the gill epithelium, mucus production is increased, trapping and transporting the toxicant away from the gills [18]. However, excessive mucus secretion also increases the oxygen diffusion distance, impairing respiration. Other nanoparticles, such as carbon nanotubes, have caused increased mucus secretion [41] and swollen mucocytes have been induced by titanium dioxide [42]. The primary target of silver ion acute toxicity for freshwater fish is, on the other hand, known to be the gills, where ionic silver accumulates and binds to the gill epithelium. These bindings lead to inhibition of Na^+ and K^+-ATPase activity, whereby the active uptake of Na^+ and Cl^- is inhibited [13, 43, 44]. Such ion regulatory disturbances may ultimately be lethal to the fish [43]. Additionally, it has been suggested that silver ions partially inhibit the carbonic anhydrase enzyme, which catalyze the hydration of CO_2 to produce H^+ and HCO_3^-, which may be exchanged for external Na^+ and Cl^- [45]. This is, however, not the primary mechanism of silver toxicity in fish [46]. Although it appears that both nanosilver and ionic silver exert their toxicity in the gills of fish, different mechanisms of toxicity are probably in play. For instance, extravasations of blood were only observed in fish exposed to nanosilver. In gram-negative bacteria, the overall effect of nanosilver also differs from the effect of silver ions [37].

The zebrafish sensed the silver ions in the water displaying an avoidance reaction, where they increased their swimming activity and were trying to escape out of the tank. This behaviour was not observed among the controls or the nanosilver-exposed fish. Most likely, the 81 nm silver nanoparticles are too big to be sensed by olfaction as opposed to the silver ions with an ionic radius of 0.137 nm [1]. A behavioural avoidance response was also observed in rainbow trout exposed to copper, cobalt [47], and chromium [48]. It has been suggested that olfactory receptors detect copper in the water [47], which may also be true of ionic silver.

The LC_{50} value of silver nanoparticles estimated in the present study is higher than present concentrations in the aquatic environment [9]. However, point discharges may result in significantly higher local nanosilver concentrations, and the expected increase in the usage of nanosilver in the nearest future will undoubtedly result in increased concentrations in the aquatic environment.

Acknowledgments

This study was supported by a grant from the Danish Strategic Research Council (NaBIIT) 216-06-0015 (SUNANO). The authors are grateful to Per G. Henriksen for technical assistance. K. Bilberg and M. B. Hovgaard contributed equally to the work.

References

[1] H. Renner, "Silver, silver compounds, and silver alloys," in *Ullmann's Encylopedia of Industrial Chemistry*, John Wiley & Sons, New York, NY, USA, 2009.

[2] T. W. Purcell and J. J. Peters, "Sources of silver in the environment," *Environmental Toxicology and Chemistry*, vol. 17, no. 4, pp. 539–546, 1998.

[3] T. Vandevelde, H. Renner, and G. Schlamp, "Silver, silver compounds, and silver alloys," in *Ullmann's Encylopedia of Industrial Chemistry*, chapter 10, John Wiley & Sons, New York, NY, USA, 2009.

[4] I. Sondi and B. Salopek-Sondi, "Silver nanoparticles as antimicrobial agent: a case study on E. coli as a model for Gram-negative bacteria," *Journal of Colloid and Interface Science*, vol. 275, no. 1, pp. 177–182, 2004.

[5] T. M. Benn and P. Westerhoff, "Nanoparticle silver released into water from commercially available sock fabrics," *Environmental Science and Technology*, vol. 42, no. 11, pp. 4133–4139, 2008.

[6] T. F. Rozan, K. S. Hunter, and G. Benoit, "Silver in Fresh Water: sources, transport and fate in Connecticut rivers," in *Proceedings of the 3th Argentum International Conference on the Transport, Fate and Effects of Silver in the Environment*, pp. 181–184, Washington, DC, USA, August 1995.

[7] L. S. Wen, P. H. Santschi, G. A. Gill, C. L. Paternostro, and R. D. Lehman, "Colloidal and particulate silver in river and estuarine waters of Texas," *Environmental Science and Technology*, vol. 31, no. 3, pp. 723–731, 1997.

[8] C. Hogstrand and C. M. Wood, "Toward a better understanding of the bioavailability, physiology, and toxicity of silver in fish: implications for water quality criteria," *Environmental Toxicology and Chemistry*, vol. 17, no. 4, pp. 547–561, 1998.

[9] K. Tiede, M. Hassellöv, E. Breitbarth, Q. Chaudhry, and A. B. A. Boxall, "Considerations for environmental fate and ecotoxicity testing to support environmental risk assessments for engineered nanoparticles," *Journal of Chromatography A*, vol. 1216, no. 3, pp. 503–509, 2009.

[10] S. A. Blaser, M. Scheringer, M. MacLeod, and K. Hungerbühler, "Estimation of cumulative aquatic exposure and risk due to silver: contribution of nano-functionalized plastics and textiles," *Science of the Total Environment*, vol. 390, no. 2-3, pp. 396–409, 2008.

[11] A. R. Lima, C. Curtis, and D. E. Hammermeister, "Acute toxicity of silver to selected fish and invertebrates," *Bulletin of Environmental Contamination and Toxicology*, vol. 29, no. 2, pp. 184–189, 1982.

[12] A. V. Nebeker, C. K. McAuliffe, R. Mshar, and D. G. Stevens, "Toxicity of silver to steelhead and rainbow trout, fathead minnows and *Daphnia magna*," *Environmental Toxicology and Chemistry*, vol. 2, no. 1, pp. 95–104, 1983.

[13] T. P. Morgan and C. M. Wood, "A relationship between gill silver accumulation and acute silver toxicity in the freshwater rainbow trout: support for the acute silver biotic ligand model," *Environmental Toxicology and Chemistry*, vol. 23, no. 5, pp. 1261–1267, 2004.

[14] R. J. Griffitt, J. Luo, J. Gao, J. C. Bonzongo, and D. S. Barber, "Effects of particle composition and species on toxicity of metallic nanomaterials in aquatic organisms," *Environmental Toxicology and Chemistry*, vol. 27, no. 9, pp. 1972–1978, 2008.

[15] R. J. Griffitt, R. Weil, K. A. Hyndman et al., "Exposure to copper nanoparticles causes gill injury and acute lethality in zebrafish (*Danio rerio*)," *Environmental Science and Technology*, vol. 41, no. 23, pp. 8178–8186, 2007.

[16] G. Oberdörster, E. Oberdörster, and J. Oberdörster, "Nanotoxicology: an emerging discipline evolving from studies of ultrafine particles," *Environmental Health Perspectives*, vol. 113, no. 7, pp. 823–839, 2005.

[17] A. Nel, T. Xia, L. Mädler, and N. Li, "Toxic potential of materials at the nanolevel," *Science*, vol. 311, no. 5761, pp. 622–627, 2006.

[18] R. D. Handy and B. J. Shaw, "Ecotoxicity of nanomaterials to fish: challenges for ecotoxicity testing," *Integrated Environmental Assessment and Management*, vol. 3, no. 3, pp. 458–460, 2007.

[19] I. Blinova, A. Ivask, M. Heinlaan, M. Mortimer, and A. Kahru, "Ecotoxicity of nanoparticles of CuO and ZnO in natural water," *Environmental Pollution*, vol. 158, no. 1, pp. 41–47, 2010.

[20] K. W. Powers, S. C. Brown, V. B. Krishna, S. C. Wasdo, B. M. Moudgil, and S. M. Roberts, "Research strategies for safety evaluation of nanomaterials. Part VI. characterization of nanoscale particles for toxicological evaluation," *Toxicological Sciences*, vol. 90, no. 2, pp. 296–303, 2006.

[21] C. Nüsselin-Volhard and R. Dahm, *Zebrafish a Practial Approch*, Oxford University Press, New York, NY, USA, 2000.

[22] E. Navarro, F. Piccapietra, B. Wagner et al., "Toxicity of silver nanoparticles to Chlamydomonas reinhardtii," *Environmental Science and Technology*, vol. 42, no. 23, pp. 8959–8964, 2008.

[23] P. Hald, J. Becker, M. Bremholm et al., "Supercritical propanol-water synthesis and comprehensive size characterisation of highly crystalline anatase TiO_2 nanoparticles," *Journal of Solid State Chemistry*, vol. 179, no. 8, pp. 2674–2680, 2006.

[24] J. I. Langford and A. J. C. Wilson, "Scherrer after sixty years: a survey and some new results in the determination of crystallite size," *Journal of Applied Crystallography*, vol. 11, pp. 102–103, 1978.

[25] J. I. Langford, "A rapid method for analysing the breadths of diffraction and spectral lines using the Voigt function," *Journal of Applied Crystallography*, vol. 11, pp. 10–14, 1978.

[26] J. R. Lead and K. J. Wilkinson, "Aquatic colloids and nanoparticles: current knowledge and future trends," *Environmental Chemistry*, vol. 3, no. 3, pp. 159–171, 2006.

[27] L. H. Heckmann, M. B. Hovgaard, D. S. Sutherland, H. Autrup, F. Besenbacher, and J. J. Scott-Fordsmand, "Limit-test toxicity screening of selected inorganic nanoparticles to the earthworm *Eisenia fetida*," *Ecotoxicology*, vol. 20, pp. 226–233, 2011.

[28] J. I. Langford and D. Louër, "Powder diffraction," *Reports on Progress in Physics*, vol. 59, no. 2, pp. 131–234, 1996.

[29] L. Kvitek, A. Panacek, and J. Soukupova, "Effect of surfactants and polymers on stability and antibacterial activity of silver nanoparticles (NPs)," *The Journal of Physical Chemistry C*, vol. 112, pp. 5825–5834, 2008.

[30] J. Alifragis, A. K. Rizos, A. M. Tsatsakis, M. Tzatzarakis, and M. Shtilman, "New polymeric systems with controlled release action: a light scattering investigation," *Journal of Non-Crystalline Solids*, vol. 307–310, pp. 882–886, 2002.

[31] J. N. Israelachvili, *Intermolecular & Surface Forces*, Academic Press, London, UK, 2nd edition, 1991.

[32] J. E. Choi, S. Kim, J. H. Ahn et al., "Induction of oxidative stress and apoptosis by silver nanoparticles in the liver of adult zebrafish," *Aquatic Toxicology*, vol. 100, no. 2, pp. 151–159, 2010.

[33] Y. J. Chae, C. H. Pham, J. Lee, E. Bae, J. Yi, and M. B. Gu, "Evaluation of the toxic impact of silver nanoparticles on Japanese medaka (*Oryzias latipes*)," *Aquatic Toxicology*, vol. 94, no. 4, pp. 320–327, 2009.

[34] C. Hogstrand, F. Galvez, and C. M. Wood, "Toxicity, silver accumulation and metallothionein induction in freshwater rainbow trout during exposure to different silver salts," *Environmental Toxicology and Chemistry*, vol. 15, no. 7, pp. 1102–1108, 1996.

[35] N. R. Bury, F. Galvez, and C. M. Wood, "Effects of chloride, calcium, and dissolved organic carbon on silver toxicity: comparison between rainbow trout and fathead minnows," *Environmental Toxicology and Chemistry*, vol. 18, no. 1, pp. 56–62, 1999.

[36] R. Foldbjerg, P. Olesen, M. Hougaard, D. A. Dang, H. J. Hoffmann, and H. Autrup, "PVP-coated silver nanoparticles and silver ions induce reactive oxygen species, apoptosis and necrosis in THP-1 monocytes," *Toxicology Letters*, vol. 190, no. 2, pp. 156–162, 2009.

[37] J. R. Morones, J. L. Elechiguerra, A. Camacho et al., "The bactericidal effect of silver nanoparticles," *Nanotechnology*, vol. 16, no. 10, pp. 2346–2353, 2005.

[38] G. Laban, L. F. Nies, R. F. Turco, J. W. Bickham, and M. S. Sepúlveda, "The effects of silver nanoparticles on fathead minnow (*Pimephales promelas*) embryos," *Ecotoxicology*, vol. 19, no. 1, pp. 185–195, 2010.

[39] N. A. Webb and C. M. Wood, "Physiological analysis of the stress response associated with acute silver nitrate exposure in freshwater rainbow trout (*Oncorhynchus mykiss*)," *Environmental Toxicology and Chemistry*, vol. 17, no. 4, pp. 579–588, 1998.

[40] T. P. Morgan, M. Grosell, K. M. Gilmour, R. C. Playle, and C. M. Wood, "Time course analysis of the mechanism by which silver inhibits active Na^+ and Cl^- uptake in gills of rainbow trout," *American Journal of Physiology*, vol. 287, no. 1, pp. R234–R242, 2004.

[41] C. J. Smith, B. J. Shaw, and R. D. Handy, "Toxicity of single walled carbon nanotubes to rainbow trout, (*Oncorhynchus mykiss*): respiratory toxicity, organ pathologies, and other physiological effects," *Aquatic Toxicology*, vol. 82, no. 2, pp. 94–109, 2007.

[42] G. Federici, B. J. Shaw, and R. D. Handy, "Toxicity of titanium dioxide nanoparticles to rainbow trout (*Oncorhynchus mykiss*): gill injury, oxidative stress, and other physiological effects," *Aquatic Toxicology*, vol. 84, no. 4, pp. 415–430, 2007.

[43] C. M. Wood, C. Hogstrand, F. Galvez, and R. S. Munger, "The physiology of waterborne silver toxicity in freshwater rainbow trout (*Oncorhynchus mykiss*) 1. The effects of ionic Ag^+," *Aquatic Toxicology*, vol. 35, no. 2, pp. 93–109, 1996.

[44] H. T. Ratte, "Bioaccumulation and toxicity of silver compounds: a review," *Environmental Toxicology and Chemistry*, vol. 18, no. 1, pp. 89–108, 1999.

[45] I. J. Morgan, R. P. Henry, and C. M. Wood, "The mechanism of acute silver nitrate toxicity in freshwater rainbow trout (*Oncorhynchus mykiss*) is inhibition of gill Na^+ and Cl^- transport," *Aquatic Toxicology*, vol. 38, no. 1–3, pp. 145–163, 1997.

[46] C. M. Wood, R. C. Playle, and C. Hogstrand, "Physiology and modeling of mechanisms of silver uptake and toxicity in fish," *Environmental Toxicology and Chemistry*, vol. 18, no. 1, pp. 71–83, 1999.

[47] J. A. Hansen, J. C. A. Marr, J. Lipton, D. Cacela, and H. L. Bergman, "Differences in neurobehavioral responses of chinook salmon (*Oncorhynchus tshawytscha*) and rainbow trout (*Oncorhynchus mykiss*) exposed to copper and cobalt: behavioral avoidance," *Environmental Toxicology and Chemistry*, vol. 18, no. 9, pp. 1972–1978, 1999.

[48] G. Svecevičius, "Avoidance response of rainbow trout *Oncorhynchus mykiss* to hexavalent chromium solutions," *Bulletin of Environmental Contamination and Toxicology*, vol. 79, no. 6, pp. 596–600, 2007.

Function of Serum Complement in Drinking Water Arsenic Toxicity

Laila N. Islam, M. Shamim Hasan Zahid, A. H. M. Nurun Nabi, and Mahmud Hossain

Department of Biochemistry and Molecular Biology, University of Dhaka, Dhaka 1000, Bangladesh

Correspondence should be addressed to Laila N. Islam, lailanislam@yahoo.com

Academic Editor: Ninoslav Djelic

Serum complement function was evaluated in 125 affected subjects suffering from drinking water arsenic toxicity. Their mean duration of exposure was 7.4 ± 5.3 yrs, and the levels of arsenic in drinking water and urine samples were 216 ± 211 and 223 ± 302 μg/L, respectively. The mean bactericidal activity of complement from the arsenic patients was 92% and that in the unexposed controls was 99% ($P < 0.01$), but heat-inactivated serum showed slightly elevated activity than in controls. In patients, the mean complement C3 was 1.56 g/L, and C4 was 0.29 g/L compared to 1.68 g/L and 0.25 g/L, respectively, in the controls. The mean IgG in the arsenic patients was 24.3 g/L that was highly significantly elevated ($P < 0.001$). Arsenic patients showed a significant direct correlation between C3 and bactericidal activity ($P = 0.014$). Elevated levels of C4 indicated underutilization and possibly impaired activity of the classical complement pathway. We conclude reduced function of serum complement in drinking water arsenic toxicity.

1. Introduction

Drinking water contamination with high levels arsenic in Bangladesh is the largest mass poisoning of a population in history, with millions of people exposed [1]. The mean arsenic concentrations in the drinking water of the exposed populations in Bangladesh are more than twenty times higher [2] than the maximum permissible limit recommended by the Environmental Protection Agency of the USA that has set the level at 10 micrograms per liter or 10 parts per billion. A total of 61 out of 64 districts in Bangladesh are already affected with high levels of arsenic in ground water. We found melanosis with black/white pigmentation on skin, keratosis, lump, and nodule formation on feet and hands in people chronically exposed to high levels of arsenic in drinking water [2]. It had been reported that symptoms of chronic arsenic toxicity develop insidiously after 6 months to 2 years or more of exposure [3].

The general adverse health effects associated with human exposure to arsenicals include cardiovascular diseases, developmental abnormalities, neurologic and neurobehavioral disorders, diabetes, fibrosis of the liver and lung, and haematological disorders [4]. We reported, that apart from the classical arsenical skin lesions, a large proportion of arsenicosis patients had breathing problems, gastric and abdominal pain, backache, headache, pain all over the body, palpitation, anemia, and weakness. Arsenic toxicity caused respiratory complications [5], modulation of serum metabolites [6], and affected the immune system with low leukocyte count [2], and elevated levels of serum immunoglobulins [5]. However, the functions of serum complements have not been studied in the arsenicosis patients suffering from such a wide range of complications.

The complement system plays an important role in defense against pyogenic infections. Complements are innate components of the immune system whose activation leads to robust and efficient proteolytic cascades, which terminate in opsonization and lysis of the pathogen as well as in the generation of the classical inflammatory response through the production of potent proinflammatory molecules [7]. Complement activation also participates in clearance of apoptotic cells and immune complexes. Recently, it was also recognized that complement plays a key role in adaptive immunity by modulating and modifying the T-cell responses [8]. Therefore, the complement systems may be regarded as a link between innate and adaptive immunity and is critically involved in the pathogenesis and prevention of immune complex diseases, such as systemic lupus erythematosus (SLE) [9].

The immunotoxicity of heavy metals has not been extensively studied. Bernier et al. [10] found that heavy metals including mercury, lead, and cadmium present in small amounts in the Great Lakes water and fish and exposure of humans to these metals via the ingestion of contaminated food especially fish alter a number of parameters of the host's immune system leading to increased susceptibility to infections, autoimmune diseases, and allergic manifestations. In another study, it was found that mercury can induce autoimmune disease both in humans and experimental animals, while cadmium treatment of rats and mice results in autoimmune responses that vary with species and inbred strain of animals [11]. The peripheral blood neutrophils of workers occupationally exposed to lead showed reduced chemotaxis and nitroblue tetrazolium dye reduction, suggesting immune dysfunction may be a sensitive indicator of lead exposure [12]. In view of lack of information on the humoral immune response, this study was designed to evaluate serum complement function in arsenicosis patients.

2. Materials and Methods

2.1. Study Area. The study areas of this investigation were the arsenic endemic rural villages of Rajarampur, Achinpara, Chandnai, and Bottola under the northwestern district of Chapainawabganj where arsenic contamination in drinking water was first detected in Bangladesh in 1993 and the village Ilumdi under Araihazar of Narayanganj that is about 35 km southeast of the capital city Dhaka.

2.2. Arsenicosis Patient Inclusion Criteria. Subjects consuming drinking water that contained arsenic levels greater than the tolerable limit recommended by the WHO (50 μg/L), not taking medicine for any illness, and having signs of arsenic toxicity were enrolled in this study as the patients. Their source of drinking water was tube well or artisan well. The signs of arsenic toxicity (arsenicosis) were assessed on the basis of appearance of skin lesions [2, 5, 6]. After informed consent, the researchers with the help of a public health nurse interviewed all the patients personally. The information on symptoms and complications of arsenic toxicity, duration of exposure, anthropometric parameters including age, height, and body weight of the patients were recorded on preformed questionnaires.

2.3. Sample Collection. Blood samples (about 3 mL) were collected from the subjects with their full consent to participate in this study. A total of 250 blood samples were collected of which 125 were from patients with arsenic toxicity (arsenicosis), 95 from unexposed subjects living in the same area as the patients but drinking safe water and with no sign of arsenic toxicity, and the remaining from unexposed subjects living in the city. Spot urine and drinking water samples were also collected from each individual. All samples were collected in fresh, sterile universals. The blood sample was allowed to clot, and serum was separated immediately after collection. The frozen sera were transported to the laboratory in ice-packed containers and stored at −80°C until analyzed.

2.4. Analyses of Arsenic. Concentrated nitric acid was mixed with the drinking water samples at 1 mL per liter and stored at 4°C until analyzed. The urine samples were frozen immediately after collection. Arsenic content in the water and urine samples were measured following the standard procedure by using a Flow Injection—Hydride Generation—Atomic Absorption Spectrophotometer, and the results were expressed in μg/L.

2.5. Assay of Complement-Mediated Bactericidal Activity. *Escherichia coli* DH5α was grown in nutrient broth for 14 hour at 37°C in an orbital shaker. The bacterial cells were harvested, washed two times using excess of PBS and then the suspension was adjusted to 0.600 O.D. at 620 nm. Immediately, aliquots of 200 μL of the bacterial cell suspensions (BCS) were taken into separate tubes, 20 μL of serum was added to each tube, and the mixture was incubated for 30 minutes at 37°C. At the end of incubation, the remaining viable cells were serially diluted with PBS to 1 : 10,000. An aliquot of 20 μL of this dilution was spread on each of 3 agar plates and incubated for 16 hours at 37°C. The number of colonies formed was counted, and the mean value for each serum was taken from the readings of 3 plates. For the negative control experiments, 20 μL of PBS (medium) was added to the BCS instead of serum, incubated, and then serially diluted with PBS to 1 : 50,000. An aliquot of 20 μL of this dilution was spread on each of 3 agar plates.

2.6. Assay of Complement-Inactivated Bactericidal Activity. Complement proteins were inactivated by heat treatment at 56°C for 30 minutes in a water bath and then used (20 μL) to test for bactericidal activity. Both the PBS (control) and bacteria treated with inactivated serum preparations were serially diluted to 1 : 50,000. The rest of the procedure was as described before.

2.7. Calculation of Bactericidal Activity. Bactericidal activity was calculated using the following formula, as described elsewhere [13, 14]. For the control, if the mean colony-forming unit (cfu) on the plate was Nc, then 1 mL of the original bacterial cell suspension contained Nc × 50 × 50,000 cfu.

For the test serum, if the mean cfu on the plate was Ns, then 1 mL of the bacterial cell suspension treated with serum complement contained Ns × 50 × 10,000 cfu. Therefore,

$$\%\text{bactericidal activity} = \frac{(\text{Nc} \times 50 \times 50{,}000) - (\text{Ns} \times 50 \times 10{,}000)}{\text{Nc} \times 50 \times 50{,}000} \times 100. \quad (1)$$

The bactericidal activity (%) of the inactivated serum for the mean cfu, Ni, was

$$\frac{(\mathrm{Nc} \times 50 \times 50,000) - (\mathrm{Ni} \times 50 \times 50,000)}{\mathrm{Nc} \times 50 \times 50,000} \times 100. \quad (2)$$

2.8. Determination of Serum C3, C4, and IgG. Quantitative estimates of serum complement components C3 and C4 were performed using a TURBOX plus Analyzer, Orion Diagnostica, Finland. The method was based on the principle of immunoprecipitation reaction of a specific antibody with its antigen. The light scattering caused by antigen-antibody complexes was measured after incubation. The intensity of the scattered light was directly proportional to the concentration of the tested complement protein present in the serum sample. IgG was measured by immunonephelometry using DADE Behring reagents (USA) and an autoanalyzer. The procedure was according to the supplier's recommended protocol. The results were expressed in g/L.

2.9. Statistical Analysis. Data analyses were carried out using the Statistical Package for Social Sciences (SPSS). The methods used were independent t-test for comparison of two groups (arsenicosis patients and control subjects), Pearson correlations, and simple statistics. The results were considered significant when P was ≤ 0.05.

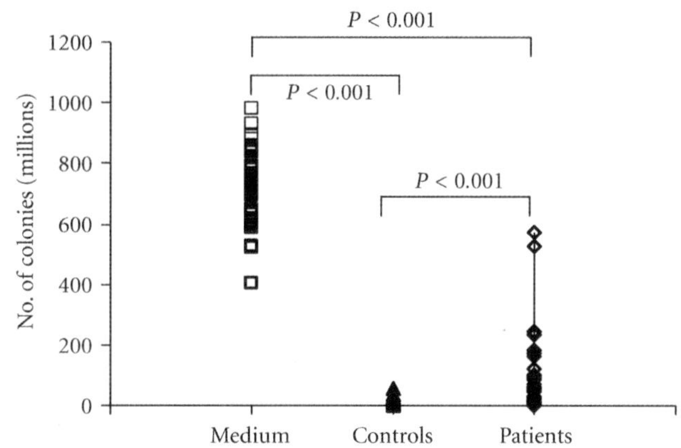

FIGURE 1: Number of *Escherichia coli* DH5α colonies (million cfu/mL) grown on agar plates from the bacterial cell suspension in PBS (Medium) and after the action of serum complements from healthy controls and arsenic patients. Before plating, the bacterial cell suspensions were diluted with PBS to 1 : 50,000 in Medium, and 1 : 10,000 both for serum samples from control subjects and arsenic patients. Compared with the Medium, complements from both the sera exhibited highly significant bacteriolytic effects ($P < 0.001$), while complements from arsenic patients showed significantly diminished bacteriolytic effects compared to the control subjects ($P < 0.001$).

3. Results

3.1. Baseline Characteristics of the Study Subjects. The baseline characteristics showed the age of the patients varied from 14–65 yrs, and the mean body mass index (BMI) was 20.9 ± 3.5. In the control subjects, the age varied from 19 to 72 yrs, and the mean BMI was 22.4 ± 2.7. The whole population of patients had a mean monthly family income of about Bangladeshi Taka 5,000 (about USD 80) that varied from Taka 1,000–16,000. About one-third of the patients had no formal education; while 30% attended primary schools and the remaining had secondary school and higher education. The number of family members of the patients varied from 2 to 9 with a mean value of 5.0 ± 1.5. Of the unexposed subjects, only about 5% were illiterate, while the education levels of the rest were from primary to higher. The monthly family income of the controls varied from Taka 1,500–25,000 with a mean of about Taka 7,000 (USD 112). Their family members varied from 2 to 6.

3.2. Clinical Symptoms and Complications of Arsenic Toxicity. The clinical symptoms based on skin manifestations were recorded on questionnaire after interviewing and careful examination of the subjects. The symptoms included diffused and spotted melanosis with black and white appearances, rough and mottled skin, keratosis or hardening of the soles and palm with often formation of nodules and cracks. Spotted melanosis was more often seen on the throat, chest, back, or limbs. The duration of exposure has been found directly related to the severity of clinical disease. About one-third of the patients suffered from severe skin irritation including itchy rash. There was high prevalence of respiratory complications including asthma, bronchitis and cough. Long-term exposure to arsenic also caused conjunctivitis, disturbances in the peripheral vascular and nervous systems, and gangrene of the limbs. The patients had the mean duration of arsenic exposure for 7.4 ± 5.3 yrs that varied from 1 to 25 yrs with a median of 6.0 yrs.

3.3. Levels of Arsenic in the Drinking Water and Urine Samples. It was found that the drinking water of the patients contained 67–875 μg/L of arsenic with the mean value of 216.2 ± 210.6 μg/L and median of 156 μg/L. The mean level of arsenic in the spot urine samples of the patients was 223.2 ± 302.4 μg/L, while the median was 114.0 μg/L and the maximum value was 1764 μg/L. On the other hand, the mean arsenic concentrations in the drinking water and urine samples of the unexposed (control) populations were 11.3 and 29.4 μg/L, respectively. Statistical analysis showed the levels of arsenic in the drinking water and urine samples of the patients were highly positively correlated ($P < 0.001$).

3.4. Complement-Mediated Bactericidal Activity. It was found that the numbers of *Escherichia coli* DH5α colonies grown on agar plates without treating the bacterial cell suspensions with serum complement (PBS alone, negative control) varied from 401–978 × 10^6 cfu/mL with a median of 714.5 × 10^6 cfu/mL. On the other hand, the numbers of colonies formed after treating the BCS with serum complements from control healthy subjects varied from 1.1–54.8 × 10^6 cfu/mL with a median of 4 × 10^6 cfu/mL, and, after treating with serum complements from arsenic patients, the number of colonies varied from 1.5–570 × 10^6 cfu/mL with a median of 47.3 × 10^6 cfu/mL (Figure 1). Compared

Table 1: Complement-mediated and complement-inactivated bactericidal activities in the serum of arsenic patients and control subjects.

Study subjects	% Bactericidal activity (mean ± SD)	
	Complement-mediated	Complement inactivated
Arsenic patients $N = 125$	92.1 ± 16.0 Median: 97.3 Range: 24.6–99.9	19.4 ± 8.6 Median: 18.6 Range: 3.3–33.0
Control subjects $N = 125$	99.1 ± 1.4 Median: 99.4 Range: 92.2–100	18.2 ± 6.9 Median: 17.1 Range: 6.2–35.3
Statistics (P value)	<0.01	NS

to the negative control experiments, complements from both healthy subjects and arsenic patients exhibited highly significant bacteriolytic effects ($P < 0.001$). However, complements from arsenic patients showed significantly diminished bacteriolytic effects (assessed by the large number of cfu) compared to the control subjects ($P < 0.001$). The bactericidal activity of complements from the arsenic patients varied widely from 24.6 to 99.9% compared to 92.2–100% in the control healthy subjects (Table 1). The complement-mediated bactericidal activity of the arsenic patients was significantly lower than that of the control subjects ($P < 0.01$).

3.5. Effect of Complement-Inactivation on Bactericidal Activity. The bactericidal activity of the complement-inactivated serum from the control subjects varied from 6.2 to 35.3% whereas that from the arsenic patients varied from 3.3 to 33.0%. These results presented in Table 1 indicated that the complement-inactivated bactericidal activity of the arsenic patients was not significantly different from that of the control subjects.

3.6. Levels of Complement Component C3. It was found that, of the total arsenic patients, about 93% had normal levels of serum complement component C3 (normal level: 0.9–2.1 g/L) whereas 5% had above normal, and only 2% had below normal levels. On the other hand, 85% of the control subjects had normal levels, and the remaining 15% had above normal levels of serum complement C3. The mean level of C3 in the arsenic patients was 1.56 ± 0.36 g/L and that in the healthy control subjects was 1.68 ± 0.35 g/L. These results showed arsenic patients had lower levels of serum complement component C3 than the healthy subjects (Table 2).

3.7. Levels of Complement Component C4. The levels of complement component C4 in about 20% of the patients were found to be above normal. The remaining patients had serum C4 levels within the normal value (0.1–0.4 g/L). Among the control subjects, 90% had normal C4, 4% had above normal and the remaining 6% had below normal levels. The whole population of patients had the mean C4 level of 0.29 ± 0.11 g/L while that in the healthy control

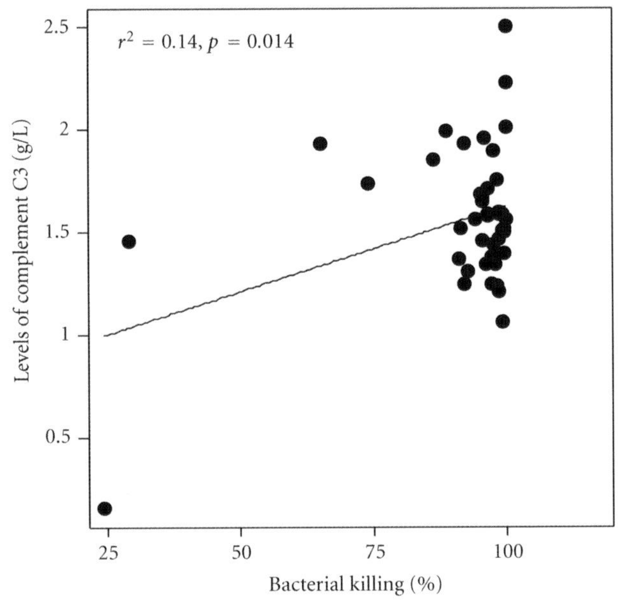

Figure 2: Correlation between the levels of serum complement C3 (g/L) from arsenicosis patients with bactericidal activity (bacterial killing, %) on *Escherichia coli* DH5α cells. The figure shows bacterial killing decreased as the levels of C3 decreased in arsenic toxicity, giving a direct correlation ($P = 0.014$).

subjects was 0.25 ± 0.11 g/L. These data showed although the differences were not significant ($P < 0.06$), the complement component C4 levels in the arsenic patients were higher than that in the control subjects (Table 2).

3.8. Correlation of the Levels of C3 with Bactericidal Activity. It was found that about one-third of the total arsenic patients tended to have lower levels of C3; however, these values were around the lower limit of the normal range showing a mean value of 1.19 ± 0.42 g/L with corresponding bactericidal activity of 67.4 ± 20.2%. Analysis of the whole population data ($N = 125$) showed a significant direct correlation between the levels of C3 and complement-mediated bactericidal activity ($P = 0.014$) among the arsenicosis patients (Figure 2).

3.9. Levels of Serum IgG. To find out an explanation whether immunoglobulin G (IgG) was responsible for enhanced killing of bacteria after complement inactivation, IgG levels were measured in the fresh serum. It was found that arsenic patients had the mean serum IgG level of 24.3 ± 7.5 g/L compared to 13.8 ± 7.8 g/L in the healthy control subjects (normal level: 7.0–16.0 g/L). Statistical analysis showed IgG levels in the arsenicosis patients were significantly higher than that in the control subjects ($P < 0.001$). The results are shown in Table 2.

4. Discussions

Millions of people worldwide are chronically exposed to arsenic through drinking water, including an estimated 35–77 million people in Bangladesh [15]. In the present study,

TABLE 2: Levels of serum complements C3 and C4 and immunoglobulin G in the arsenic patients and control subjects.

Study subjects	Concentration in serum: (Mean ± SD) g/L		
	Complement C3 NV: 0.9–2.1	Complement C4 NV: 0.1–0.4	Immunoglobulin G NV: 7.0–16.0
Arsenic patients $N = 125$	1.56 ± 0.36 Median: 1.56 Range: 0.16–2.50	0.29 ± 0.11 Median: 0.27 Range: 0.1–0.57	24.3 ± 7.5 Median: 22.7 Range: 7.7–49.3
Control subjects $N = 125$	1.68 ± 0.35 Median: 1.67 Range: 0.9–2.64	0.25 ± 0.11 Median: 0.22 Range: 0.05–0.49	13.8 ± 7.8 Median: 10.8 Range: 4.2–31.6
Statistics (*P* value)	NS	NS (0.06)	<0.001

NV: normal value; NS: not significant.

skin manifestations have been found as the prime and common features of arsenic toxicity that has been considered as definite exposure [2]. About 27% of the enrolled patients had BMI lower than 18.5 compared to only 6% of the control subjects. Thus, a relation between arsenic toxicity and poor nutritional status (low BMI) was confirmed in the present study, as described earlier [2]. It had been reported that infection could rapidly lead to nutritional stress and weight loss, thereby worsening nutritional status and immunologic function [16–18]. In a prospective cohort study on 14 patients with severe anorexia nervosa having BMI less than 14.0, serum complement C3 levels were found significantly lower than in the healthy controls [19]. We found a direct correlation, though marginally insignificant, between nutritional status (BMI) and serum complement protein C3 in the arsenicosis patients ($P = 0.057$). Poor nutritional status of the affected subjects might have a role in high retention of arsenic in the body.

Measurements of complement proteins C3 and C4 aid in the diagnosis of immunologic disorders, especially those associated with deficiencies of complement components. The proteins of complement system play important role in the innate immune response. The results of some clinical studies have suggested that complement activation exacerbated myocardial defect following ischaemic injury [20], has been involved in the generation of spontaneous atherosclerotic lesions, and may indeed be an initiating factor in lesion formation [21]. Assessment of the complement C3 and C4 concentration ratio (C3/C4 ratio) in serum has been suggested as a potential measurement to predict cardiovascular attacks [22]. New studies point to the complex interplay between the complement cascade and adaptive immune response, and complement is also being studied in association with ischemic injury as a target of therapy [9].

Escherichia coli DH5α used in this study is a non-pathogenic bacterium, and, therefore, no appreciable levels of specific antibody should be present in the sera of human subjects against this organism. Therefore, killing of bacteria would be solely due to serum complement. We found that the complement-mediated bactericidal activity in the patients was significantly lower than that in the control group. We also found the concentration of C3 in the arsenicosis patients was lower but that of C4 was higher, although none was significantly different than in the control subjects. However, about one-third of the arsenic patients had significantly lower values of C3 compared to the controls ($P < 0.001$). These sera containing lower levels of C3 showed highly significantly reduced bactericidal activity (67.4 ± 20.2%) compared to the healthy controls (99.1 ± 1.4%) and showed a value of $P < 0.001$.

The lower levels of C3 in the arsenic patients might be the reason for reduced complement function since a significant direct correlation was found between the levels of C3 and complement-mediated bactericidal activity ($P = 0.014$). The complement-inactivated bactericidal activity of the patients was similar to that of the control group. We reported earlier that the arsenic patients had significantly elevated levels of serum IgG, IgA, and IgE [5]. Since the arsenic patients suffer from melanosis, keratosis, cracks on foot soles and palms that might harbor bacterial infections, their sera might contain high levels of IgG antibodies against these organisms. These IgG antibodies might play a role in enhanced killing of bacterial cells, while the serum complements had been destroyed by heat inactivation. We reported similar findings in the pulmonary tuberculosis patients who had chronic lung infection [14].

The role of serum complement in immunotoxicity of heavy metals remains poorly understood. It had been reported in an old study that the lead workers had lower serum complement C3 and immunoglobulins IgG, IgM and IgA levels, as well as lower salivary IgA levels than the reference subjects [23]. In another study, the effects of gallium arsenide (GaAs) exposure as a single intratracheal dose on immunocompetence of B6C3F1 female mice were investigated and found that GaAs affected both humoral and cellular immune parameters in the mice and impaired the ability of the immune system to protect against B16F10 tumor challenge [24]. It had been found that bivalent nickel or cobalt at concentrations below 100 micro-M could stimulate the conversion of complement protein C3 to C3b faster than magnesium, which was the natural cofactor in the alternative pathway of complement activation, suggesting that the increased rate of C3-fragment production induced by nickel or cobalt ions was central for the immunotoxicity of these metals [25].

Deficiencies of complement proteins are frequently associated with an immunodeficiency state in which the patients suffer with recurrent bacterial infections from organisms that are normally susceptible to opsonization or lysis by complement. A recent study has shown low serum complement level in chronic liver disease significantly increases the risk of spontaneous bacterial peritonitis in children [26]. In patients with nonalcoholic liver cirrhosis, serum bactericidal activity had been found to be reduced and complement proteins C3 and C4 were found to have significantly low values [27]. In the arsenicosis patients, suppressed complement function might be a direct effect of chronic arsenic toxicity. It may be recalled that zymogen forms of complement protein C3 are activated both by the alternative and classical complement pathways, thereby making the activated fragment C3b takes part in bactericidal activity by either or both of these pathways. On the other hand, complement C4 takes part only in the classical pathway. Our finding of elevated levels of C4 in about 20% of the patients indicated underutilization of complement C4 and hence possibly suppressed activity of the classical complement pathway in drinking water arsenic toxicity.

5. Conclusion

Lower levels of serum complement protein C3 in the arsenicosis patients and reduced complement-mediated bactericidal activity reveal serum complement functions are suppressed in drinking water arsenic toxicity. The findings from this preliminary study show immunotoxicity of arsenic resulting impaired complement function that requires further investigation on a large population.

Acknowledgments

This work was supported by research grants from the Ministry of Science and Information & Communication Technology, Government of Bangladesh, and the University Grants Commission of Bangladesh. The authors thank Dr. M. M. Hoque Bakul and Ms. Nasima Begum of Chapainawabganj for helping them collecting arsenic samples from the northwestern region; Mr. M. Shafiul Alam for helping them collecting arsenic samples from Araihazar; Mr. Mahfuzur Rahman, Scientific Officer, BCSIR, Dhaka, Mr. M. Aktar Hossain of Bangladesh Medical College Hospital, and Mr. M. Saiful Islam of BIRDEM Hospital, Dhaka, and all the participants of this study.

References

[1] A. H. Smith, E. O. Lingas, and M. Rahman, "Contamination of drinking-water by arsenic in Bangladesh: a public health emergency," *Bulletin of the World Health Organization*, vol. 78, no. 9, pp. 1093–1103, 2000.

[2] L. N. Islam, A. H. M. N. Nabi, M. M. Rahman, M. A. Khan, and A. I. Kazi, "Association of clinical complications with nutritional status and the prevalence of leukopenia among arsenic patients in Bangladesh," *International Journal of Environmental Research and Public Health*, vol. 1, no. 2, pp. 74–82, 2004.

[3] M. M. Rahman, U. K. Chowdhury, S. C. Mukherjee et al., "Chronic arsenic toxicity in Bangladesh and West Bengal, India—a review and commentary," *Journal of Clinical Toxicology*, vol. 39, no. 7, pp. 683–700, 2001.

[4] C. H. Tseng, "Metabolism of inorganic arsenic and non-cancerous health hazards associated with chronic exposure in humans," *Journal of Environmental Biology*, vol. 28, no. 2, pp. 349–357, 2007.

[5] L. N. Islam, A. H. M. N. Nabi, M. M. Rahman, and M. S. H. Zahid, "Association of respiratory complications and elevated serum immunoglobulins with drinking water arsenic toxicity in human," *Journal of Environmental Science and Health*, vol. 42, no. 12, pp. 1807–1814, 2007.

[6] A. H. M. N. Nabi, M. M. Rahman, and L. N. Islam, "Evaluation of biochemical changes in chronic arsenic poisoning among Bangladeshi patients," *International Journal of Environmental Research and Public Health*, vol. 2, no. 3-4, pp. 385–393, 2005.

[7] J. R. Dunkelberger and W. C. Song, "Complement and its role in innate and adaptive immune responses," *Cell Research*, vol. 20, no. 1, pp. 34–50, 2010.

[8] H. Rus, C. Cudrici, and F. Niculescu, "Defective neutrophil function in workers occupationally exposed to lead," *Immunologic Research*, vol. 33, pp. 103–112, 2005.

[9] R. K. Chaganti and R. A. Schwartz, "Complement deficiencies," in *Drug, Diseases and Procedures*, 2009.

[10] J. Bernier, P. Brousseau, K. Krzystyniak, H. Tryphonas, and M. Fournier, "Immunotoxicity of heavy metals in relation to Great Lakes," *Environmental Health Perspectives*, vol. 103, no. 9, pp. 23–34, 1995.

[11] P. E. Bigazzi, "Autoimmunity and heavy metals," *Lupus*, vol. 3, no. 6, pp. 449–453, 1994.

[12] M. L. S. Queiroz, M. Almeida, M. I. Gallao, and N. F. Hoehr, "Defective neutrophil function in workers occuptionally exposed to lead," *Pharmacology and Toxicology*, vol. 72, no. 2, pp. 73–77, 1993.

[13] L. N. Islam, M. Hossain, and M. S. H. Zahid, "Complement mediated bactericidal activity and humoral immune response in type 2 diabetes mellitus," *International Journal of Diabetes and Metabolism*, vol. 14, no. 2, pp. 92–97, 2006.

[14] K. J. Ferdous, R. Sultana, M. Hossain, M. S. H. Zahid, and L. N. Islam, "Evaluation of the humoral immune response in pulmonary tuberculosis patients," *Research Journal of Immunology*, vol. 1, pp. 36–44, 2008.

[15] M. Argos, T. Kalra, P. J. Rathouz et al., "Arsenic exposure from drinking water, and all-cause and chronic-disease mortalities in Bangladesh (HEALS): a prospective cohort study," *The Lancet*, vol. 376, no. 9737, pp. 252–258, 2010.

[16] G. T. Keusch, "Nutrition and infection," in *Current Clinical Topics in Infectious Diseases*, J. S. Remington and M. N. Swartz, Eds., pp. 106–133, McGraw-Hill, New York, NY, USA, 1984.

[17] G. T. Keusch, "Nutrition and infection," in *Modern Nutrition in Health and Disease*, M. E. Shils, J. A. Ol-son, and M. Shike, Eds., pp. 1241–1258, Lea & Febiger, Philadelphia, Penn, USA, 1994.

[18] R. K. Chandra, "Nutrition and immunity: lessons from the past and new insights into the future," *American Journal of Clinical Nutrition*, vol. 53, no. 5, pp. 1087–1101, 1991.

[19] M. A. Flierl, J. L. Gaudiani, A. L. Sabel, C. S. Long, P. F. Stahel, and P. S. Mehler, "Complement C3 serum levels in anorexia nervosa: a potential biomarker for the severity of disease?" *Annals of General Psychiatry*, vol. 10, pp. 16–20, 2011.

[20] M. Gardinali, L. Conciato, C. Cafaro, and A. Agostino, "Complement system in coronary heart disease: a review," *Immunopharmacology*, vol. 30, no. 2, pp. 105–117, 1995.

[21] J. Torzewski, R. Oldroyd, P. Lachmann, C. Fitzsimmons, D. Proudfoot, and D. Bowyer, "Complement-induced release

of monocyte chemotactic protein-1 from human smooth muscle cells: a possible initiating event in atherosclerotic lesion formation," *Arteriosclerosis, Thrombosis, and Vascular Biology*, vol. 16, no. 5, pp. 673–677, 1996.

[22] A. Palikhe, J. Sinisalo, M. Seppänen et al., "Serum complement C3/C4 ratio, a novel marker for recurrent cardiovascular events," *American Journal of Cardiology*, vol. 99, no. 7, pp. 890–895, 2007.

[23] U. Ewers, R. Stiller Winkler, and H. Idel, "Serum immunoglobulin, complement C3, and salivary IgA levels in lead workers," *Environmental Research*, vol. 29, no. 2, pp. 351–357, 1982.

[24] E. E. Sikorski, J. A. McCay, K. L. White, S. G. Bradley, and A. E. Munson, "Immunotoxicity of the semiconductor gallium arsenide in female B6C3F1 mice," *Fundamental and Applied Toxicology*, vol. 13, no. 4, pp. 843–858, 1989.

[25] F. Acevedo and O. Vesterberg, "Nickel and cobalt activate complement factor C3 faster than magnesium," *Toxicology*, vol. 185, no. 1-2, pp. 9–16, 2003.

[26] B. Fatemeh, P. Simin, K. H. Reza, M. H. Reza, and M. Toktam, "Evaluation of complement function in children with chronic liver disease," *Middle-East Journal of Scientific Research*, vol. 5, pp. 498–502, 2010.

[27] H. E. Akalin, Y. Laleli, and H. Telatar, "Serum bactericidal and opsonic activities in patients with non-alcoholic cirrhosis," *Quarterly Journal of Medicine*, vol. 56, no. 220, pp. 431–437, 1985.

16

Phospholipogenic Pharmaceuticals Are Associated with a Higher Incidence of Histological Findings than Nonphospholipogenic Pharmaceuticals in Preclinical Toxicology Studies

Linda R. Barone,[1] Scott Boyer,[2] James R. Damewood, Jr,[3] James Fikes,[4] and Paul J. Ciaccio[4]

[1] *Biologics Research, Janssen Research and Development, LLC, 145 King of Prussia Road, Radnor, PA 19087, USA*
[2] *Safety Assessment, AstraZeneca Pharmaceuticals, Pepparedsleden 1, 431 83 Mölndal, Sweden*
[3] *Haskell Global Centers for Health and Environmental Sciences, DuPont Central Research and Development, Newark, DE 19711, USA*
[4] *Safety Assessment, AstraZeneca Pharmaceuticals, 35 Gatehouse Drive, Waltham, MA 02451, USA*

Correspondence should be addressed to Paul J. Ciaccio, paul.ciaccio@astrazeneca.com

Academic Editor: J. J. Stegeman

While phospholipidosis is thought to be an adaptive response to chemical challenge, many phospholipogenic compounds are known to display adverse effects in preclinical species and humans. To investigate the link between phospholipogenic administration and incidence of preclinical histological signals, an internal AstraZeneca *in vivo* toxicology report database was searched to identify phospholipogenic and nonphospholipogenic compounds. The datasets assembled comprised 46 phospholipogenic and 62 nonphospholipogenic compounds. The phospholipogenic potential of these compounds was confirmed by a pathologist's interpretation and was supported by well-validated *in silico* and *in vitro* models. The phospholipogenic dataset contained 37 bases, 4 neutral compounds, 3 zwitterions, and 1 acid, whereas the nonphospholipogenic dataset contained 9 bases, 34 neutrals, 1 zwitterion, and 18 acids. Histologic findings were tracked for adrenal gland; bone marrow; kidney; liver; lung; lymph node; spleen; thymus; and reproductive organs. On average, plasma exposures were higher in animals dosed with the nonphospholipogenics. Phospholipogenics yielded proportionally more histologic changes (exclusive of phospholipidosis itself) in all organs. Statistically significant higher frequencies of liver necrosis, alveolitis/pneumonitis, as well as lymphocytolysis in the thymus, lymph nodes, and spleen occurred in response to phospholipogenics compared to that for nonphospholipogenics.

1. Introduction

Drug-induced phospholipidosis (PLD) is a lipid storage disorder characterized by the intralysosomal accumulation of polar lipids, membranous lamellar inclusions, and drug. The cytological features of PLD mimic inherited lipidoses [1]. Common primary tissue targets are alveolar macrophages, hepatic Kupffer cells, bile duct epithelia, and peripheral blood mononuclear cells, although numerous other cellular targets have been reported. Many marketed and experimental drugs have been reported to cause PLD preclinically [2]. Most have basic and hydrophobic physicochemical properties (amphiphilic cations) that enable binding with phospholipids, crossing of biological membranes, and lysomotropism (partitioning of drug into lysosomes once it is protonated at acidic intralysosomal pH) [3]. Lysomotropic properties and drug accumulation potential are underscored by studies employing lysosomal modulators which have a demonstrated ability to abolish the pH gradient from cytoplasm to lysosome, preclude accumulation of drug in the lysosome (depot effect), and/or rescue cells *in vitro* [4–6].

There is a consensus view that PLD itself is largely an adaptive rather than an adverse response to xenobiotics as a number of *ex vivo* studies have failed to consistently reveal specific functional detriment in responding phospholipidotic tissues [2, 7–9]. Yet there is suggestive evidence that

TABLE 1: Nominal doses and exposures from both the nonphospholipogenic compound (NP) and phospholipogenic compound (P) datasets. Averages and standard deviations (in parentheses) shown. Data from mid-doses are not shown. Average phospholipogenic plasma exposures were lower for all species across all doses than exposures from the negative dataset, but differences were not statistically significant.

Species	Low dose (μmol/kg)	Low C_{max} (μM)	Low AUC (μM·hr)	High dose (μmol/kg)	High C_{max} (μM)	High AUC (μM.hr)
Dog (NP)	89 (124)	52 (71)	297 (429)	936 (1266)	253 (334)	2561 (4457)
Dog (P)	47 (67)	9 (13)	102 (177)	467 (614)	27 (20)	335 (345)
Mouse (NP)	323 (182)	15 (16)	52 (60)	2018 (1437)	56 (71)	322 (519)
Mouse (P)	117 (83)	6 (5)	65 (80)	958 (635)	62 (108)	320 (446)
Rat (NP)	162 (356)	25 (51)	224 (671)	1351 (2659)	204 (390)	1377 (2607)
Rat (P)	235 (384)	9 (21)	117 (324)	737 (802)	26 (32)	372 (485)

phospholipogenic compounds are associated with concurrent toxicities preclinically and clinically. These toxicities include liver necrosis (amiodarone), motor neuropathies (imipramine, amitriptyline), proximal tubule kidney injury (gentamicin), pulmonary alveolitis that can progresses to fibrosis (amiodarone), pneumonitis (fluoxetine), peripheral neuropathies (suramin, amiodarone, chloroquine, perhexiline), and corneal opacity (chloroquine, amiodarone) [10–15]. Despite this potential association, to date, there have been no comprehensive published reviews of pharmaceutical industry data that enumerate these risks or that probe the statistical connection between phospholipogenic compounds and concurrent toxicities. Understanding whether such a connection exists would help define the relative importance of thorough pathological characterization of phospholipidosis and concurrent toxicities in early drug discovery and assist in reducing attrition in drug development.

To investigate the link between phospholipogenic compound administration and the incidence of preclinical histological signals, phospholipogenic and nonphospholipogenic compounds were identified in an internal AstraZeneca *in vivo* toxicology report database and their histological results annotated. We herein report on a robust, unbiased analysis revealing that *in vivo* phospholipogenic compounds are statistically more likely to demonstrate non-PLD histologic changes in all organs investigated. This observation is even more compelling when one considers that, in these studies, the nominal dose (or exposures) for nonphospholipogenic compounds typically exceeded that for phospholipogenic compounds.

2. Methods

2.1. Compound Identification. An internal AstraZeneca database containing repeat-dose *in vivo* toxicology reports was searched to identify phospholipogenic compounds using the common PLD indicator terms phospholipidosis, histiocytosis, foamy macrophages, lamellar lysosomes, and myeloid bodies. To identify reports on nonphospholipogenic compounds, the database was searched for the absence of these PLD indicator terms. Species, study duration, histological findings, nominal doses, and plasma exposures were the key data extracted. We focused on nine responding organs: adrenal gland; bone marrow; kidney; liver; lung; lymph node; reproductive organs; spleen; thymus. (While we have observed nervous and muscle tissue phospholipidosis in our studies, reports were not archived in time, or search terms were inadequate for the purpose of performing an unbiased analysis.)

Reports were individually read to verify the presence or absence of indicator terms, and both PLD and all non-PLD histologic findings were recorded and annotated. Although PLD often presents as vacuolation by light microscopy, due to its common occurrence, by itself, this finding was not considered sufficient for PLD classification. One or more of the following was considered an additional confirming measure for membership in the phospholipogenic dataset: a positive result in an *in vitro* PLD assay [16], a positive prediction from our in-house *in silico* PLD model, a pathologist interpretation/description of PLD in the report (PLD had to be considered by the pathologist a familiar and salient finding and not that of background), or an electron microscopic finding of PLD, the latter being the gold standard for detecting lysosomal phospholipid-laden myeloid inclusions indicative of PLD. One or more of the following was considered an additional confirming measure of a compound having a nonphospholipogenic status: a negative result in an *in vitro* PLD assay or a negative result in our *in silico* PLD predictive model.

2.2. Pharmacokinetic Properties. Nominal dose (μmol/kg), $AUC_{\mu m \cdot hr}$ and C_{max} (μM) plasma exposure data for the two compound classes were extracted from the study reports if available (Table 1). The majority of the study reports had three dose groups. If a study had four dose groups, the second lowest dose was designated as the low dose. AUC exposure information for at least two doses was available for 77% of the phospholipogenic reports and 86% of the negative's reports; C_{max} exposure information for at least 2 doses was available for 73% of the phospholipogenic compounds and 79% of the nonphospholipogenic compounds. Exposures were not adjusted for plasma protein binding as complete measurements were not available for a majority of the studies.

2.3. Statistical Analysis. Statistically significant differences between the two datasets for organ histological findings were assessed using Chi Square analysis at a 95% confidence level. Statistically significant differences are indicated by Chi Square values greater than 3.84 in Table 2.

TABLE 2: Incidence of nonphospholipidosis histological findings (HFs) for liver, kidney, lung, adrenals, and lymphoid tissues for 46 phospholipogenics and 62 nonphospholpogenics. Results are presented as the total number of compounds exhibiting (or not exhibiting—"No findings") the given histological finding and the percentage of the total number of compounds in that category. ChiSquare values of ≥3.84 conferred statistical significance at $P < 0.05^*$. Statistical significance was achieved for select histological findings in liver, lung, thymus, lymph node, and spleen but not kidney and adrenal glands. HF: histological findings.

	Phospholipogenics		Nonphospholipogenics		Chi-Sq*
	Total number	Percent of total compounds	Total number	Percent of total compounds	
Liver					
Necrosis/degeneration	22	48	13	21	8.7*
Hypertrophy	12	26	11	18	1.1
Reduced glycogen vacuolation	8	17	5	8	2.2
No findings	14	30	32	52	4.8*
Kidney					
Necrosis/degeneration	8	17	6	10	1.4
Nephropathy	5	11	5	8	0.25
No findings	27	59	40	65	0.28
Lung					
Pneumonitis	5	11	0	0	7.1*
Oedema	3	7	1	2	1.8
Alveolitis	3	7	0	0	4.2*
No findings	34	74	61	98	14.9*
Adrenal gland					
Hypertophy	5	11	5	8	0.25
Necrosis	4	9	2	3	1.5
No findings	30	65	46	74	1.1
Thymus					
Lymphocytolysis, lymphoid depletion	16	35	6	10	10.3*
Atrophy/involution	13	28	16	26	0.08
No findings	22	48	43	69	5.1
Lymph node					
Lymphocytolysis, lymphoid depletion	12	26	1	2	14.9*
Atrophy	2	4	5	8	0.6
No findings	28	61	52	84	7.3*
Spleen					
Lymphocytolysis, lymphoid depletion	8	17	0	0	11.7*
Altered hematopoiesis	4	9	6	10	0.01
Atrophy	4	9	3	5	0.65
Apoptosis	3	7	0	0	4.2*
No findings	30	65	52	84	5.0*

3. Results

3.1. Source Data for Phospholipogenic and Nonphopholipogenic Compounds. *In vivo* data extracted from an internal *in vivo* toxicology report archive resulted in compilation of forty-six phospholipogenic compounds and sixty-two nonphospholipogenic compounds. To obtain the forty-six phospholipogenic compound set, fifty-three compounds initially identified as phospholipogenics based on verbal descriptors in the study reports were tested in our *in vitro* PLD assay [16], found to be positive, and selected for further analysis. The majority of these compounds exhibited *in vitro* EC_{50} values less than 50 μM (mean 44 μM, sd 66; ranging from 2.4 to 273 μM). For comparison, the phospholipogenics amiodarone, chloroquine, and citalopram yield 4.8, 12, and 38 μM EC_{50} values in this assay, demonstrating that many positives selected for analysis were intrinsically weaker in their phospholipidosis inducing potential than these standard reference drugs.

3.2. Physiochemical Properties Analyses. The 107 compounds in the phospholipogenic and nonphospholipogenic datasets were structurally diverse. Clustering based on 2-dimensional molecular fingerprints resulted in seventy-five sets of compounds, with the largest cluster containing eight compounds. Physical and computed molecular properties also revealed this diversity, with molecular weights (MW) ranging from 139 to 696 (mean 434, sd 115), polar surface area (PSA) between 20.5 and 194.9 (mean 85.9, sd 33.4), and ClogP between −2.53 and 8.95 (mean 3.0, sd 2.0). The number of hydrogen bond donors ranged from 0 to 4 (mean 1.7, sd 1.2) and hydrogen bond acceptors from 2 to 14 (mean 6.9, sd 2.4). At pH 7, the phospholipogenic compounds were predicted to contain 37 bases, 4 neutrals, 3 zwitterions, and 1 acid, while the nonphospholipogenic compounds contain 9 bases, 34 neutrals, 1 zwitterion, and 18 acids. This is consistent with the generalization that many phospholipogenic compounds are amphiphilic cations. The MW for the phospholipogenic compounds ranged between 256 and 645 (mean 476, sd 85) and 139 and 695 (mean 404, sd 124) for the negative compounds. ClogP for the phospholipogenic compounds range between 0.67 and 8.95 (mean 3.8, sd 1.6) and for the negative compounds between −2.53 and 7.46 (mean 2.4, sd 2.0). PSA for the phospholipogenics ranged between 30.6 and 138.1 (mean 76.4, sd 25), while, for the nonphospholipogenic compounds it ranges between 20.5 and 194.9 (mean 92.8, sd 37.2). The number of hydrogen bond donors ranges between 0 and 4 (mean 1.5, sd 1.1) and the number of hydrogen bond acceptors between 3 and 12 (mean 6.9, sd 1.8) for the phospholipogenic compounds and between 0 and 4 (mean 1.8, sd 1.2) and 2 and 14 (mean 6.9, sd 2.7), respectively, for the negatives. Aside from the obvious difference in the ionization characteristics of the two sets, these simple physical chemical parameters alone do not appear to effectively distinguish between phospholipogenic and nonphospholipogenic compounds.

3.3. Species, Study Durations, and Plasma Exposures. Mouse, rat, and dog are the three species represented in the compound datasets. Study durations ranged from five days to two years, with the majority of repeat dose studies having been conducted for 1 to 4 weeks duration. Figure 1 shows the percentage of study reports by species. Figure 2 shows the percentage of study reports by study duration. There were on average 4.8 (4.6 sd) and 3.2 (2.3 sd) reports per compound in the phospholipogenic and nonphospholipogenic datasets, respectively. Where there were multiple study reports for a compound tested in the same species, reports were counted as a single "report" to minimize weighting bias. There were some notable differences in the distribution of study species and duration for both compound classes. There were 29% (of the total) (or 1.6-fold) more rat study "reports" available in the phospholipogenic dataset than the negatives

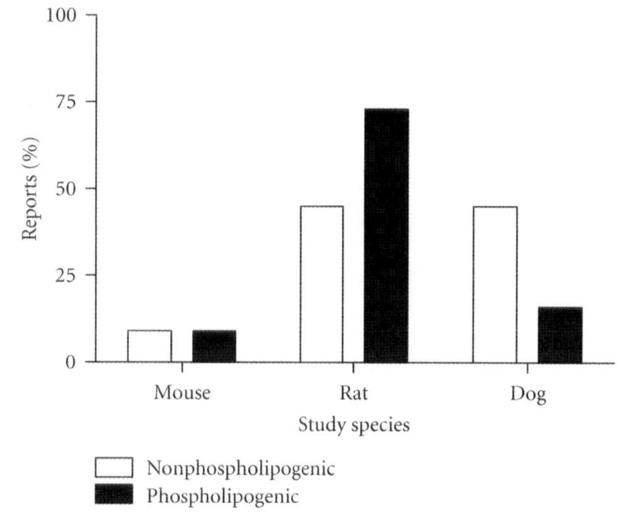

FIGURE 1: Percentage of study reports by species for both phospholipogenic and nonphospholipogenic datasets. Where there were multiple study reports for a compound tested in the same species, reports were counted as a single "report" to minimize weighting bias. There were 29% (of the total) (or 1.6-fold) more rat study "reports" available in the phospholipogenic dataset than the negatives dataset, whereas there were 28% (of the total) (or 2.8-fold) more dog study "reports" available in the negative dataset than the phospholipogenic dataset. Phospholipidosis potential (descriptors and pathologists interpretation) identified in study reports for all compounds was also confirmed *in silico* or *in vitro*.

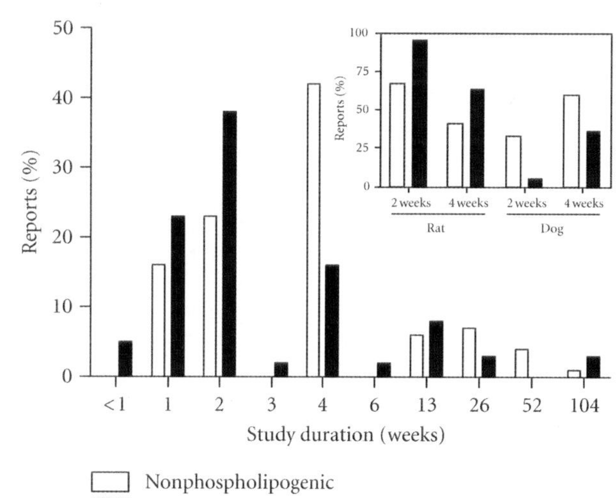

FIGURE 2: Percentage of study reports for both nonphospholipogenic and phospholipogenic datasets by study duration. Where there were multiple study reports for a compound tested in the same species, reports were counted as a single "report" to minimize weighting bias. There were 15% (of the total) (or 1.7-fold) more 2-week "reports" available for the phospholpogenic dataset than for the negatives; there were 26% (of total) (or 1.7-fold) more 4-week "reports" available for the negative dataset than for the phospholpogenics. The larger figure reflects data pooled from the three species. The *inset* shows the breakdown of two-week and four-week studies by dog and rat species.

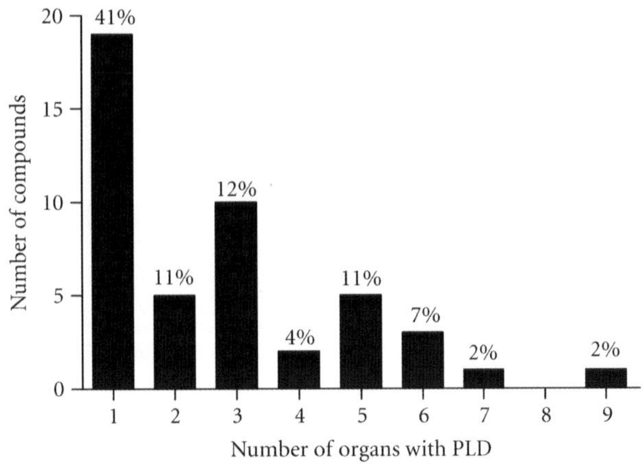

FIGURE 3: Number of phospholipogenic compounds by incidence of organ phospholipidosis responses. The values above the bars represent proportions of the compounds yielding a phospholipidosis response descriptor (i.e., "phospholipidosis," "histiocytosis," "foamy macrophages," "lamellar lysosomes," and "myeloid bodies" and where phospholipidosis potential was confirmed by *in silico* or *in vitro* testing). Approximately half of the compounds caused multiorgan PLD (i.e., ≥3 organs) phospholipogenics. The data represent that pooled from three species and all study durations.

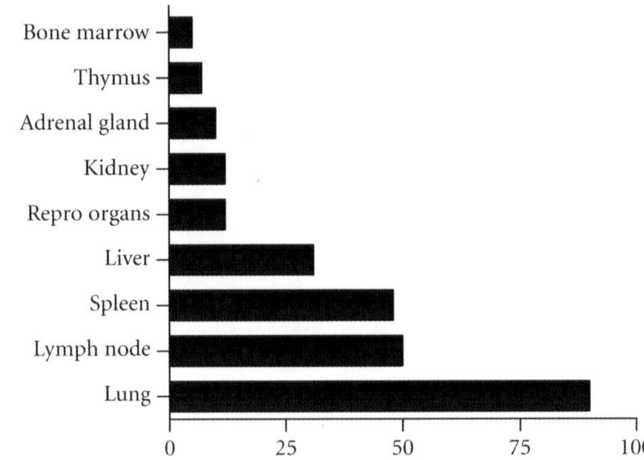

FIGURE 4: Percent phospholipogenics giving histological findings consistent with phospholipidosis, by organ. In response to phospholipogenic administration, lung and lymph node presented with the greatest number of histological findings that matched phospholipidosis descriptors whereas bone marrow and thymus presented with the least. The data represent that pooled from three species and all study durations.

dataset, whereas there were 28% (of the total) (or 2.8-fold) more dog study "reports" available in the negative dataset than the phospholipogenic dataset. The percentage of mouse reports was equivalent for both compound classes. The two-week and four-week groupings had the greatest variation in study duration distribution. There were 15% (of the total) (or 1.7-fold) more 2-week "reports" available for the phospholpogenic dataset than for the negatives; there were 26% (of total) (or 1.7-fold) more "reports" available for the negative dataset than for the phospholpogenics. Except for mouse where $AUC_{\mu m \cdot hr}$ and C_{max} (μM) exposure data were similar between datasets at high nominal doses, nominal dose (μmol/kg), $AUC_{\mu m \cdot hr}$, and C_{max} (μM) values for the negative compounds were on average higher for the other two species (Table 1). C_{max} exposures from the nonphospholipogenic bin on average well exceeded 10 μM.

3.3.1. Phospholipogenic Compound Incidence of Organ PLD versus Non-PLD Findings. Compound treatments yielding three or more organ PLD responses were deemed multi-organ phospholipogenic compounds. Approximately 50% of phospholipogenic compounds caused multiorgan PLD (Figure 3). Multiorgan PLD was more likely to occur when predicted percent free compound (free of protein binding) was greater than ~10%, whereas PLD more often occurred in only one to two organs when the predicted percent free was less than 10%. PLD incidence by organ is illustrated in Figure 4. Lung, lymph node, and spleen presented with the highest incidence, bone marrow, and thymus the lowest. The liver PLD incidence was approximately 35%. In contrast, the rank order of non-PLD histologic findings incidence for this dataset differed from that of organ PLD ranking (Figure 5). Liver and thymus exhibited the highest incidences of non-PLD findings, lung, and bone marrow the lowest.

3.4. Incidence of Organ Non-PLD Histologic Findings, Comparing Phospholipogenic, and Nonphospholipogenic Datasets. To ascertain which dataset was associated with more histologic findings, frequencies of non-PLD histologic findings were compared. Phospholipogenic compounds consistently exhibited more non-PLD histologic changes for all organs (Figure 6), and among these the liver exhibited the highest percentage of histologic findings for both datasets. Compared to nonphospholipogenic compounds, phospholipogenic compounds yielded a statistically significant higher percentage of liver necrosis findings (Table 2). For those phospholipogenic compounds in this subset where exposure data were available (i.e., 11 of 22 compounds that caused necrosis), top plasma exposures did not on average exceed those phospholipogenics that did not cause necrosis (data not shown). A statistically significant, higher frequency of lymphocytolysis/lymphoid depletion in lymphoid organs increased apoptosis in spleen, and alveolitis/pneumonitis in lung were observed with this subset of compounds. No differences were apparent for adrenals or kidney. Finally, statistically significant higher levels of "no histologic findings" in the liver, lung, thymus, lymph nodes, and spleen were reported for the nonphospholipogenic compounds.

4. Discussion and Conclusions

The purpose of this study was to test whether pharmaceutically relevant phospholipogenic compounds were associated with a higher frequency of histologic changes in repeat dose *in vivo* preclinical toxicology studies than that for non-phospholipogenic compounds. For the comparison, forty-six phospholipogenic compounds were identified; sixty-two negative compounds were identified. Results of the analysis may be summarized as follows. Phospholipogenic administrations were found to yield proportionally more

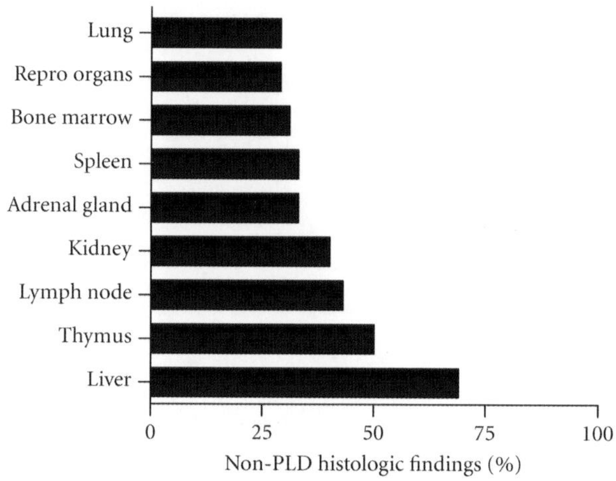

Figure 5: Percent phospholipogenics with nonphospholipogenic histological findings by organ. The data represent that pooled from three species and all study durations.

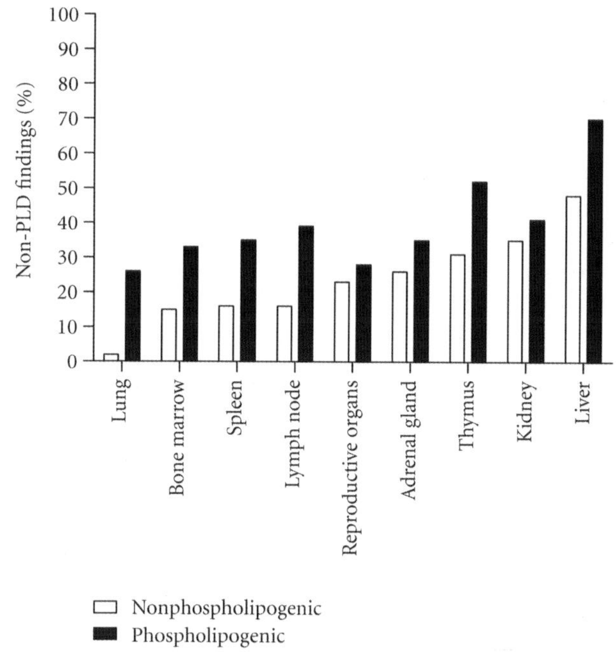

Figure 6: Percent nonphospholipogenic and phospholipogenic compound administrations yielding non-PLD histological findings, by organ. For every organ, on average, phospholipogenic administration resulted in more non-PLD histological findings than did negative compound administration. The data represent that pooled from three species and all study durations.

non-PLD histologic changes in general in all organs examined and for select histological findings in liver, lung, thymus, lymph node, and spleen but not for kidney and adrenal glands. Nonphospholipogenic compounds exhibited a higher incidence of "no findings" for several organs. Phospholipogenic compounds exhibited statistically significant increases in lung alveolitis/pneumonitis and in true toxicities relating to liver necrosis. Not surprisingly, phospholipogenic compounds demonstrating "no liver findings" tended to exhibit fewer histological findings across the 9 organs overall (data not shown). Increased incidences of lymphocytolysis and/or lymphoid depletion in three lymphoid tissues (thymus, lymph nodes, and spleen) were also observed in the phospholipogenic dataset. Lymphocytolysis/lymphoid depletion is often attributed to high-dose-mediated stress responses; but they may in some instances represent a true toxicological response. Without other hematologic correlates it is not possible to shed light on this matter, and for this reason labeled these results conservatively simply as excess histological findings. Finally, it also appears from the study duration analysis that two-week study designs and the rat model are typically sufficient to capture phospholipidotic signals *in vivo*. Although concurrent toxicities were not specified, it is of interest that a recent report indicates that a 24 h duration may be sufficient to detect/predict phospholipidosis accurately by employing a small biomarker set in toxicogenomic evaluation [17].

Several additional comparisons were made for the phospholipogenic dataset, particularly regarding physical-chemical properties and toxicokinetic behavior. Consistent with the well-described cationic amphiphilic nature of phospholipogenic compounds, the phospholipogenic dataset was comprised mostly of amphiphilic bases and the negative dataset contained primarily neutrals and acids with only a few bases. Plasma exposures tended to be lower in animals dosed with phospholipogenic compounds. For the dog and mouse, this pharmacokinetic behavior can be explained in part by the selection of lower phospholipogenic compound nominal doses in the study designs but not entirely since relative exposures are still lower if dose-normalized (data not shown). Nominal doses for rat were on average higher than that of the nonphospholipogenic dataset, but plasma exposures in the phospholipogenic dataset were considerably lower. There is an acknowledged general tendency for bases, and particularly lipophilic bases, to have higher volumes of distribution [18], although it has recently been demonstrated that this property alone does not differentiate phospholipogenics from nonphospholipogenics [19]. Finally, it should be noted that not only were the average doses and exposures of the nonphospholipogenic compounds higher, but, as can be seen in Figure 2, the average duration of their studies is somewhat longer as well. All of these factors should bias the number of nonphospholipidosis histological findings profile towards the higher dose, higher exposure, longer study duration group, but, as demonstrated in this study, we see the opposite.

This thorough and systematic analysis of a large preclinical toxicology dataset containing both confirmed phospholipogenics and nonphospholipogenic compounds indicates that phospholipogenic administration is likely to be associated with more and various histological findings, including liver toxicities, than do nonphospholipogenic administrations. The data, while compelling, are correlative and cannot be used to prove causality between phospholipidosis and toxicities. It should also be noted that speculation on functional compromise cannot be made and that histologic findings identified in this exercise were not equal in severity. Findings ranged from relatively benign to severe, and we did not apply risk assessment analysis where it may be found that compounds could proceed normally through the drug development process, taking concurrent toxicities, tissues affected, severity, and safety margins (therapeutic window) into account. Even with these caveats, it is clear that phospholipogenic compounds tend to produce more histological findings and may require additional monitoring and risk assessment, thereby increasing the overall burden on a drug development project.

Acknowledgment

The authors are grateful to Sherri Matis-Mitchell for her assistance in obtaining the negative compound dataset from the AstraZeneca report archives.

References

[1] R. Lullmann-Rauch, "Drug-induced lysosomal storage disorders," in *Lysosomes in Applied Biology and Thereapeutics*, J. T. Dingle, P. J. Jacques, and I. H. Shaw, Eds., pp. 49–128, North-Holland Publishing, Amsterdam, The Netherlands, 1979.

[2] M. J. Reasor, K. L. Hastings, and R. G. Ulrich, "Drug-induced phospholipidosis: issues and future directions," *Expert Opinion on Drug Safety*, vol. 5, no. 4, pp. 567–583, 2006.

[3] U. P. Kodavanti and H. M. Mehendale, "Cationic amphilic drugs and phospholipid storage disorder," *Pharmacological Reviews*, vol. 42, no. 4, pp. 327–354, 2001.

[4] W. A. Daniel and J. Wójcikowski, "The role of lysosomes in the cellular distribution of thioridazine and potential drug interactions," *Toxicology and Applied Pharmacology*, vol. 158, no. 2, pp. 115–124, 1999.

[5] A. D. Wladyslawa, J. Wójcikowski, and A. Palucha, "Intracellular distribution of psychotropic drugs in the grey and white matter of the brain: the role of lysosomal trapping," *British Journal of Pharmacology*, vol. 134, no. 4, pp. 807–814, 2001.

[6] J. J. Shacka, B. J. Klocke, M. Shibata et al., "Bafilomycin A1 inhibits chloroquine-induced death of cerebellar granule neurons," *Molecular Pharmacology*, vol. 69, no. 4, pp. 1125–1136, 2006.

[7] N. Anderson and J. Borlak, "Drug-induced phospholipidosis," *FEBS Letters*, vol. 580, no. 23, pp. 5533–5540, 2006.

[8] M. J. Reasor and S. Kacew, "Drug-induced phospholipidosis: are there functional consequences?" *Experimental Biology and Medicine*, vol. 226, no. 9, pp. 825–830, 2001.

[9] M. E. Cartwright, J. Petruska, J. Arezzo et al., "Phospholipidosis in neurons caused by posaconazole, without evidence for functional neurologic effects," *Toxicologic Pathology*, vol. 37, no. 7, pp. 902–910, 2009.

[10] R. J. Gonzalez-Rothi, D. S. Zander, and P. R. Ros, "Fluoxetine hydrochloride (Prozac)-induced pulmonary disease," *Chest*, vol. 107, no. 6, pp. 1763–1765, 1995.

[11] D. Laplane and M. G. Bousser, "Polyneuropathy during perhexiline maleate therapy," *International Journal of Neurology*, vol. 15, no. 3-4, pp. 293–300, 1981.

[12] M. Mäntyjärvi, K. Tuppurainen, and K. Ikäheimo, "Ocular side effects of amiodarone," *Survey of Ophthalmology*, vol. 42, no. 4, pp. 360–366, 1998.

[13] M. P. Mingeot-Leclercq and P. M. Tulkens, "Aminoglycosides: nephrotoxicity," *Antimicrobial Agents and Chemotherapy*, vol. 43, no. 5, pp. 1003–1012, 1999.

[14] S. L. Vonderfecht, M. L. Stone, R. R. Eversole et al., "Myopathy related to administration of a cationic amphiphilic drug and the use of multidose drug distribution analysis to predict its occurrence," *Toxicologic Pathology*, vol. 32, no. 3, pp. 318–325, 2004.

[15] E. A. Tengstrand, G. T. Miwa, and F. Y. Hsieh, "Bis(monoacylglycerol)phosphate as a non-invasive biomarker to monitor the onset and time-course of phospholipidosis with drug-induced toxicities," *Expert Opinion on Drug Metabolism and Toxicology*, vol. 6, no. 5, pp. 555–570, 2010.

[16] J. K. Morelli, M. Buehrle, F. Pognan, L. R. Barone, W. Fieles, and P. J. Ciaccio, "Validation of an *in vitro* screen for phospholipidosis using a high-content biology platform," *Cell Biology and Toxicology*, vol. 22, no. 1, pp. 15–27, 2006.

[17] H. T. Yudate, T. Kai, M. Aoki et al., "Identification of a novel set of biomarkers for evaluating phospholipidosis-inducing potential of compounds using rat liver microarray data measured 24-hours after single dose administration," *Toxicology*, vol. 295, no. 1–3, pp. 1–7, 2012.

[18] F. Lombardo, R. S. Obach, M. Y. Shalaeva, and F. Gao, "Prediction of volume of distribution values in humans for neutral and basic drugs using physicochemical measurements and plasma protein binding data," *Journal of Medicinal Chemistry*, vol. 45, no. 13, pp. 2867–2876, 2002.

[19] U. M. Hanumegowda, G. Wenke, A. Regueiro-Ren, R. Yordanova, J. P. Corradi, and S. P. Adams, "Phospholipidosis as a function of basicity, lipophilicity, and volume of distribution of compounds," *Chemical Research in Toxicology*, vol. 23, no. 4, pp. 749–755, 2010.

17

Clinical Validation of a Highly Sensitive GC-MS Platform for Routine Urine Drug Screening and Real-Time Reporting of up to 212 Drugs

Hari Nair,[1] Fred Woo,[1] Andrew N. Hoofnagle,[1,2] and Geoffrey S. Baird[1,3]

[1] *Department of Laboratory Medicine, University of Washington, P.O. Box 357110, 1959 NE Pacific Street, Seattle, WA 98185, USA*
[2] *Department of Medicine, University of Washington, Seattle, WA 98150, USA*
[3] *Department of Pathology, University of Washington, Seattle, WA 98150, USA*

Correspondence should be addressed to Geoffrey S. Baird; gbaird@u.washington.edu

Academic Editor: Steven J. Bursian

An important role of the clinical toxicology laboratory is to provide continuous diagnostic testing for patients with altered mental status and for other medical indications. To meet these needs, we have developed a new Gas Chromatography-Mass Spectrometry (GC-MS) platform that facilitates routine screening and automated reporting of 212 drugs by laboratory technologists around the clock without the need to sign out by an on-site mass spectrometry-trained toxicologist. The platform uses a programmable temperature vaporizer (PTV) injector for large sample volume injection and the free software Automated Mass Spectral Deconvolution and Identification System (AMDIS) for data reduction and spectral matching that facilitates rapid library searching and analyte identification. Method comparison with 118 patient samples demonstrated that this platform and data searching algorithm independently provided improvements in sensitivity compared to an established GC-MS platform. Further examination of the role of the data processing software and the in-house databases used in the established versus the new platform demonstrated that the improved analytical sensitivity of the new platform was attributed to both the technical superiority of the new GC-MS instrumentation and the use of AMDIS in conjunction with the newly generated in-house library for data processing.

1. Introduction

Screening patients for toxins, including prescription and/or illegal drugs, is a key function of a clinical toxicology lab. In our hospital, we perform comprehensive toxicological screening of a patient population with a high pretest probability of use, abuse, and overdose of prescription, over-the-counter (OTC), and illegal drugs using a combination of immunoassays and Gas Chromatography-Mass Spectrometry (GC-MS). Clinicians are advised to use this comprehensive urine drug screen to evaluate possible accidental or intentional overdose or poisoning, to assess the type of prescribed and/or illicit drugs used by a patient, or to determine the cause of acute drug toxicity. The assay is also used in specific clinical contexts to investigate whether specific drugs are present in a patient's urine before starting a medical procedure.

Most clinical toxicology laboratories employ one or more of a variety of analytical and immunological approaches such as Liquid Chromatography-Tandem Mass Spectrometry (LC-MS/MS) [1–4], GC-MS [5, 6], and immunoassay (i.e., EMIT) [7] to screen patient urine samples for a variety of drugs. While immunoassays are fast and fully automated, the technique is prone to moderate-to-severe assay interference from structurally similar members of drug families. Therefore, an immunoassay result is only presumptive and not considered confirmatory. Electron Impact Ionization (EI) GC-MS, on the other hand, is the historical gold standard approach for both qualitative identification and quantitation of a large number of drugs in urine, due to its ability to efficiently separate drugs chromatographically and thereafter produce structurally rich mass spectra that are generally unique to a specific drug [8, 9]. LC-MS/MS in a selective reaction monitoring (or multiple reaction monitoring) mode allows for highly specific qualitative drug identification and highly sensitive drug quantitation, but it is difficult, in practice, to design an effective comprehensive screen based on a large number of transitions because many drugs are not adequately resolved by liquid chromatography. This problem has partly been resolved by the use of high-resolution mass analyzers coupled to LC [4], but this approach requires significant expertise in assay design, an extremely expensive mass spectrometer (~5–10 times more expensive than a GC-MS instrument), and usually a specifically trained staff of operators and clinical interpreters. For these reasons, therefore, we chose to develop a highly sensitive EI GC-MS comprehensive drug screen for use in our clinical laboratory, employing programmable temperature vaporization (PTV) [10] sample injection to increase analyte sensitivity and an automated data analysis algorithm based on free software—Automated Mass Spectral Deconvolution and Identification System (AMDIS) [11–13]—to allow operation by generalist clinical technologists. PTV allows the introduction of a sample into a cold system followed by a temperature ramp that selectively evaporates the injection solvent prior to introduction onto the column, instead of direct injection into a hot oxidative environment of the default injector. This, in turn, allows for the injection of larger volume of sample for enhanced sensitivity. We have characterized the platform using 118 patient samples. Although data analysis strategies similar to ours have been demonstrated in metabolomics [14, 15] and environmental applications [16], clinical validation of such an approach has not been reported previously. Our approach encompasses an effective platform for routine toxicology applications.

2. Materials and Methods

2.1. Experimental

2.1.1. Chemicals and Reagents. Pharmaceutical drugs and reagents were purchased from Sigma-Aldrich (St. Louis, MO, USA), Grace Davison Discovery Sciences (Columbia, MD, USA), and PhytoLab GmbH & Co. KG (Vestenbergsgreuth, Germany).

2.1.2. Urine Samples. Samples used for the method comparison study were accrued from leftover clinical specimens, stored at −20°C, that had been submitted to the laboratory for comprehensive drug screen analysis on a previous GC-MS platform. Urine for comprehensive drug screens was submitted without preservatives. Specimens were used in accordance with procedures approved by the local Institutional Review Board.

2.1.3. Sample Preparation. Five mL of urine was pipetted into a 13 × 100 mm disposable glass tube. To this, 50 μL of internal standard (0.35 mg/mL of allobarbital and 0.2 mg/mL cyheptamide in methanol) was added and vortexed. The urine/internal standard mixture was transferred to a ToxiLab (Agilent Technologies, Santa Clara, CA, USA) tube and mixed on rotator for 5 min and centrifuged for 5 min at 2500 rpm. The upper organic layer was transferred into a glass 20 mm × 150 mm culture tube to which 50 μL of 0.025 mol/L HCl had been added, and the mixture was vortexed for 10 minutes. The tube contents were evaporated to dryness at 40°C in a water bath under a stream of air (10 minutes). The dried extract residue was reconstituted with 1 mL methanol and vortexed briefly to redissolve the extract. The sample was finally transferred to a labeled 2 mL snap cap vial, capped, and transferred to the instrument autosampler.

2.2. GC-MS

2.2.1. Instrumentation. The GC-MS platform was a Thermo-Scientific ISQ Mass Spectrometer with Trace GC Ultra Gas Chromatograph, TriPlus RSH automated sample injector, and a computer workstation with X-calibur software (Waltham, MA, USA). The GC column was a Restek capillary column, 30 m × 0.25 mm ID × 0.25 μm, Restek Rtx-5MS Cross bond 5% diphenyl-95% dimethyl polysiloxane (Restek, Bellefonte, PA). GC conditions were as follows: PTV splitless injection mode, 3 μL injection; crosslinked methyl silicone, film thickness 330 nm; injection port temperature ramped from initial 65°C for 1.5 minutes, 280°C for 30 s, and then to 300°C for 35 min; helium carrier gas flow-rate 1 mL/min; and column oven temperature programmed from 150 to 300°C at 14.5°C/min, initial 150°C for 20 min, 250°C for 15 min, and then to 300°C for 5 min. The MS conditions were as follows: electron ionization mode, ionization energy 70 eV, ion source temperature 220°C, capillary direct interface 290°C, and full-scan mode *m/z* 33–550, 1 scan/s with a dwell time of 0.2 s.

2.2.2. Method. Three μL of urine extract was injected into the PTV liner at 60°C for solvent evaporation, and the residue was transferred to the capillary GC column without split by ramping to 280°C. GC column eluents were directly ionized and analyzed by full-scan EI-MS. For validation experiments, samples run on the new platform were compared with the results from the established GC-MS platform used in the clinical laboratory (see Section 2.2.3). The sample preparation and extraction used prior to analysis on the previous HP system were identical to the current procedure.

Carryover from injection to injection was tested using a urine sample spiked with mixtures of drugs containing 50 μg/mL of each drug (high sample). The injection of this mixture of drugs was preceded and followed by the injection of a negative urine sample. Carryover was quantified using mass spectra generated from the negative urine samples injected before and after the high sample.

2.2.3. Reference GC-MS: Instrumentation and Method. Hewlett Packard 6890 Gas Chromatograph was combined with an HP 5973 MSD Mass Spectrometer. An HP MS Chem-Station (DOS series) was used with HP G1034C software version C03.00 (Agilent Technologies, Santa Clara, CA, USA). The GC column was a Restek capillary column, 30 m × 0.25 mm ID × 0.25 μm, Restek Rtx-5MS Crossbond 5% diphenyl-95% dimethyl polysiloxane (Restek, Bellefonte, PA). GC conditions were as follows: Hewlett-Packard 7683 series automated sample injector, 1 μL injection; 5% diphenyl-95%

dimethyl polysiloxane; injection port temperature ramped from initial 65°C to 280°C to 300°C; helium carrier gas flow-rate 1 mL/min; and column temperature programmed from 100 to 310°C at 30°/min, initial time 3 min, final time 8 min. The MS conditions were as follows: electron ionization mode, ionization energy 70 eV, ion source temperature 220°C, capillary direct interface 290°C, and full-scan mode *m/z* 33–550, 1 scan/s with a dwell time of 0.2 s.

2.3. In-House Library and Data Analysis. Full-scan data files acquired by the GC-MS system from injecting pure compounds in methanol solution were analyzed by the Automated Mass Spectral Deconvolution and Identification System (AMDIS) [11–13] in simple mode. An AMDIS-readable library of 212 drugs was compiled from using the Lib2NIST converter software version 1.0.0.13 included in the NIST MS-search software version 2.0a. For this, mass spectra for each of the 212 drugs were acquired by injecting 1 mg/mL of the drug in neat methanol. The final settings of the deconvolution and search parameters derived from the results of a series of optimization experiments were as follows: width, 12; adjacent peak subtraction, 2; sensitivity, medium; resolution, medium; and shape requirement, medium. Relative retention time (RRT) was calculated for each drug based on the retention time difference between the drug and the internal standard cyheptamide (RT of the drug/RT of internal standard; RRT of cyheptamide = 1). A relative retention time range of ±0.2 minute window was assigned to each drug in the library to account for sample-to-sample variation in retention times. RRT matching was accomplished using a simple Microsoft Excel macro developed in-house. Only the drugs whose retention times matched the preset RRT range are considered reportable.

2.4. Analytical Sensitivity. Analytical sensitivity of the platform was evaluated using dilutions of urine containing spikes of multiple drug standards at various concentrations which were extracted as aforementioned in Section 2.1.3 and injected into the GC-MS. The lowest concentration of a drug in the mixture examined was 1 ng/mL. If the drug could not be detected at the lowest concentration tested, the next higher concentration of the drug was analyzed. In this manner, the concentration of undetected drugs increased in folds (1, 10, 100, and 1000 ng/mL) until the concentration was detectable by the platform. Figure 1 shows the lowest concentration at which each of the 212 drugs was detected.

2.5. Clinical Correlation. Ninety-nine retrospective patient samples were used for clinical correlation of the results generated by the new platform. The list of drugs identified per patient by the new platform was compared with the number of drugs reported by the reference platform for each patient. Discrepancies between the two platforms were adjudicated by chart review, corroborating the analytical results with the patient's history by looking for drugs that were known to have been administered or suspected to have been self-administered based on documented risky behavior. A drug was called positive by the new platform when the

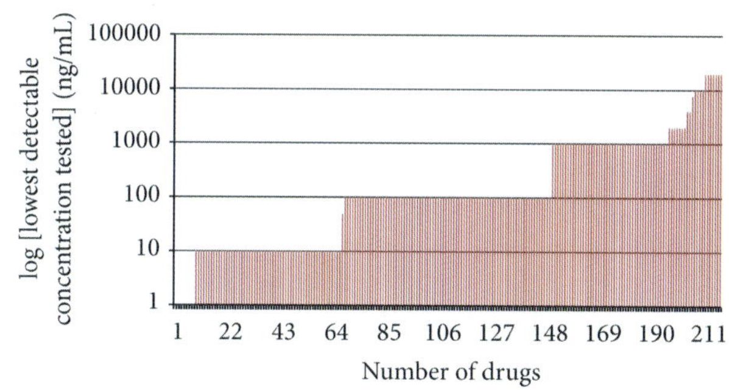

Figure 1: Lowest concentration of each of the 212 drugs detected by the new GC-MS platform. Dilutions of urine containing spikes of drug standards prepared by spiking 1, 10, 100, and 1000 ng/mL into negative urine were used to determine the analytical sensitivity of the platform. If the drug could not be detected at the lowest concentration tested, the next higher concentration of the drug was analyzed. Analytical sensitivity of the drug was recorded as the lowest formulated concentration at which the drug was detected (see Supplementary Material available online at http://dx.doi.org/10.1155/2013/329407 for the list of all drugs along with the lowest concentrations at which each drug was detected).

analytical criteria (Section 3.1) were met and the clinical records supported the presence of the drug in the patient sample.

3. Results and Discussion

3.1. Optimization of the New GC-MS Platform. Our objective in introducing a new GC-MS platform in our clinical toxicology laboratory was to enable nonexpert generalist operators to run the assay at all hours, generate reports, and communicate results directly to physicians without the need for verification by a doctorate-level toxicologist with experience in MS-based compound identification. Because the clinical samples for this assay often come from patients with high urine drug concentrations after overdoses, and because the platform was highly sensitive, it was all the more important to evaluate the extent of injection-to-injection carryover first and if necessary to optimize the GC method to minimize carryover (described in 2.4.2). AMDIS parameters were optimized to further ensure that any lingering carryover peaks or potential false positives are excluded from the final report.

AMDIS extracts pure ion chromatograms from complex compound spectra and deconvolutes noise, peak shape, and retention time and subsequently matches the pure and deconvoluted spectra with those of the in-house reference library (target) consisting of 212 drugs. AMDIS uses two match factors [11, 12], forward search and reverse search, to qualify a match and generate a preliminary list of matched drugs. The AMDIS spectral matches are thus *qualified hits* that can be reported if the RRTs match the preset retention time range in the in-house library. While RRT matching can be performed by AMDIS using a library of external standards (a mixture of commercially available alkanes), such an approach would significantly interfere with the current quality control and daily operating procedures in our laboratory, and it would likely require that RRT bounds be redefined if the GC column needed to be shortened. Thus, we chose instead to assess an acceptable RRT for each individual drug relative to a single internal, rather than external, standard so that laborious external recalibrations were not needed.

Using the optimized GC-MS parameters, data was generated for 99 retrospective patient samples. Using these data, AMDIS deconvolution settings for resolution and sensitivity were first optimized such that maximum numbers of target drugs were generated using a low minimum match factor (MMF) of 60 for both forward and reverse search approaches. At an MMF of 60, some low-level carryover peaks as well as potentially false positive drugs were detected in some samples. Next, the optimal MMF was identified that excluded low-level carryover peaks as well as any false positives that may be present in the report. For this, a range of MMFs (60, 70, 80, and 90) were examined; an example of which is shown in Table 1 for one patient. Table 1 lists the number of drugs reported using each of the 4 MMFs examined. Based on the evaluation of a number of datasets and correlating the results with patient's clinical and prescription histories, it was observed that reports generated with a combined MMF of 80 (or higher) contained no verifiable false positive results. Therefore, an MMF of 80 was used for further validation of the new GC-MS platform.

TABLE 1: List of drugs reported (X) by AMDIS for four MMFs for a patient sample. Number of drugs reported reduced from 15 with an MMF of 60 to 12 (MMF = 70) to 10 (MMF = 80 and 90). Based on such investigation, an MMF of 80 was identified to exclude all verifiable false positives and low-level carryovers from previous injection from the target list.

Target list	60	70	80	90
Methyl salicylate	X	X	X	X
Nicotine	X	X	X	X
Ecgonine methyl ester	X	X	X	X
Cotinine	X	X	X	X
Diphenhydramine	X	X	X	X
Etomidate	X	X	X	X
Levamisole	X	X	X	X
Cocaine	X	X	X	X
Benzoylecgonine	X	X	X	X
Midazolam	X	X	X	X
Propofol	X	X		
Mepivacaine	X	X		
Caffeine	X			
Acetaminophen	X			
Butalbital	X			

3.2. *Clinical Validation: Retrospective Study.*

Reports were generated for 99 retrospective patient samples using optimized GC-MS and AMDIS parameters. No evidence for false positive test results was observed for any of the 99 reports validated with clinical data. However, in some instances, drugs expected based on the prescription history were not reported at MMF of 80 (see, e.g., Table 1). Because the primary goal of the assay was to ensure that the reported results are true and not to determine every drug present in the patient sample, the extent of false negative results was not examined. The comparison of the number of drugs reported for each of the 99 patients by each platform is plotted in Figure 2. The figure clearly demonstrates that the new platform reported an increased number of drugs per patient compared to the reference platform. In only two patients did the reference platform report more drugs (in fact, a single additional drug) than the new platform. For most patients, the new platform reported more drugs per patient while for a few patient samples both platforms reported equal number of drugs. Figure 3 shows that for the 99 patient samples the new platform reported, on average, 6–8 drugs per patient while the reference platform reported, on average, 3–5 drugs per patient.

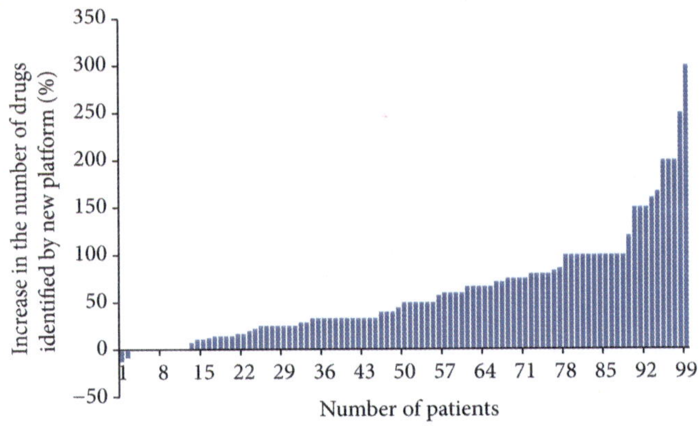

FIGURE 2: Percentage increase in the number of drugs reported for each patient for the new platform (>0) over the number of drugs reported by the reference platform (<0). The number of drugs reported per patient for the 99 retrospective patient samples was compared with the number of drugs reported for these patients by clinical testing using the reference platform. The % excess (or deficit) in the number of drugs reported by the new platform compared to the reference platform is plotted for each patient. For 2 patients, the reference platform reported one drug each (Clonidine and Clozapine) in excess of the number of drugs reported by the new platform for those patients. For 10 patients, both platforms reported equal number of drugs per patient while for all other patients (N = 87) the new platform reported more drugs per patient.

3.3. *Prospective Study.*

Because the retrospective study compared data from fresh versus frozen samples and used different urine extracts of the same specimen, a second smaller prospective clinical validation study was performed using 19 fresh patient samples. In this study, drugs were extracted from patient samples for clinical analysis and aliquots of these extracts were analyzed by both the reference platform (for clinical testing) and the new platform (for this study). GC-MS data generated by the new platform and the established platform were processed by their respective software and libraries as well as by compatible configurations of software and libraries across platforms. Five different configurations of analytical components were used in this

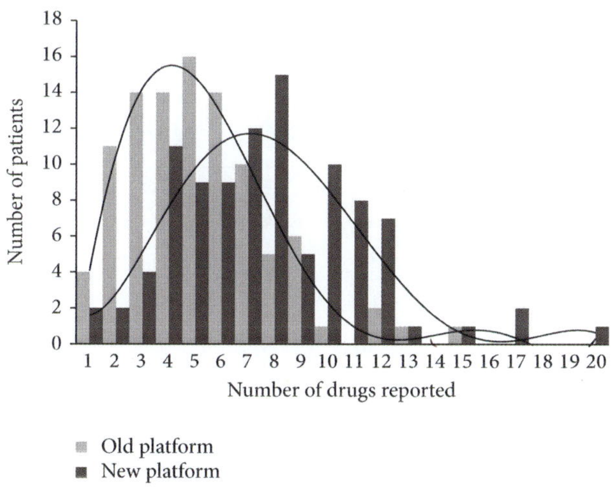

FIGURE 3: Distribution of qualified hits across 99 retrospective patient samples used for clinical validation. The reference platform reported up to 15 drugs per patient while the new platform reported up to 20 drugs per patient. On an average, the reference platform reported 3–5 patients per sample while the new platform reported 6–8 patients per sample.

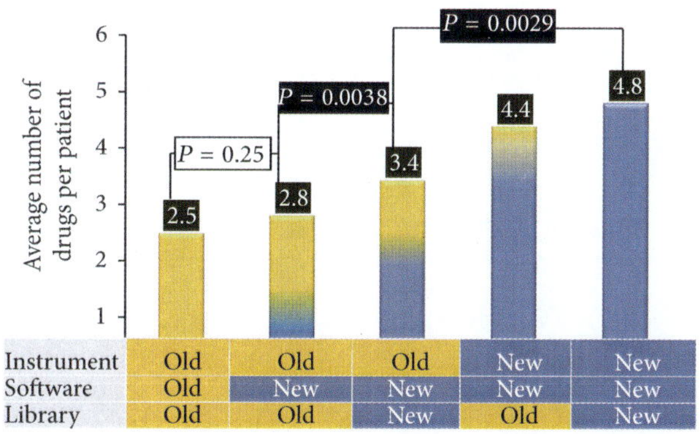

FIGURE 4: Comparison of the number of drugs identified by the new, reference, and mixed configuration platforms. The number of drugs reported per patient is shown against each configuration, and the statistical significance (P value) in the differences in the number of drugs reported for three configurations compared is provided. Statistically valid (P value = 0.0038) increment in the number of drugs was reported when the data from the reference GC-MS instrument is analyzed using AMDIS in conjunction with the new in-house library compared to the use of the default data analysis approach. In-addition, both data generated using the reference instrument and that by the new platform were analyzed using AMDIS in conjunction with the new in-house library. The results from this comparison show that an even higher and statistically significant (P value = 0.0029) increment in the number of drugs was reported from the data generated by the new platform compared to the data generated by the reference platform.

study and are described in Figure 4 along with the number of drugs reported per patient by each possible configuration of analyzers and software. When data from the reference platform were processed using AMDIS, the number of drugs increased modestly but nonsignificantly (15%, $P = 0.25$) compared to the number of drugs reported by using the default software for data analysis. However, when the new in-house library, was used in conjunction with AMDIS to analyze data from the reference GC-MS instrument, the number of drugs reported increased significantly (50%, $P = 0.0038$). When data generated by the new and the reference instruments were both analyzed by AMDIS in conjunction with the new in-house library, a further significant ($P = 0.0029$) increase in the number of drugs (40%) was reported per patient. Table 2 lists the drugs reported by each of the 5 platform configurations for a subset (three) of patient samples examined by this approach. An increased number of drugs were identified from the data generated by the reference platform when a combination of AMDIS and new in-house library is used. When the data generated by both the new GC-MS instrument and the reference instrument are both processed by AMDIS in conjunction with the new library, the new platform consistently reported a larger number of drugs. The new platform uniquely identified drugs in most patient specimens analyzed (see Table 2). For example, for patient 1 in Table 2, the new platform uniquely identified trazodone, morphine, and gabapentin in the patient's urine, all three of which were missed by the established platform. The patient was prescribed trazodone and gabapentin while he was not prescribed morphine. In this case, the patient who has a history of illicit drug abuse (and hence positive for morphine) was presented to the clinic in altered mental status. Therefore, the physician relied upon the lab results for clinical management. It is conceivable that the knowledge of the presence of these drugs could have altered the management.

Results from both retrospective and prospective studies clearly reveal that the new platform significantly enhanced the range of drugs reported by the toxicology laboratory. Based on the results of the prospective study, we found that the improvement in the clinical performance of the new GC-MS platform resulted partly from the data analysis pipeline but more significantly from the new instrumentation, likely because of the use of PTV injection (allowing increased sample volume and a wider range of drugs to be sampled by GC-MS) and from the improved ion transmission offered by the new quadrupole mass analyzer. Based on our chart review, no verifiable or suspected false positive results were reported for any of the 118 patient samples processed by the new GC-MS platform.

The ability to detect many drugs with our new analytical platform has already aided clinicians in complex toxicology cases. In the case in Table 3, a 71-year-old female patient was admitted to the emergency room for altered mental status. The patient lived in a nursing home and shared a room with another patient who had a similar name. Table 3 shows the list of drugs prescribed to the patient, the list of drugs identified by the new GC-MS platform in her urine specimen, and the list of drugs prescribed to her roommate. As demonstrated in the table, the urine drug screen identified a completely different panel of drugs in her urine compared to the list of drugs prescribed to her. A preanalytical error such as a sample swap was suspected in this case, but the fact that the lengthy

Table 2: List of drugs identified by the five platform configurations for three patient specimens. More drugs were detected by the new platform compared to the reference platform and the mixed configurations.

	Reference platform	Reference GC-MS with AMDIS and old spectral library	Reference GC-MS with AMDIS and new spectral library	New GC-MS with old spectral library	New platform
Patient 1	Acetaminophen	Acetaminophen	Acetaminophen	Acetaminophen	Acetaminophen
	Caffeine	Caffeine	Caffeine	Caffeine	Caffeine
	Venlafaxine	Venlafaxine	Venlafaxine	Venlafaxine	Venlafaxine
	Codeine	Codeine	Codeine	Codeine	Codeine
	Trimethoprim	Trimethoprim	Trimethoprim	Trimethoprim	Trimethoprim
			Gabapentin	*Morphine*	*Gabapentin*
				Trazodone	*Morphine*
				Theophylline	*Trazodone*
Patient 2	Nicotine	Nicotine	Nicotine	Nicotine	Nicotine
	Cotinine	Cotinine	Cotinine	Cotinine	Cotinine
	Caffeine	Caffeine	Caffeine	Caffeine	Caffeine
	Diphenhydramine	Diphenhydramine	Diphenhydramine	Diphenhydramine	Diphenhydramine
				Cocaine	*Cocaine*
Patient 3	Oxycodone	Oxycodone	Oxycodone	Oxycodone	Oxycodone
	Methadone	Methadone	Methadone	Methadone	Methadone
	Theophylline	Theophylline	Theophylline	Theopylline	Theophylline
	Gabapentin	Gabapentin	Gabapentin		*Gabapentin*
	Caffeine	Caffeine	Caffeine	Caffeine	Caffeine
			Paraxanthine	Paraxanthine	Paraxanthine
				Morphine	*Morphine*

drug list derived from the GC-MS analysis matched perfectly to the panel of drugs prescribed to her roommate led the clinical team to determine unequivocally that the cause of the patient's altered mental status was a medication error in the nursing home.

4. Conclusion

We have demonstrated that a highly sensitive GC-MS platform employing PTV injection technology for sample injection coupled with a public data analysis package (AMDIS) can be used for routine screening of a large number of drugs in urine in a semiautomated fashion. The newly designed workflow together with a new in-house library of pure compound mass spectra allows for routine analysis of a large number of drugs in urine with superior sensitivity compared to an established platform. By employing higher match quality thresholds, the platform generates qualified (true positive) hits that can be reported in an unsupervised manner by a lab technician around the clock without the need to sign out by an on-site doctoral-level toxicologist. The workflow has been clinically validated for qualitative analysis of urinary drugs and is currently employed for routine toxicological screening of up to 212 drugs in urine.

Table 3: List of drugs detected in the patient specimen, list of drugs prescribed to the patient and the list of drugs prescribed to the patient's roommate. From this comparison it was clear that the patient was administered the drugs of her roommate which potentially caused the altered mental status for the patient.

Drugs detected in the patient specimen by GC-MS	Drugs prescribed to the patient	Drugs prescribed to the patient's roommate
Valproic acid	Fluphenazine	Valproic acid
Desipramine	Benztropine	Desipramine
Citalopram	Atenolol	Citalopram
Clozapine	Lisinopril	Clozapine
Caffeine	Lovastatin	
	Metformin	
	Oxybutynin	
	Cogentin	

By the use of appropriately designed calibrators, the platform and the analytical approaches described herein can also be used for quantitative analysis.

Abbreviations

GC-MS:	Gas Chromatography-Mass Spectrometry
PTV:	Programmable temperature vaporizer
AMDIS:	Automated Mass Spectral Deconvolution and Identification System
OTC:	Over the counter
LC-MS/MS:	Liquid Chromatography-Mass Spectrometry/Mass Spectrometry
EMIT:	Enzyme multiplied immunoassay Technique
RRT:	Relative retention time
MMF:	Minimum match factor.

Conflict of Interests

The authors declare that they have no conflict of interests. They would like to clarify that the commercial entities mentioned in the materials section are only intended as additional information regarding the sources of materials and instrumentation used in the study. They have no financial or other interests in the entities listed in the section.

Acknowledgment

The authors are grateful to Dr. Gary Mallard (NIST) for the many discussions and helpful recommendations during the implementation of AMDIS in their workflow.

References

[1] F. T. Peters, "Recent advances of liquid chromatography-(tandem) mass spectrometry in clinical and forensic toxicology," *Clinical Biochemistry*, vol. 44, no. 1, pp. 54–65, 2011.

[2] A. H. Wu and D. French, "Implementation of liquid chromatography/mass spectrometry into the clinical laboratory," *Clinica Chimica Acta*, vol. 420, pp. 4–10, 2013.

[3] S. K. G. Grebe and R. J. Singh, "LC-MS/MS in the clinical laboratory—where to from here?" *Clinical Biochemist Reviews*, vol. 32, no. 1, pp. 5–31, 2011.

[4] A. H. Wu, "Role of liquid chromatography-high-resolution mass spectrometry (LC-HR/MS) in clinical toxicology," *Clinical Toxicology*, vol. 50, no. 8, pp. 733–742, 2012.

[5] H. H. Maurer, "Current role of liquid chromatography-mass spectrometry in clinical and forensic toxicology," *Analytical and Bioanalytical Chemistry*, vol. 388, no. 7, pp. 1315–1325, 2007.

[6] H. H. Maurer, "Hyphenated mass spectrometric techniques—indispensable tools in clinical and forensic toxicology and in doping control," *Journal of Mass Spectrometry*, vol. 41, no. 11, pp. 1399–1413, 2006.

[7] M. D. Krasowski, A. F. Pizon, M. G. Siam, S. Giannoutsos, M. Iyer, and S. Ekins, "Using molecular similarity to highlight the challenges of routine immunoassay-based drug of abuse/toxicology screening in emergency medicine," *BMC Emergency Medicine*, vol. 9, article 5, 2009.

[8] E. L. Schymanski, M. Meringer, and W. Brack, "Automated strategies to identify compounds on the basis of GC/EI-MS and calculated properties," *Analytical Chemistry*, vol. 83, no. 3, pp. 903–912, 2011.

[9] F. W. McLafferty and F. Turecek, *Interpretation of Mass Spectra*, USB, 4th edition, 1993.

[10] E. Matisová and M. Dömötörová, "Fast gas chromatography and its use in trace analysis," *Journal of Chromatography A*, vol. 1000, no. 1-2, pp. 199–221, 2003.

[11] S. E. Stein, "An integrated method for spectrum extraction and compound identification from gas chromatography/mass spectrometry data," *Journal of the American Society for Mass Spectrometry*, vol. 10, no. 8, pp. 770–781, 1999.

[12] http://chemdata.nist.gov/mass-spc/amdis/index.html.

[13] M. R. Meyer, F. T. Peters, and H. H. Maurer, "Automated mass spectral deconvolution and identification system for GC-MS screening for drugs, poisons, and metabolites in urine," *Clinical Chemistry*, vol. 56, no. 4, pp. 575–584, 2010.

[14] V. Behrends, G. D. Tredwell, and J. G. Bundy, "A software complement to AMDIS for processing GC-MS metabolomic data," *Analytical Biochemistry*, vol. 415, no. 2, pp. 206–208, 2011.

[15] S. Choea, S. H. WooDong, W. K. Park et al., "Development of a target component extraction method from GC-MS data with an in-house program for metabolite profiling," *Analytical Biochemistry*, vol. 426, no. 2, pp. 94–102, 2012.

[16] S. O. Callaghan, D. P. Souza, A. Isaac et al., "PyMS: a Python toolkit for processing of gas chromatography-mass spectrometry (GC-MS) data. Application and comparative study of selected tools," *BMC Bioinformatics*, vol. 13, article 115, 2012.

Permissions

The contributors of this book come from diverse backgrounds, making this book a truly international effort. This book will bring forth new frontiers with its revolutionizing research information and detailed analysis of the nascent developments around the world.

We would like to thank all the contributing authors for lending their expertise to make the book truly unique. They have played a crucial role in the development of this book. Without their invaluable contributions this book wouldn't have been possible. They have made vital efforts to compile up to date information on the varied aspects of this subject to make this book a valuable addition to the collection of many professionals and students.

This book was conceptualized with the vision of imparting up-to-date information and advanced data in this field. To ensure the same, a matchless editorial board was set up. Every individual on the board went through rigorous rounds of assessment to prove their worth. After which they invested a large part of their time researching and compiling the most relevant data for our readers. Conferences and sessions were held from time to time between the editorial board and the contributing authors to present the data in the most comprehensible form. The editorial team has worked tirelessly to provide valuable and valid information to help people across the globe.

Every chapter published in this book has been scrutinized by our experts. Their significance has been extensively debated. The topics covered herein carry significant findings which will fuel the growth of the discipline. They may even be implemented as practical applications or may be referred to as a beginning point for another development. Chapters in this book were first published by Hindawi Publishing Corporation; hereby published with permission under the Creative Commons Attribution License or equivalent.

The editorial board has been involved in producing this book since its inception. They have spent rigorous hours researching and exploring the diverse topics which have resulted in the successful publishing of this book. They have passed on their knowledge of decades through this book. To expedite this challenging task, the publisher supported the team at every step. A small team of assistant editors was also appointed to further simplify the editing procedure and attain best results for the readers.

Our editorial team has been hand-picked from every corner of the world. Their multi-ethnicity adds dynamic inputs to the discussions which result in innovative outcomes. These outcomes are then further discussed with the researchers and contributors who give their valuable feedback and opinion regarding the same. The feedback is then collaborated with the researches and they are edited in a comprehensive manner to aid the understanding of the subject.

Apart from the editorial board, the designing team has also invested a significant amount of their time in understanding the subject and creating the most relevant covers. They scrutinized every image to scout for the most suitable representation of the subject and create an appropriate cover for the book.

The publishing team has been involved in this book since its early stages. They were actively engaged in every process, be it collecting the data, connecting with the contributors or procuring relevant information. The team has been an ardent support to the editorial, designing and production team. Their endless efforts to recruit the best for this project, has resulted in the accomplishment of this book. They are a veteran in the field of academics and their pool of knowledge is as vast as their experience in printing. Their expertise and guidance has proved useful at every step. Their uncompromising quality standards have made this book an exceptional effort. Their encouragement from time to time has been an inspiration for everyone.

The publisher and the editorial board hope that this book will prove to be a valuable piece of knowledge for researchers, students, practitioners and scholars across the globe.

List of Contributors

Marie-France Martin-Eauclaire and Pierre E. Bougis
Aix-Marseille University, CNRS, UMR 7286, CRN2M, Faculte de Medecine secteur Nord, CS80011, Boulevard Pierre Dramard, 13344 Marseille Cedex 15, France

Chensheng Lu
Department of Environmental Health, Harvard School of Public Health, 401 Park Drive, Boston, MA 02215, USA

Leo Andres
Atlanta Clinical and Translational Science Institute, School of Medicine, Emory University, 1440 Clifton Road, Atlanta, GA 30322, USA

Sanah Sadiq, Zena Ghazala, Arnab Chowdhury and Dietrich Busselberg
Weill Cornell Medical College in Qatar, Qatar Foundation—Education City, P.O. Box 24144, Doha, Qatar

Maria Stankiewicz and Marcin Dąbrowski
Biophysics Laboratory, Institute of General and Molecular Biology, N. Copernicus University, 87-100 Torun, Poland

Maria Elena de Lima
Departamento de Bioquımicae Imunologia, Instituto de Ciencias Biologicas, Universidade Federal de Minas Gerais, Belo Horizonte, 31270-901 MG, Brazil

Frank J. Lebeda
Integrated Toxicology Division, US Army Medical Research Institute of Infectious Diseases (USAMRIID), 1425 Porter Street, Fort Detrick, MD 21702, USA USAMRMC, Combat Casualty Care Research Program, ATTN: MCMR-RTC, 504 Scott Street, Fort Detrick, MD 21702-5011, USA

Zygmunt F. Dembek
Division of Medicine, USAMRIID, 1425 Porter Street, Fort Detrick, MD 21702-5011, USA

Michael Adler
Neurobehavioral Toxicology Branch, Analytical Toxicology Division, US Army Medical Research Institute of Chemical Defense, Aberdeen Proving Ground, Edgewood Area, MD 21010, USA

Mario Nizzari, Stefano Thellung, Alessandro Corsaro, Valentina Villa and Tullio Florio
Section of Pharmacology, Department of Internal Medicine and Center of Excellence for Biomedical Research, University of Genova, 16132 Genova, Italy

Carola Porcile and Claudio Russo
Department of Health Sciences, University of Molise, 86100 Campobasso, Italy

Aldo Pagano
IRCCS Azienda Ospedaliera Universitaria San Martino-Istituto Nazionale per la Ricerca sul Cancro (IST), Universita di Genova, 16132 Genova, Italy

Tanvir Abir and Abul Hasnat Milton
Centre for Clinical Epidemiology and Biostatistics (CCEB), The School of Medicine and Public Health, Faculty of Health, The University of Newcastle, Newcastle, NSW 2008, Australia

Bayzidur Rahman
The School of Public Health and Community Medicine, Faculty of Medicine, The University of New South Wales, Sydney, NSW 2052, Australia

Catherine D'Este
Biostatistics, School of Medicine and Public Health, The University of Newcastle, Newcastle, NSW 2008, Australia

Farooq A.
Research and Education Department, ASPETAR-Qatar Orthopaedic and Sports Medicine Hospital, P.O. Box 29992, Doha, Qatar

Wayessa Amasa
Department of Eco-Bology, Addis Ababa Science and Technology University, P.O. Box 16417, Addis Ababa, Ethiopia

Dante Santiago and Seblework Mekonen
Department of Environmental Health Sciences and Technology, College of Public Health and Medical Sciences, Jimma University, P.O. Box 378, Jimma, Ethiopia

Argaw Ambelu
Department of Environmental Health Sciences and Technology, College of Public Health and Medical Sciences, Jimma University, P.O. Box 378, Jimma, Ethiopia Department of Environmental Health Sciences and Technology, College of Public Health and Medical Sciences, Jimma University, P.O. Box 807, Jimma, Ethiopia

James J. Galligan
Department of Pharmacology, University of Colorado Anschutz Medical Campus, Aurora, CO 80045, USA

Rebecca L. Smathers, Colin T. Shearn, Kristofer S. Fritz, Donald S. Backos, Christopher C. Franklin and Dennis R. Petersen
Department of Pharmaceutical Sciences, University of Colorado Anschutz Medical Campus, Aurora, CO 80045, USA

Kenneth N. MacLean and Hua Jiang
Department of Pediatrics, University of Colorado Anschutz Medical Campus, Aurora, CO 80045, USA

David J. Orlicky
Department of Pathology, University of Colorado Anschutz Medical Campus, Aurora, CO 80045, USA

L. Manzo
Laboratory of Clinical Toxicology, Salvatore Maugeri Foundation IRCCS, Institute of Pavia, 27100 Pavia, Italy Department of Internal Medicine and Therapeutics, Division of Toxicology, University of Pavia, 27100 Pavia, Italy

T. Coccini and E. Roda
Laboratory of Clinical Toxicology, Salvatore Maugeri Foundation IRCCS, Institute of Pavia, 27100 Pavia, Italy

S. S. Agrawal and R. S. Ray
Department of Pharmacology, Delhi Institute of Pharmaceutical sciences and Research (DIPSAR), University of Delhi, Pushp Vihar, Sector 3, M.B. Road, New Delhi 110017, India

Ratna Tantra, Alex Cackett, Roger Peck and Jacqueline Snowden
Nano analysis Group, National Physical Laboratory, Hampton Road, Teddington, Middlesex TW11 0LW, UK

Dipak Gohil
Advanced Engineered Materials Group, National Physical Laboratory, Hampton Road, Teddington, Middlesex TW11 0LW, UK

Thomas Peyret and Kannan Krishnan
Departement de Sante Environnementale et Sante au Travail, Universite de Montreal, C.P. 6128, Succursale Centre-Ville, Montreal, QC, Canada

Katrine Bilberg
Interdisciplinary Nano science Center (iNANO) and Department of Physics and Astronomy, Aarhus University, 8000 Aarhus C, Denmark Section of Zoo physiology, Department of Biological Sciences, Aarhus University, C.F. Moellers Alle 3, Building 1131, 8000 Aarhus C, Denmark

Mads Bruun Hovgaard and Flemming Besenbacher
Interdisciplinary Nano science Center (iNANO) and Department of Physics and Astronomy, Aarhus University, 8000 Aarhus C, Denmark

Erik Baatrup
Section of Zoo physiology, Department of Biological Sciences, Aarhus University, C.F. Moellers Alle 3, Building 1131, 8000 Aarhus C, Denmark

Laila N. Islam, M. Shamim Hasan Zahid, A. H. M. Nurun Nabi and Mahmud Hossain
Department of Biochemistry and Molecular Biology, University of Dhaka, Dhaka 1000, Bangladesh

Linda R. Barone
Biologics Research, Janssen Research and Development, LLC, 145 King of Prussia Road, Radnor, PA 19087, USA

Scott Boyer
Safety Assessment, AstraZeneca Pharmaceuticals, Pepparedsleden 1, 431 83 Molndal, Sweden

James R. Damewood Jr.
Haskell Global Centers for Health and Environmental Sciences, DuPont Central Research and Development, Newark, DE 19711, USA

James Fikes and Paul J. Ciaccio
Safety Assessment, AstraZeneca Pharmaceuticals, 35 Gatehouse Drive, Waltham, MA 02451, USA

Hari Nair and Fred Woo
Department of Laboratory Medicine, University of Washington, P.O. Box 357110, 1959 NE Pacific Street, Seattle, WA 98185, USA

Andrew N. Hoofnagle
Department of Laboratory Medicine, University of Washington, P.O. Box 357110, 1959 NE Pacific Street, Seattle, WA 98185, USA Department of Medicine, University of Washington, Seattle, WA 98150, USA

Geoffrey S. Baird
Department of Laboratory Medicine, University of Washington, P.O. Box 357110, 1959 NE Pacific Street, Seattle, WA 98185, USA Department of Pathology, University of Washington, Seattle, WA 98150, USA